Listening to the Whispers

Interpretive Studies in Healthcare and the Human Sciences

VOLUME V

Listening to the Whispers

Re-thinking Ethics
in Healthcare

Christine Sorrell Dinkins

and

Jeanne Merkle Sorrell

Volume editors

THE UNIVERSITY OF WISCONSIN PRESS

The University of Wisconsin Press
1930 Monroe Street
Madison, Wisconsin 53711

www.wisc.edu/wisconsinpress/

3 Henrietta Street
London WC2E 8LU, England

1   3   5   4   2

Printed in the United States of America

Library of Congress Cataloging-in-Publication Data
Listening to the whispers : re-thinking ethics in healthcare /
edited by Christine Sorrell Dinkins & Jeanne Merkle Sorrell.
p.;   cm.—(Interpretive studies in healthcare and the human sciences ; v. 5)
Includes bibliographical references and index.
ISBN 0-299-21650-0 (hardcover: alk. paper)
ISBN 0-299-21654-3 (pbk.: alk. paper)
1. Medical ethics.   2. Clinical medicine—Moral and ethical aspects.
[DNLM: 1. Delivery of Health Care—ethics.
2. Ethics, Clinical. W 50 L773 2006]
I. Title: Re-thinking ethics in healthcare.
II. Dinkins, Christine Sorrell.
III. Sorrell, Jeanne Merkle.   IV. Series.
R724.L57   2006
174.2—dc22   2005021509

Stories hold a saving power of their own:
the power to invite us to listen to voices
that might otherwise have been unheard whispers
in the margins of modern healthcare.

From Editors' Response to
"Corporatization and the Institutional Aspects of
Morality in Home Care"

To the participants of the Institutes for Interpretive Phenomenology—
who gather stories from the margins
and invite us to listen to otherwise unheard whispers

Contents

Acknowledgments

We gratefully acknowledge the many persons whose contributions have made the completion of this book possible. We cannot possibly list all of these special individuals but would like to specifically acknowledge the following:

Nancy and John Diekelmann for their constant guidance;

Steve Salemson for his knowledgeable editorial and administrative support;

Susan Crocker for her careful compilation of language for the index;

Our patient authors who never said, "You want me to revise this *again*?";

Our loyal reviewers who never said, "I don't have time";

Our always-encouraging husbands, Christopher Dinkins and Gregory Sorrell, who never said, "How many more hours are you going to spend discussing this?";

Those who whispered their stories in the hope that we would listen;

And each other, for the mentoring that goes between mother and daughter, daughter and mother, as our lives and learning overlap.

Listening to the Whispers

Introduction

CHRISTINE S. DINKINS and
JEANNE M. SORRELL

Ethics is a pause to wonder, to question, to step back, to notice.

And this teacher . . . did that through her being open to the angst that the silence brought, through a willingness to let it sit, through a knowingness that ethics are
Always, and necessarily, inhabited by silence.

This is what I saw.
This is my participant observation.

Nancy J. Moules, March 5, 2004

This fifth volume of the Series on *Interpretive Studies in Healthcare and the Human Sciences* gives voice to scholars in philosophy, medical anthropology, physical therapy, and nursing, gathering together each scholar's understandings of ethics in his or her own discipline. The studies contained herein reflect different interpretive methodologies to help us rethink ethics in the context of today's healthcare system. The diverse voices of these authors encourage us to enlarge the circle of our ethical concerns, step back from the pressures of our personal and professional lives, and take time to notice, to question, and to wonder. Contained in these essays, too, are stories told by voices often unheard, alongside silences that provide an eternal challenge to the understanding of ethics.

The story of ethics in this volume opens with a poem, *A Whispered Story*, which came forth as an intuitive response from Nancy Moules, a reviewer of one of the manuscripts for the volume. During the period of time Nancy was reviewing the manuscript, she was also teaching a qualitative research class. Brenda Paton, a guest for her class, presented a research ethical dilemma, paused, and then invited the class into a discussion of pauses as ethics. It created a wonderful discussion with the students, and Nancy felt called to write about it. She read her writing to the class, and one person suggested that it was an invitation to hermeneutics. Thus, it is presented here also as an invitation to hermeneutics. The poem invites us to listen to the essays in the volume, reminding us that we can listen best in the pauses and silences of ethics. The poem beckons us on as participant observers to five diverse studies of ethics.

The first essay, by Tobie Olsan, opens up for the reader some of the central problems facing healthcare today, particularly in the context of corporatization and a managed care environment. "Corporatization and the Institutional Aspects of Morality in Home Care," an ethnographic study, uncovers and unconceals the moral problems experienced by a group of community health nurses at one home care agency. Expressions of personhood can raise individual and group consciousness about changing contexts in healthcare and the significance of new circumstances. To understand how to improve the whole institution, we must listen to the individuals within it, even those who at first may be difficult to hear. Giving these persons a voice in home care policy reform is essential in addressing the moral problems created by corporate healthcare.

The second essay, "Ethics of Articulation: Constituting Organizational Identity in One Catholic Hospital," may offer a possible solution to the problems uncovered in Olsan's study. Simon Lee's ethnographic study brings us an inside out picture of how values in a Catholic hospital system guide the functions of the organization. The historical overview of the women religious in healthcare provides a valuable description of their unique contribution. The study juxtaposes business and religious values and considers the question of "no margin, no mission," observing that while it may be the margin that makes the mission possible, the mission makes the margin necessary. Findings of the study demonstrate that even in a Catholic hospital system, dominant conversations contain silences, and the social practice of ethics is inherently political. The re-thinking of ethics requires that ethical spaces be created in healthcare organizations to articulate their values and sustain themselves as ethico-political entities in today's managed care environment.

Given the problems and concerns revealed in the first two essays, John Paul Slosar's "Teleology, the Modern Moral Dichotomy, and Postmodern Bioethics in the 21st Century" offers a possible philosophical framework with which to approach these problems. Slosar looks between and beyond traditional categories of ethics to recover the approach of the ancients, primarily Aristotle, for contemporary healthcare. The dominant paradigms in modern ethics are inadequate for guiding moral decisions in the face of the complexities of 21st-century healthcare, and they are also troubling simply because of their overwhelming dominance. This author's revisiting and reinterpretation of Aristotelian ethics is therefore quite timely, and he offers compelling suggestions for re-thinking ethics in an ancient yet also truly contemporary way.

In the next study, "Reflections of Moral Dilemmas and Patterns of Ethical Decision Making in Five Clinical Physical Therapists," Bruce Greenfield brings us into the world of physical therapy practitioners as they describe ethical dilemmas they face in their practice. These dilemmas illustrate the failures of the same traditional ethical systems Slosar finds to be unsatisfactory. Healthcare professions embody similar codes of ethics, but these may be of limited use in guiding practitioners as moral agents in clinical practice. Greenfield's study raises the questions: What is the moral responsibility of practitioners of healthcare? Is it ethical to bend, or even break, the rules? Greenfield finds that we need to listen to experiences of healthcare practitioners to understand the moral dilemmas they face and the ethical decision-making processes undertaken. His study also shows that practitioners may need to rely on their own individual values and upbringing, as Slosar via Aristotle would suggest, rather than adhering to a strict code.

The final study in this volume, "Beyond the Individual: Healthcare Ethics in Diverse Societies," illustrates quite dramatically where we are right now in terms of healthcare ethics and challenges us to find the best and most fruitful path from here. In this study, Kathryn Kavanagh begins with a thorough examination of the state of healthcare, ethics, and society today. She then challenges the fundamental values of society as they directly but silently impact on healthcare. Drawing examples from diverse cultures, Kavanagh brings us to understand that in caring for others, we must move beyond "side-by-side-ness." We must question and attempt to understand each person's context in society, and we must advocate for and empower diverse others.

The volume concludes with "An Ethics of Diversity," calling us to listen to stories from the margins of healthcare. This volume, along with the four previous volumes in the series, gathers together substantive scholarship from diverse disciplines into what is hoped will be continued conversations of interpretive research in healthcare. The editors have added responses at the end of each chapter to help readers reflect on various interpretations and applications of the research. In focusing on the need to re-think ethics in today's system of healthcare, it becomes apparent that the best possibilities for healthcare in the 21st century lie between and beyond traditional and mainstream thought. We cannot make progress in ethical healthcare without questioning our assumptions and questioning the path we may not even realize we're already on. One of the participants in Tobie Olsan's study was hopeful that this important research would reach others. Mrs. B. says:

"I'm hoping you just don't keep this to yourself. I hope that this gets to somebody." (Corporatization and the Institutional Aspects of Morality in Home Care, p. 42)

To create an ethical healthcare system, we need to listen to the whispers and the silences in the margins, which may be muffled by the more centralized shouts of concern. We hope that readers who journey through this volume will find opportunities to step back, to question, to wonder, and to listen.

1

A Whispered Story

NANCY J. MOULES

She started off differently than I expected.

With a story.
(And yet, why should that surprise me, lover of stories? Maybe
because somehow I forgot that stories lie here in this topic of ethics.)

She started with a story.

A story that called us in.
And there was this quietness that permeated the room, the night.
Almost a reverence that I recall in church as a young child, a call, not an
expectation (I once asked my dad, a minister, why we had to whisper in
church and he said, "We don't").
Yet . . . somehow, despite permission to do otherwise, there was a call
to speak softly, reverently, respectfully . . . because . . . why?

Because something was important, was to be honored. Something was
worthy of respect.

Ethics.

Did you notice our voices became quiet and we had to "speak up" to be
heard?

In my moments of most reverent and sacred conversations, I notice that
kind of quietness,

softening, stilling. It is palpable;
embodied, Merleau-Ponty might suggest.

And in our class—that quietness as our voices simultaneously and curi-
ously softened—
something remarkable happened . . .

More voices emerged, voices that had not been heard before, and there
in the middle of all that, another layer was added.

A pause.

An asking of a question; a waiting for response . . .
And in that deliberately and exquisitely crafted pause lay everything.
Ethics, moments, memories, reflections, questions, breathlessness,
reverence.

I waited, perhaps somewhat anxiously, for the pause to end, guessing and
second-guessing what
everyone else thought, feeling responsible for this class that I bear the
obligation toward.

Ethics. Mine.

And in that waiting, ethics landed—its huge berth filling, talking over,
consuming . . .

Yet calling, as Caputo suggests the young child on the beach, lost, calls for
something and we are obligated to answer.
Calling . . .

Calling Amie to talk about a last heartbeat in such a way that her description took my breath away; Christine to question hope and her love of it, in
such a way that made *me* almost even love hope more; Karen to think of
moments of community and decision and obligation with such passion
and experience and expertise and artistry; Blaine to ponder *Dasein* and

Being and money and larger and smaller commitments in a witty articulation that almost belies the softness of his heart; Rich to enter into intentionality, politics, drives, and yet, fundamentally, losses; Violet to move
into her question of learning and knowing; Lorraine to move back and
forth between living and dying and *that* moment and to find herself as a
young woman compassionately and passionately drawn to *that* moment;
Lisa, in her thoughtful, kind-ful, and mind-ful manner to speak of piece-
ing and peace-ing; Stacey to quietly smile, nod, bring it in, respectfully
making space for these new ideas; Tanya to passionately bring it all consistently back to practicing living moments of birth, and choice, and decisions, and questions; Julian to remind us that it matters and that it is
never that simple—as he takes the taken-for-granted and infuses it with
heart and rhythm and mindfulness; Ruth to bring it to children and to
lean into the questions with the passion and perseverance I have come to
understand infuse her practice and life; Eileen to offer the gracious wide-
eyed wonder and intelligence that seeps from her very presence . . .

Calling us all to . . . what?

To an *Ethics* of obligations of everyday practices, of bearers of names,
and filler of pauses.

Ethics cannot be empty words—ethics is a pause to wonder, to question,
to step back, to notice.

And this teacher, Dr. Paton; this nurse, B. Paton, RN, PhD; this woman,
Brenda, my colleague, my friend, my sister in many ways, did that
through her being open to the angst that the silence brought, through a
willingness to let it sit, through a knowingness that ethics are
Always, and necessarily, inhabited by silence.

This is what I saw.

This is my participant observation.

2

Corporatization and the Institutional Aspects of Morality in Home Care

TOBIE H. OLSAN

When I approached the community health nurses[1] at the Riverside Home Care Agency[2] about participating in an ethnographic analysis of the institutional aspects of morality in home care, they interpreted my work as being a study about "the other stuff." They were referring to the workplace domain as they understood it, namely, business principles, bureaucracies, formal rules, regulations, expectations, and work group relationships. The other stuff was distinct from, but intertwined with, "patient care," a second domain in the nurses' work world. Caregiving, professional obligations, and relationships with patients were included in patient care, as was the nurses' agentive capacity for professional judgment and nursing practice.

Put another way, when I asked a case manager whom I will call Eva, "What does it mean to be a nurse at the Riverside Home Care Agency?" she responded, "That's too generic a question. You've got to be more specific. What do you mean? Is it the organization or is it the community health part of it, or what?"

Eva's questions, like the two workplace domains, patient care, and the other stuff, demonstrate the moral force of institutions in healthcare. Institutions classify thinking, acting, and systems of social relations (Douglas, 1986), and as such they construct moral problems and influence moral judgments and actions in a work group. Institutions are defined here sociologically as a legitimized social grouping and the associated history, values, purpose, roles, rules, relationships, and moral comportment of members of the group. Examples include a work group, profession, managed care organization, and government entity. Institutional arrangements define, shape, and reshape the picture of morality that occurs in them (Wolgast, 1992), yet the sociocultural study of moral life in the workplace is largely unaccounted for in the bioethics literature.

Bioethics primarily connotes medical ethics and philosophical analysis from abstract principles to gain insights into questions about what *should be* in healthcare. The entire body of work in bioethics has little to say about *what is,* including the particulars of experience in organizations and the relationship of persons to other structures in the workplace. Descriptive ethics offers a corrective approach and is a good fit with this research, which is concerned about morality and culture.

Morality is part of culture (Jameton, 1990), and the moral aspects of market-driven healthcare cannot be adequately understood without examining the social dimensions of the workplace (Potter, 1999). When institutions are in a state of flux, the upheaval from change and uncertainty can be accompanied by competing conceptions of persons and work. Ethnographic analysis exposes those conflicts and brings the institutional aspects of the dilemmas they generate into view.

The aim in this chapter is to raise awareness of the role institutions play in morality by naming and describing dilemmas the nurses encountered at Riverside during a change in governance from the public to the private sector. In the sections that follow, the larger ethnographic study about morality in market-driven healthcare, from which the workplace dilemmas were derived, is described. Analytic concepts from personhood theory that guided fieldwork and analysis are explained next. Examples of the dilemmas appearing in the nurses' work life are excerpted from their reflective work narratives. A discussion of the implications of the nurses' encounter with corporatization for healthcare reform concludes the chapter.

Riverside Home Care Agency

The larger ethnographic study was conducted with a group of community health nurses at the Riverside Home Care Agency. The rich history of

Riverside is too detailed to recount here, but briefly, the life cycle of the organization largely reflects the shape of public health during the 19th and 20th centuries. Riverside was established as a Public Health Bureau in the late 19th century during urbanization and the proliferation of community-based public health services for immigrants and the poor. Around 1950, Riverside was restructured as a public health home care agency to provide illness care to patients discharged from hospitals. Throughout the 1970s public health nursing included a mix of preventive health services and illness-focused care. Working at a distance from mainstream acute care secured in a safety net of public funding throughout the 1980s, the nurses at Riverside were initially protected from the corporate transformation of healthcare occurring at that time. But eventually, the frenzied wave of acquisitions and mergers sweeping the country in the private sector (Todd, 1999) penetrated the public sector too.

In the mid-1990s Riverside was purchased by UniCare, a private, nonprofit integrated health system (IHS) located in the northeast United States. There are 23 distinct operating affiliates at UniCare with a total of $500 million in operating revenues. The largest UniCare affiliates include two community hospitals, one rural hospital, a network of community-based services for older adults, and the Riverside Home Care Agency (see Figure 2.1). About 7,000 people are employed at UniCare.

UniCare was one of three highly competitive nonprofit IHSs in the region formed from freestanding organizations and physician groups. A win-at-all-costs mentality deeply divided the region into fractious camps along the lines of organization affiliation. Collegial relationships between physicians were tense and efforts to develop services across health systems faltered. In some cases, physicians left one IHS to join another.

During this time, the nurses at Riverside were facing their own struggles with healthcare restructuring. The magnitude of disruption that converged on them when Riverside was sold to UniCare cannot be overstated. Steeped in the values and traditions of public health nursing, the nurses were forced to confront a particularly intense and ruthless corporatization for the first time in their careers.

From the outset the nurses were situated in the turmoil of an affiliation agreement with unrealistic time frames for accomplishing objectives. Within the first year of operation, Riverside was expected to be profitable and to offer an array of services comparable to the well-established private home care agencies in the region. Riverside was envisioned as the

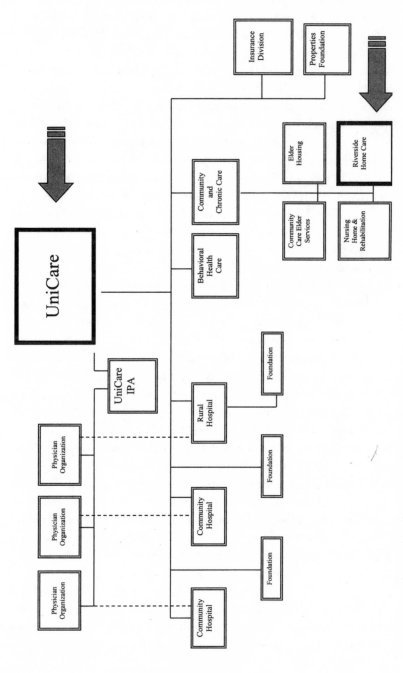

Figure 2.1. Organizational chart of the UniCare health system (1997)

preferred home care provider for UniCare, but referral patterns of physicians and social workers were not easily changed. Even after affiliation, patients were regularly referred outside of UniCare to home care agencies in competing IHSs. From the advantage of hindsight, the complexities of incorporating a traditional public sector home care agency into a private IHS were vastly underestimated.

Every month for the first two years following affiliation there were unexpected financial losses at Riverside. Year-end operating deficits exceeded $500,000. UniCare executives and trustees wavered in their support for the home care affiliate. Top executives at Riverside foundered in their efforts to redesign the home care agency to meet the demands of a competitive marketplace. Ineffective quick fixes of outdated operating systems aggravated problems they were intended to address. Hasty implementation of a consultant's recommendations to restructure clinical services heightened the disarray. At the end of two years all the top executives at Riverside had resigned from the agency.

By 1999, other affiliates at UniCare were facing financial losses. Culture clashes occurred between affiliates, and cooperation was rare. Distrust among segregated work groups and governing boards was rampant. A vision for integration was not clearly articulated, and anticipated cost savings were never realized. Administrative expenditures added millions of dollars to the losses at UniCare, with no tangible benefits for patient care. A crisis of confidence in leadership prompted a series of abrupt resignations among top executives at UniCare.

As the entire IHS reeled from a vulnerable position in the marketplace, new top executives were hired at UniCare and Riverside. Widespread organizational dysfunction, however, would not be easily overcome. Financial losses continued into 2001, but eventually small gains in operations were realized. In time, Riverside received accreditation with commendation from the Joint Commission on Accreditation for Healthcare Organizations. Some of the nurses who resigned during the early years of the affiliation came back to work at Riverside, but there was a notable human cost of the affiliation. By 2001, 83 (75%) of the 110 nurses who came over to UniCare from the public sector agency had resigned.

The nurses referred to home care negatively as "a business" and often said, "It is a difficult time to be at Riverside." They referred to themselves as "corporate entities." They described their work as being about "making visits and making money." One nurse equated the "corporatization of healthcare" with the "systematic destruction of nursing." And in response to my question, "What color is Riverside?" another nurse said, "It is the color of turmoil, a painting made with two paint brushes, a Rorschach test, because everything is changing. It is whatever color turmoil would be."

Corporatization loomed large in the nurses' work world. I was concerned they would be too preoccupied to include a researcher in their day, but the disruption may actually have facilitated my entrée to the group. The nurses wanted to talk about what was going on, and I was poised to listen.

The Ethnographic Approach

According to Van Maanen (1988), ethnography is a way of representing the social reality of others. As a research process, ethnography is useful for examining "the intricate ways individuals and groups understand, accommodate, and resist a presumably shared order" (Van Maanen, 1988, p. xiv). As a product of research, ethnography is a written account of culture that fundamentally involves interpretation. Ethnography is not about scientific precision and objectivity, but rather, as Mauss remarked to fellow anthropologist Fortes (1987), ethnography is like fishing with a net: "All you need is a net, any kind of net; and then if you step into the sea and swing your net about, you are sure to catch some kind of fish" (p. 247). This metaphor illuminates the interpretive project for the ethnographer, which is to see parts as connected to larger wholes and to try to grasp the contexts and frameworks within which people learn, experience, act, and render their lives meaningful (Peacock, 1986).

One assumption in ethnography is that understanding culture requires sorting, comparing, and integrating "insider" (emic) perspectives with "outsider" (etic) perspectives. In order to arrive at a coherent representation of a group, it is further assumed that insiders know more than they realize (Dombeck, Markakis, Brachman, Dalal, & Olsan, 2002). The researcher's immersion in the group is fundamental to her ability to link the emic and the etic perspectives so that she may learn how persons understand and navigate structural relationships and changes in their everyday lives.

Data Collection and Analysis

My close contact with the nurses at Riverside occurred through field-work and extensive participant observation over four years from 1997 to 2001. Data were also derived from in-depth interviews with nurses, administrators, and support staff at the agency. Patients and family members were also interviewed. Photographs and various kinds of agency records were additional sources of data useful for tracking changes over time and for learning about the flow and content of information communicated among members of the work group. The complete data set included 119 home visits, 66 interviews, 62 meetings and educational sessions, 9 work-related social functions, and many casual conversations with members of the work group.

The verbatim transcriptions and field notes were analyzed using an inductive iterative process (Emerson, Fretz, & Shaw, 1995; Huberman & Miles, 1994; Taylor & Bogdan, 1984), which can be thought of as a conversation between researcher, participants, and texts. The ethnographer begins by carefully and reflectively reading and rereading the data, dwelling in the details to become intimately familiar with what participants have expressed and what has been observed in the field. Words, ideas, events, topics, and themes are identified, respectfully sorted, and arranged in relational graphic displays. As the nuances of morality are uncovered in the analysis, insights are gained about what is happening in the work group and what is meaningful to the members. No effort is made to force the data to fit predefined categories. Understanding is generated inductively by moving from the particular to the general and back and forth between data analysis and data collection. The dialectic interplay between text and interpretation forms a general picture of human experience as meaning and relationships emerge. In this research, all of these aspects of data analysis and the storage and retrieval of data were managed using QSR N5 software.

The Nurses

Fifty highly experienced and educated case managers were the primary participants in this research. Their combined years in nursing totaled 932 (mean = 18.64 years) with 451 years of experience in home care (mean = 9.02 years). Twenty-four percent (n = 12) of the nurses were educationally prepared with a Master's degree. The other nurses held a Bachelor's degree (56%; n = 28), Associate degree (18%; n = 9), and a diploma in nursing (2%; n = 1).

Case managers had a vast range of job responsibilities. They oversaw a caseload of 25 to 45 patients whose care needs ranged from post-acute hospital care to long-term chronic care and hospice care. They provided direct care to patients and managed all aspects of coordinating patient care. They arranged referrals to therapists, communicated with physicians, and made decisions about when to admit and discharge patients from home care. They authorized insurance payments for services, supervised home health aides, and continually integrated a never-ending flow of new regulations and insurance rules into their practice. Case managers were expected to meet a productivity target of visiting six patients each day.

In addition to their responsibilities for patients, case managers collected and delivered specimens to the lab, picked up medical supplies for patients, attended required mandatory in-service education programs, and attended meetings at the agency. They oriented and taught classes for new case managers, and they precepted student nurses. On behalf of Riverside, they worked as volunteers for local health and wellness events to keep the agency visible in the community. Considered the best representatives for Riverside from a marketing perspective, the case managers acted as liaisons to physicians' offices to foster long-term referral relationships.

These nurses' jobs were daunting. Long hours were expected, and work responsibilities regularly overflowed into personal time. When insurers refused to authorize official reimbursable visits for nursing care, the nurses made unofficial visits to patients in need of support. They took donated clothes and furniture to patients who otherwise would not have had the basics for living. Some nurses went so far as to describe community health nursing as a calling, work they were destined to do. Despite changes in their work world, the nurses were committed to Riverside and were hopeful for what could be achieved in the marketplace. One nurse, Fran, said, "With all that is going on in home care between competition and reimbursement, if any agency can make it, we can."

The Researcher

My part in the study was to approach the nurses as an active learner (Creswell, 1998). I was a stranger to home care, so it was not difficult for me to be attentive to the nurses' activities and words. The vast majority of my 21 years in nursing have been in acute care, which is a long distance from the natural setting of patients' homes and the independence of working in the community.

During the ten years that I worked in executive positions in hospitals, I grappled with the tensions between priorities in the boardroom and my responsibilities to nurses on the front line of healthcare. As corporatization advanced during the 1990s my questions included, "What is going on here?" "How does decision-making in the boardroom influence caregiving on the front line?" "What matters in healthcare?" and "How will my actions change nurses' ability to fulfill their professional obligations to patients?" Budget summaries, position control reports, and quality improvement reports were permanent fixtures in my administrative life, but they were vastly insufficient for informing my questions about the role of institutions in morality. Eventually I resigned my position as a nurse executive for a student career in doctoral studies. My intent was to understand changing healthcare values and structures in human terms that fall outside of productivity and efficiency measures.

I chose to spend time with nurses in home care in part because of my long-standing curiosity about community health nursing. It was also important to be in an unfamiliar setting so I would not be tempted to take words, practices, and meanings for granted. I had to learn the specialized words of community health nursing in home care—"485s," "homebound status," "choicing," "OASIS," "IMO," "caseload," "off-loading," and "recerts." The nurses taught me that at the core of their institutional dilemmas were matters of personhood. They asked questions such as, "Who are we?" "What will it take to survive in the corporate world of healthcare?" and "How much can we sacrifice and still be true to who we are as nurses?"

Institutions and Professional Personhood

The etymology of the word *person* is from the Latin *persona* (Ayto, 1990). It means mask, like the dramatic masks worn by an actor responsible for playing an assigned role in a play (Dombeck & Olsan, 2002). Masks signify identity and give meaning to social relationships. Mauss (1989) traced the evolution of the concept of person from this early meaning to the notion of a personal self with social standing and rights and obligations conferred by the larger society. *Person* is an empowering moral concept. It connotes being a "significant somebody" with a face and a voice, endowed by the larger society with the agentive capacity to make choices about one's roles and relationships with others.

Nurses are professional persons, with professional duties and entitlements added to their other social obligations (Dombeck, 1997). Their knowledge, practice, and moral agency is constituted at the intersection of professional nursing culture and healthcare institutions. Changes in nurses' professional personhood are linked to changing values and structures in local healthcare cultures. In that sense, persons and institutions are a set (Harris, 1989); the larger society ascribes capacities and qualities to persons, and personhood is accompanied by an expectation to act purposefully and to do the right things in relations with others.

Persons, however, do not solely interact and respond with others as deliberate strategic thinkers and calculating automatons. They possess reflective awareness of the standards they are living by (or failing to live by). Persons have freedom to choose among possible lines of action, albeit in a web of opposing demands and limited options (Harris, 1989; Wolgast, 1992). The way in which persons understand themselves is shaped by culture and by interactions with others. As an analytic concept, *person* stimulates explorations of culture (Allen, 1989), and as the nurses taught me through their questions and dilemmas, person is the starting point for morality (Thompson, Melia, & Boyd, 2000).

Institutional Dilemmas and Nurses' Professional Personhood

Analysis of community health nurses' work narratives functions partly to set their reflections and actions in a professionally coherent context, but more broadly, the nurses' moral problems reveal structural features and relationships in institutions. Nurses' daily work provides an interpretive context for shedding light on the moral dimensions of changing values and structures in healthcare. Learning to see the authority of institutions in morality is not only important to nurses, it points to avenues for guiding future reform efforts. Naming and describing the dilemmas affords people willing to engage in the nurses' stories an authentic connection between private moments on the front line of healthcare and the institutional forces that construct the moments in the first place. These dilemmas are named and described in the following pages.

Liminality and the Moral Reference Group Dilemma

Liminality is one aspect of a typology for passage through social change (Turner, 1974), the significance of which is frequently underestimated and, worse, often ignored during organizational restructuring (Gross, Pascale, & Athos, 1993). When the governance of Riverside changed from the public to the private sector, the nurses at Riverside found themselves in a liminal, or threshold, state, and they struggled to find their footing in an unfathomable web of shifting and overlapping institutional structures. The lengthy but only partial list of shifting structures noted in Table 2.1 shows the magnitude and the depth of disruption created for the nurses. Essentially, the nurses' public-sector social, cultural, and moral maps were outdated, irrelevant, and unusable in the marketplace. Accustomed to knowing their workplace and how to act in it, the nurses were not yet sure who they were or what was expected of them at UniCare.

The deeper moral problem of the nurses' liminality arose from being county nurses in the private sector. As marginals at UniCare, they were simultaneously members of two groups "whose social definitions and cultural norms were distinct from, and often even opposed to, one another" (Turner, 1974, p. 233). Resolution of the moral tension between the public and private sector was difficult at Riverside, because the nurses could not agree about which group was the structural reference group.

Sonia, a mid-level manager, explained her thinking behind choosing the private sector as the prestigious reference group, leaving the county in the so-called inferior group:

When you hear people say county nurse, it is meant to be a negative. . . . There is a sense that if you were a county agency you were incompetent, you didn't know what you were doing, you were not the experts. The private agencies got all the paying insurances, or a majority of the paying insurances; the HMOs, the Blues, the Medicare cases. They serviced the higher socioeconomic groups. The county got the Medicaid clients, the lower socioeconomic groups, the underserved, the underinsured.

Table 2.1. A Web of Shifting Structures at Riverside

PUBLIC SECTOR	PRIVATE SECTOR
Freestanding facility	Integrated health system
Charity care	Reimbursement for care
Uninsured populations	Insured populations
Medicaid	Medicare and commercial insurers
Cost unaware	Cost aware
Public health nursing	Home care nursing
Socially at-risk populations	Socially advantaged populations
Chronic care	Post-hospital care
Low-tech care	High-tech care
Unchanging organizational structure	Frequent reorganizations
Stable work group	Unstable work group
Open and common offices	Private and separate offices
Loose work practices	Data-driven systems
Low expectations	High expectations
Low to moderate workload	High workload
Emphasis on social relationships	Emphasis on efficiency
Somebody	Nobody

Holly also expressed a preference for the private sector as the structural reference group but was cautious about the erosion of nursing values at UniCare:

In terms of what it means to be here rather than at the county [pause], how do I want to put it [long pause]? I think, for myself personally, I feel a lot more a part of the healthcare system in general at this point. It's the integration with the hospitals, the idea of the county versus UniCare, and that expectations have changed. . . . We have to be more efficient and we have to learn to do things differently and that's challenging. It's stressful, but as a nurse I can look confident, because I have had to integrate more information and be able to provide care in a way that's more cost effective. I hate to use that term, but I think it's part of doing things differently.

I equate it with a train coming at us. We can either stand on the tracks and be run over, we can step aside and run away and go do something else, or we can just jump on board. Even though I don't agree with everything, I have chosen to jump on board, but the most important parts of this job are the relationships I develop with my clients and acting as an advocate. These are the things that I love the most, and if I lose them, I won't be able to stay on the train.

Holly was inclined toward supporting IHSs, but was uncertain about what integration meant for her professional life over the long term.

In contrast to Sonia and Holly, who cautiously considered the private sector to be the more prestigious group in which to aspire, other nurses saw the public sector as the higher status reference group. April chose public health nursing as the best moral guide for nurses:

I think they [UniCare] bought us because that was the thing to do, but I don't think they have respect for us as county nurses. A visiting nurse doesn't get a lot of respect in a private agency, but a county nurse is respected in community health. It sounds really bad for me to say, but nurses in the private agencies come to community health because they need a job change, or they were too long at another job, or they were burnt out. They really don't belong in community health. So we had a bad reputation at first, not because we were county nurses, but because we had to prove ourselves as nurses as well as being money producers. It was a big burden.

Barbara, an executive, similarly saw public health nursing as higher in status than home care nursing in the private sector. Her perception was based on two hallmarks of public health nursing: a holistic approach to care and providing charity care for the poor.

In public health, we looked at a patient's care as the family's care. We focused on creating wellness and doing prevention so that the person gets well and stays well and the rest of their family doesn't get sick around them. It is different than what I picture home care nursing. That to me is what our procedure nurses do. They go in, they change a dressing, they fill a medi-set, and they do an assessment. A public health nurse takes a look at the entire picture and treats the entire family, whoever is in that person's support system, . . . regardless of their ability to pay. We never even thought about looking at how many reimbursable visits nurses made.

As she often did, Alice poignantly captured the nurses' reference group dilemma. She saw the tension between the public and private sector values in the larger scope of nursing practice: "If we end up letting go of our nursing values in order to survive in a corporate environment, it will be equivalent to selling our soul."

Her reflection takes on additional significance in light of the Latin for corporation, *corporalis*, which refers to a tangible material body that is exterior to the spirit, an abode of the soul (Little, Fowler, & Couslon, 1955; Neilson, 1947). Alice was concerned that doing what was expected on the job in the private sector might satisfy the corporate *body*, but it would risk nurses' souls, destroying their public health identity and the embodied experience of nursing. Alice also understood the realities of market-driven healthcare in terms of a commitment to patients: "We need to keep in business so we can serve the public." The nurses at Riverside perceived they could not meet the expectations of the private sector and be faithful to public health nursing ideals. On the other hand, if they acted on their public health ideals they feared Riverside would go out of business. In this no-win dilemma, solace eluded them.

Loss of Nurses' Personhood

Residing in a turbulent liminal zone where the framework for judging nurses and the good of their work in a corporate context was so different from the framework in the public sector, the nurses concluded, "We can't be nurses anymore." It was a disturbing phrase, signaling a loss of personhood, or as Marge referred to it, "a lack of humanness at work."

From an institutional perspective, when nurses are depersonalized they are no longer respected as moral agents in the workplace (Harris, 1989). Their professional roles, obligations, and relationships are disregarded (Scott, 1995). They are stripped of their identity and the freedom to act on their obligations to patients. They are socially dismantled and incapable of being persons in the full sense (Taylor, 1985).

Depersonalization occurs through social processes that separate persons from factors that would otherwise attach them to the social systems (Henry, 1973). Depersonalization is the loss of the sense of identity that follows when people are treated with indifference, as if they have no value and are of no significance (Kayser-Jones, 1981). Depersonalization occurred at Riverside when the nurses' professional and personal lives were gradually eclipsed by their economic purpose for Riverside. Nurses' relationships with patients were disregarded, and the nurses' right to respect was ignored. Unable to do what they perceived was right, the nurses believed they could not be good nurses. Five dilemmas of depersonalization were analyzed in the nurses' narratives.

1. Depersonalization through symbolic means (Henry, 1973). A situation Donna described involved depersonalization through acts that deprive nurses of the symbols that attach them to their professional systems:

There is a corporate policy [at UniCare] that we cannot put the letters RN after our name on the name badges we are required to wear. Below the UniCare logo is our name, but no credentials. It does say nurse in small letters but no one can see it. By making us all healthcare workers we are generic, we are all the same to the higher-ups. Doctors, housekeepers, nurses, we are all healthcare workers. They can move us around and make changes without seeing us. They can just take away one of us and get another. Who we are doesn't matter. They say too many letters after our name will confuse patients, but patients want to know who is taking care of them. Someone comes in wearing a white coat and takes blood, patients think it is a nurse. We worked hard to become nurses. The letters matter to us. . . . Nurses in other health systems have them, but we can't use them.

Credentials legally represent nurses' educational qualifications and ability to provide specialized healthcare services (Hall, 1996). Credentials connect nurses to the history of their profession and symbolize acceptance of responsibility, obligations, and trust accrued to them from the larger society. In encounters with competitors, credentials affirm comparable professional status. Thus, the corporate "no credentials" policy promulgated to standardize the corporate image ignored the nurses' professional personhood and blurred their identity in the eyes of patients.

2. Depersonalization through mechanized routinization (Henry, 1973). After the changeover to UniCare, the nurses faced pervasive workaholism. Workaholism is defined here not as a behavior resulting from personal variables, but sociologically, as a response to situational variables and expectations (Scott, Moore, & Miceli, 1997). As a form of depersonalization through mechanized routinization, the nurses were viewed as identical and interchangeable. The rhythm of their lives was governed by the time demands of the job.

Workaholism was the manifestation of a corporate attitude that the needs of the agency were paramount. Taking on the expectation that it was their responsibility to "keep the agency afloat," the nurses reported thinking about and dreaming about work when not on the job. Voice-mail messages were accessed remotely even on weekends and in the evening before going to bed. Work interfered in social relationships each time the nurses set aside commitments to family and friends to do paperwork at home or make additional visits to patients during periods of short staffing.

Complicating the situation further, top executives at Riverside considered long hours and personal sacrifice for the agency a desirable quality in employees. There was no distinction between work time and personal time (Steinfelds, 2001). An hour worked on Wednesday afternoon was treated the same as an hour of family time on Sunday morning. Special requests for time off to coach a friend through labor or to attend a mid-week religious service were viewed as inappropriate trade-offs for work and lost opportunities for meeting weekly productivity. Sacrificing professional and personal interests for the agency was treated as routine.

An agency rife with exhausted and overworked nurses illustrates the powerful influence of institutional norms on the standing of persons in a work group. When time is treated solely as instrumental for earning revenue for the agency, the value of nurses' professional time with patients is muted and the joy of doing meaningful work is denied (Steinfelds, 2001). From the perspective of depersonalization, when workplace norms are integrated into identity to the point where actions are no longer guided by role obligations, individuals can no longer be persons (Durkheim, 1947).

3. Depersonalization by deprivation of individuality (Henry, 1973). At UniCare, nurses were redefined as competitors, exposing them to a form of deprivation of individuality wherein there is no acknowledgment of the characteristics that distinguish one nurse from another. Being viewed as a competitor was particularly difficult for home care coordinators. Coordinators arrange home care for patients leaving the hospital, which requires working face-to-face with professionals from competing organizations. Tamar described how competition changed her relationships at a hospital affiliated with an IHS competing with UniCare:

It is like being an unwanted guest in the competitor's house. . . . We are the same bunch of nurses as we always were. We take care of babies and sick people. But with all that is happening we are now competitors. We are politically incorrect. It is a hurtful thing.

Donna recalled a petty incident that illustrates how the corporate persona deprived nurses of individuality and reduced them to one level, treating them like things (Henry, 1973):

I stopped by the cafeteria [located in an IHS in competition with UniCare] the day they announced the rollout of their new insurance plan. I got in a line where they were giving out free water bottles and cookies. When I got up to the front the person handing out water bottles saw my UniCare name tag. She had been handing everyone a water bottle as they were going through the line, but when she realized that I was from UniCare she hesitated. It wasn't real obvious, but she held back her hand. She wasn't sure if she should give me a water bottle or not. I helped her out. I said, that's okay, I don't want a water bottle anyway, I just want a cookie. So, I took a cookie and went over to sit at our table.

I walked by a group of people in white coats, maybe administrators, I'm not sure, but I know they worked there. When one woman saw I had a cookie she actually said to me, "I didn't know we gave free cookies to *those* people from Uni-Care." I got angry—she really made me mad—so I said back to her, "Why not? If you were at UniCare we would give you cookies!"

The whole thing made me feel like the enemy. I was not there to harm anyone. I thought, we're all here for patient care. Aren't we all here to take care of patients? Why divide us like we are in separate camps? Before the merger everybody loved us. We took care of the high-risk cases, the babies with cocaine, and the poor people. Within hours, or at least it seemed that way, we were the enemy, the competitor. Maybe as nurses we are naïve, maybe we are not here for the same purpose, but we should be here for everyone. We take care of patients.

Through these deprivations of individuality, the nurses' corporate persona was changing what it meant to be a nurse. Distressed about their new roles as generic healthcare worker, workaholic, and competitor, nurses raised questions about rules and expectations that did not fit with their own image of who they were as nurses. They were reflective about the expectations imposed upon them by the workplace. They spoke about their obligation to patients and envisioned a more harmonious community where professionals worked together for the welfare of patients. Unfortunately, these efforts alone were insufficient for assuring effective moral agency and overcoming features of the workplace that constrained their moral actions.

4. Depersonalization through inconsistency and flawed systems (Henry, 1973). Depersonalization also occurred when systems in the workplace failed to function and prevented nurses from practicing according to professional nursing norms. Deborah was assigned to care for a patient she did not know and explained what happened to her during a home visit:

I looked at the chart and there was no information, no diagnosis, surgery, no treatment, none of that information. I knew the patient needed a dry dressing change, but I didn't know where her wound was. In a roundabout way I asked her what surgery she had done without her thinking I was a complete idiot and didn't know what I was doing. Trust with patients is important when you make a home visit. Probably, ethically, I should have said, you know I didn't get all the information on you, could you tell me what surgery you had. You want to do that, but on the other hand, it's embarrassing.

To compensate for an ineffective medical record information system, Deborah and other nurses perfected ways to gather information indirectly in order to figure out what they needed to do during the visit. They were understandably concerned about making mistakes, and they also struggled with not being truthful with patients. Mary Pat described the situation as "going in blind. I use my best judgment, but I have to rely on what the patient and family say about how things are done." The inconsistency in this and similar situations occurred repeatedly and predictably throughout the workday. Flawed systems disrupted professional relationships (Henry, 1973) and required nurses to put aside professional standards in order to be useful for the agency (Wolgast, 1992).

5. Depersonalization through deprivation of social protection. A social system must protect its members from threats to their obligations to others and to themselves; when that protection is not given, the unprotected feel like "nobody cares" (Henry, 1973). Social protection in the workplace frees nurses to act on professional judgments and fulfill obligations to patients. But at Riverside, the nurses felt that their leaders had abandoned them. No one was listening to their need for support or responding to their concerns. Drawing intentionally on a biblical metaphor, Alice recalled, "We were voices crying in the wilderness."

A problem behind the nurses' lack of protection was segmentalism, a dysfunctional organizational paradigm created by mechanistic divisions between different hierarchical levels, functions, roles, and people in the workplace (Morgan, 1997). Segmentalism creates barriers and stumbling blocks that interfere with working and acting morally. Complex problems float up the organizational hierarchy as members of each level find in turn that they are unable to solve them. Information often gets distorted; interdepartmental communication and coordination are often poor. The work group has a myopic view of what is occurring, so that often no member of the group has an overall grasp of the situation facing the enterprise as a whole.

Segmentalism at Riverside occurred in many forms and rose to the highest levels within UniCare. Three of these forms are particularly illustrative of the nurses' situation. First, segmentalism separated nurses from patients. To maximize efficiency and productivity, the nurses were pressured to "off-load," or delegate, some of their visits to procedure nurses. Because public health nurses learn to care for patients from a holistic perspective, a stratified staffing plan requiring them to think of patients as an intravenous antibiotic to be administered or a heart to be monitored was morally problematic. Holly explained:

There are legitimate reasons not to off-load your cases. It is not just because nurses like to see their patients, it has to do with the intricacies of case management. The plan is very specific to my care. Part of case management, as far as for me, is to have hands-on, visual visiting. It involves taking your coat off, sitting down, establishing rapport, and being emotionally available to patients. If I send out a procedure nurse, I will not see the patient for another two weeks. The patients need to know who their nurses are. So much of healing is feeling cared for. . . . I am not just caring for a leg.

Second, segmentalism separated nurses from their leaders. As the crisis grew at Riverside, the well-respected top executives, who had espoused a commitment to total quality management and open communication in the public sector, now adopted a harsh autocratic stance for communication and decision making. When nurses fell short of performance targets, feedback was ruthless and punitive. During one staff meeting where the assembled nurses were voicing concerns about the workload and their fears about making mistakes, an executive said, "If you can't keep up with the work, it's better that you leave. We'll find people who can."

Gradually, communication, shared problem solving, and teamwork across levels of the agency's organizational hierarchy disappeared. The nurses, separated from their managers and from each other, were left to fend for themselves about matters involving patient care and professional issues. Ginny, a new nurse and new to community health nursing, recounted her experience:

I knew I was over my head, but we're all so overwhelmed and busy with our own problems there is really no one to help you. Everyone is willing to listen but nobody's willing to take an active role. They're restructuring everything, but I need to know who my supervisor is. I need a resource, someone to call and ask questions to when I'm out there and don't have the answers. Everyone said I was doing a great job, but I needed someone to back me up.

Cameron commented:

I actually lost some power because I was not getting any supervision. Empowerment comes from supervision and input, and from learning as well. If we asked for it, we would probably get it, but if you don't, it doesn't happen.

Marge had an insightful grasp of the work group's deteriorating moral situation:

I think the agency was under more pressure than we realized. Administratively, they were probably running scared a lot longer than we knew. . . . I see supervisors overwhelmed, who can't get complicated cases assigned to a primary nurse. It is a hodgepodge of things; there is no continuity. . . . We also don't have a support system here. We are human beings, we have lives and needs, and I don't see that being addressed. . . . Self-esteem is being lost. . . . People are being lost, and I don't like that.

Georgianna, a respected manager, recalled her frustration with her inability to see the bigger picture and to help stabilize day-to-day operations:

We were out there on a limb with no support . . . and we were going downhill. We couldn't figure out why things were not working. I'm a manager and I couldn't figure out what was wrong. None of us were quite sure how to fix it. I didn't even see that the nurses were having trouble with what I was doing.

Third, segmentalism separated Riverside executives from UniCare executives. The problem was traced to the highest executive ranks and the governing bodies in the health system. Abby, an executive at Riverside, told me:

It is really hard here. When we came over from the county, UniCare told us they would give us unlimited support. Now we need them to help us financially, until we can get things in order, and they want to sell us.

Segmentalism also appeared in a UniCare executive's description of what was happening at the top of the IHS with executives and board members. Ronald explained:

The ideal way would be that everybody who was creating this system would come together and say . . . this is the vision of the future and let's invest in it by starting a partnership. That wasn't the case at all. . . . Everything has got to stand on its own, not as a system, but as individual pieces.

Amy provided a final vivid example of segmentalism. She was a member of the support staff at Riverside and one of few people able to see the structural defect contributing to the work group's feelings of abandonment:

Coming over here [from the public sector] was sold to us as a positive thing with lots of opportunities. I think that was true, but coming here was a lightning change. We came over and we plowed ahead, but we didn't do the people work. We weren't clear about our mission then, and we still don't know what it is now.

We are not clear about our standards either, and for certain, we are not dealing with the emotional problems that have developed because of it.

They [members of the work group] have worked so hard and given so much. The problems we are having are not from lack of trying on their part. It is hard to imagine that they could do more than they do, but the reality is that we are not thriving. We are in a survival mode. We are terrified to risk anything, and we don't feel safe asking for help. It is every man for himself.

It is like each one of us is in a separate car on a deserted road in the dark and the car breaks down. We are stuck, congealed, paralyzed. We are afraid to get out of the car and we are afraid to stay in the car. We believe good things are outside of the car, things that will make us the best home care agency in Arlen County, but we don't know if we will be mugged or fall into a pit, so we feel like we have to defend ourselves. There is no innovation. I see this scenario played out at all levels of the health system, from the bottom to the top, and it pushes us into a survival mode.

We are a system on paper, but integration has not occurred. It is every man for himself. I know I keep saying that, but it is true. We are all here but we are in separate cars, and it makes me feel ineffective. Some days it is like I am standing in the parking lot, surrounded by all these cars and watching things happen, but I am all alone.

This entire situation is fundamentally a reflection of leadership. If we are going to overcome it we need to start all over and build a new culture, probably with new people who can see the things that others have missed. We have to find out where people are, what they know, and what they feel about the system. If we are going to be successful we have to attend to the structures. We have to understand what values are driving our decisions. From my perspective, we need to make substantive changes if we are to overcome the disillusionment with being part of a health system.

To peer inside UniCare was to see institutional affiliates and people working in isolated pods. Segmentalism was so deeply rooted in the work group's understanding of institutional life that it existed at all levels of the hierarchy. At the top, segmentalism defeated seeing affiliates as part of a larger system; functional integration at the level of the health system could not occur. At Riverside, competing values and outdated infrastructures hampered group members' ability to reach out across an abyss of separateness to help each other. Stability was impossible. On the front line, nurses and others were abandoned in a contentious work world. The nurses' public health culture, ideology, norms, relationships, and identity were rendered irrelevant for changing healthcare structures and care delivery. And worse, when nurses can't be nurses any more, it follows that dilemmas will arise for patients who need nursing care at home.

Institutional Dilemmas in Patient Care

In this section, four institutional dilemmas the nurses encountered in the context of caring for patients are presented. There were certainly more than four dilemmas described by the nurses, but the ones discussed here were the most prominent and pervasive. The nurses at Riverside found that institutional dilemmas imposed constraints ranging from "bothersome" to "destructive" in their efforts to care for patients. The latter term represents situations so distorted by the marketplace that nursing work was unrecognizable as nursing.

The Dilemma of Home Care as a Business

The market model pervaded every aspect of patient care at Riverside, which inevitably created moral dilemmas when business principles were appropriated to individual patient situations and professional judgment. Maria described a dilemma that illuminates the problem with treating persons like commodities:

I have one guy who has cardiac problems, but he also has Alzheimer's. PCI [a nonprofit health plan] told me they would pay for me to do a cardiopulmonary assessment only, nothing about the Alzheimer's. Well, I had to laugh. They will pay for me to do cardiopulmonary assessment, but won't pay me to teach about his Alzheimer's disease or work with the family about making plans. It's a joke. His dementia affects his cardiac status. How can you not deal with it? He doesn't take his medication, he is angry, and he has rages, but I think Friday will be my last visit because cardiacwise he is stable. I let the doctor know how I felt and that I was going to call PCI today to see if we can get a few more social work visits out there. There isn't much else we can do . . . but I am going to get the case back, I know it. Something is going to happen. Either this guy is going to hit his wife or he is going to have an MI [Myocardial infarction] and he's going to be in the hospital. I understand that we have to get paid for what we do, we can't do it for nothing, so you do the best you can.

Restricting Maria's visits to cardiopulmonary assessments ignores the patient's Alzheimer's disease and works against the goal of cost control by subverting the nursing principle of treating the whole patient. Vladeck

(1996) casts this dilemma more broadly as short-term profit maximization (e.g., denying visits) that can harm patients when caregiving is truncated. Good nursing in home care is an example, because it requires time for change and developing relationships. Rehabilitation from an acute illness and watchful waiting during exacerbations of chronic illness requires time and persistence. These aspects of home care nursing do not fit a corporate framework for judging bottom-line results on a quarter-to-quarter basis.

The Dilemma of Productivity

When productivity is used to measure nurses' contribution to the bottom line, nurses face the limits of reducing nursing practice solely to a measure of performance. One of the nurses at Riverside explained productivity and efficiency as "the number of visits set by the hierarchy to generate money for the organization," a definition that cannot capture the complexity of caregiving and the meaning of nurse–patient relationships.

One glaring measurement problem at Riverside was that visit productivity targets were not adjusted for case mix. Managers and case management nurses used their best judgment to adjust overall caseloads daily, but the approach contributed to uneven workloads and ultimately undermined teamwork necessary for dealing with fluctuations in referrals and patient needs. Jane explained some of her stress and frustration with productivity:

Our productivity is expected to be 6 [visits] a day, 30 a week, so when we have an opening [admission] it creates a conflict with time and other situations I have to deal with. When I first started, it was 2 to 3 openings a week and then I would finish up with other visits. But now we're doing an opening a day, sometimes 2. On the weekend I did 3. The bottom line is that I did 9 or 10 openings in 7 or 8 days. It's rather overwhelming and I am really getting burnt with this. It's a productivity issue.

An opening takes anywhere from 2 to 3 hours, start to finish, as far as documentation, phone calls, and everything else goes. To help out a manager, I did two openings then three revisits, which means I've only done five visits for the day. Five visits is not productivity, six is, so I was short a visit but not short on hours. For two openings I've got about 5 hours. Then to meet productivity I've got to do another four patients, plus I'm driving. Add in an IV Vanco [intravenous antibiotic] visit with peaks and troughs [blood draws], which is another 2 hours, and I'm always doing overtime. But it is not paid overtime. I am up to 10 to 12 hours, and I don't want to spend that much time working every day.

So you do this for a while. But after the first year it is "ah ha," I see how this is working. I'm not going to be dealing into this sucker business any more. Either I'm going to make a stink or else I'm not going to take these cases anymore.

Do you see what I am saying? The difference is a 30-minute visit versus 2 to 3 hours for an opening. . . . Both are counted as one visit, but they are not the same.

The unrelenting stress of meeting productivity constantly strained cooperation. When I mentioned the obvious, that referrals were linked to reimbursement and the financial success of home care, Sam pointed out the other side of the story:

Right, it is their [managers'] job [to accept and assign referrals], but it's our job to make sure it's not more than we can handle. People never go home, they are here all the time. Some days nurses come in here at 9:00 p.m. to get their morning assignment, rather than come in before 6:00 a.m. Managers do it too. You have to protect yourself or you can't do this job. You get pushed as far as you can get pushed and then I open my mouth wide and scream. I tell them [managers] the truth, "No, I can't do that." I've never said no unless I meant no, ever, ever, ever, ever.

Productivity not only contributed to work speedup and overload, it affected attitudes about patients and patient care. In a system oriented toward productivity and efficiency, chronically ill, complex patients who take time to care for become undesirable patients in a nurses' case load. April, a nurse, explained productivity as a system of perverted incentives to "focus on equipment" and to categorize people as if they were a medical condition and a health plan. "When people are grouped together as wheelchair bound or chronic Medicaid people, you can say you don't want anything to do with them."

A problem with productivity also showed up in the nurses' efforts to keep up-to-date with new research and the demand for new skills. Inservice education and case conferences were cancelled and rescheduled time and time again because the nurses could not take time out for education with the looming requirement to "make productivity." It got to the point where Mary Pat said, "I am starved for professional development." One day I spoke with Fran, who was emotionally worn out from trying to schedule time for education and still meet her home visit productivity:

Sometimes I get so frustrated. Most of the time we deal with it, we put in extra hours, but I feel a little beat up this week. I took my calendar into my manager to show her that I had an in-service, my six patients, and a meeting. Productivity is six and she told me I'd have to get it all done in 8 hours. I said it would be close, because I knew I'd have paperwork left over. So she said that she would take away a patient, but then I said I wouldn't make productivity. She looked at me and said, "Well, I guess you'll have to decide." And then I said, "Wait, you guys tell us you want us to go to classes, to stay current, but then you want us to make productivity and do it all in 8 hours." She just leaned back and she said, "You'll have to figure it out." I just wanted to choke her. I was looking for a little guidance, "Can I help you?" "Let's figure out the priorities." So I thought, "Wait a minute—education or productivity." It was a real battle in my mind, because I was trying to stay within 9 hours, 10 tops, but I still need to thrive and grow. It was really awful.

A theme in the experiences of Jane, Sam, April, Mary Pat, and Fran was that under the pretext of their productivity, for the sake of keeping the agency afloat, they were pushed to their limit. Distressed that nurses were being exploited for the bottom line, Fran concluded, "The company runs on the backs of the nurses." Bypassing the complex human dimensions of caregiving, productivity measured in terms of visits took a toll on the work group. When a supervisor's feeble reference to empowerment, "you'll have to figure it out," fell short for resolving the gap between work and the time available to do it, there was no plan or process in place for making a decision about what *not* to do. Looking for support, Fran subtly raised the issue of how best to handle the situation, but found no way out of her dilemma when she sensed that "everything is a priority."

The Dilemma of Regulatory Paperwork

Regulatory paperwork, one component of productivity, is consuming nurses' time and energy for patient care (PricewaterhouseCoopers, 2001). Paperwork is an accepted feature of bureaucracy, but it raises serious moral questions when scarce nursing resources are used for administrative purposes, while patient access to adequate nursing care is diminishing (Bowers, Lauring, & Jacobson, 2001; Fagin, 2001). The paperwork burden in home care, like other settings in healthcare, is generated from federal regulations, myriad state and local laws, requirements of commercial insurers, and accreditation bodies. The burden is excessive, and while efforts are under way to address the problems (HR107: *Health Care Financing Administration paperwork burdens,* 2001), no changes are anticipated in the short term.

Typically, paperwork is so important that there is a tendency to value documentation over the clinical judgment of experienced nurses, especially in matters of reimbursement. For example, unlike HMOs, where home care visits are approved prior to the nurse making the visit, Medicare auditors conduct retrospective medical record reviews to determine if care provided to patients was in compliance with federal regulations. Medicare reimbursement can be denied if any findings in the medical record are not consistent with regulations.

During an audit cycle of 100 claims submitted to Medicare for reimbursement, a glitch in the internal process of documentation at Riverside was discovered. There was a discrepancy on the government-required "485" form, whereby the date the case management nurse signed the form in the signature box did not always match two other related dates—the date when the patient's home care started and the date when the nurse notified the physician of the patient's admission to home care. The discrepancy in dates did not affect patient care, but it appeared in the medical record that the patient was admitted to the home care without a physician's order.

At a summation meeting, open to everyone at Riverside, the Medicare auditors identified the medical records that contained the documentation discrepancy. Following a careful review of the questionable records, the auditors reported that the patients met the eligible criteria for home care, and in fact were provided with "medically necessary" clinical care. Nevertheless, the auditors denied reimbursement in each case because of the signature box and date mix-up. The denial decision resulted in about $60,000 of lost reimbursement to Riverside.

The example shows why paperwork required for regulatory compliance is a growing concern. PricewaterhouseCoopers (2001) studied the regulatory burden faced by professionals and found that as more time is spent on regulatory paperwork, less time is devoted to patient care across healthcare settings. Every hour of patient care in home care generates 48 minutes of paperwork.

One of the greatest regulatory burdens in home care is the Medicare Outcomes and Assessment Information Set (OASIS). Nurses collect extensive information from every home care patient at regular intervals. According to the Centers for Medicare and Medicaid Services (HR107: *Health Care Financing Administration paperwork burdens*, 2001), home care agencies nationally spend approximately 800,000 hours per year collecting OASIS data at a cost of approximately $30 million. The data collection burden created by OASIS was added to the existing 850,000 hours and $17 million required to comply with the other conditions of participation required by Medicare. Thus, the Medicare paperwork burden alone costs home care agencies approximately $50 million annually.

The OASIS form at Riverside included questions required by Medicare and additional agency-specific questions. When fully compiled, their OASIS was a 25-page document consisting of 170 multipart questions with multiple-choice answers. The document, filled out by hand, required 40 to 90 minutes to complete; then it was processed by clerical staff and data entry personnel and entered into an electronic record. The computerized version of the document was returned to the nurse for approval and then transmitted to several agencies. Eva understandably concluded, "This nursing job is not nursing. It's 65% paperwork, 25% patient care, 10% driving."

If there can be compassionate acts involving paperwork, I observed one such act during a home visit with April. She gently worked her way through the opening (admission) process with a 71-year-old woman discharged from the hospital following surgery for an abdominal aortic aneurysm. April conducted a thorough physical assessment, responded knowledgeably to the woman's questions, spoke with her husband, and explained to them both how home care worked. April inconspicuously jotted notes on the OASIS form out of sight of the patient and then, without fanfare, obtained the required signatures from the patient on a number of government-required forms. The visit lasted 50 minutes.

April conducted the visit like an accomplished artist. The minimal shuffling of paper struck me as peculiar, so when I commented later about how little the paperwork intruded on the visit, April explained:

Oh that [knowingly, gently laughing]. Several months ago I was admitting an older woman, who had just come home from the hospital. She was exhausted and in pain. I pulled out the OASIS and when she saw the length of it and all the questions she started to cry. She couldn't face it. She just wanted to get into her own bed and go to sleep. That night I went home and memorized the whole form, so I wouldn't have to pull it out in front of a patient during a visit again. Patients have enough on their minds without being upset by paperwork.

April shouldered an unreasonable burden for her compassion when she consistently worked overtime to complete the OASIS form she refused to take into her relationship with a patient. While it is reasonable to expect a nurse to try and shield a patient from cumbersome bureaucratic processes, April's altruistic approach struck me as an example of shadow nursing. I use the term *shadow nursing* to refer to nursing work provided in the shadow of the corporate ethos. It is work systematically hidden from routine assessments and reporting about home care services, because there is no box or service code for recording compassionate acts in patient care. April's skillful approach to OASIS is not reimbursed and is uncompensated work.

The range of unbilled nursing work can range from as high as 88 unbilled visits for one episode of care and as many as 99 unbilled care-related activities, including phone calls, conferences, and special errands (Phillips, Cloonan, Irvine, & Fisher, 1990). In a home care system where what counts as skilled nursing care is only what is reimbursed, Deborah most clearly expressed the corporate eclipsing of patient care: "No one really sees the results of the work you do." Shadow nursing is troubling morally because it is largely altruistic work, and altruistic work is assumed to be natural for nurses. It is expected to be given limitlessly to patients and institutions and abets the objectification of patients.

The Dilemma of Treating Patients as Objects

The shifting of professionals' attention from patients to paperwork is just one way patients are treated as objects in home care. Listed as records in a database, patients are viewed as a medical record number, a health plan contract number, and a series of diagnoses and visit codes. And although nurses are committed to patients, the objectification of patients puts nurses in the peculiar position of both contributing to and mitigating their objectification.

Mrs. B., a patient, explained her skepticism about nurses: "The problem is the bureaucracy. I become a number and the nurses become part of the business plan and forget what they went into nursing for." In other words, in the business of home care, business models are all-encompassing. Four of these models are described below: marketplace language, cost-control strategies, hierarchical authority, and prescribed home care services.

1. Marketplace language. By the time patients are in need of home care, most have already been in other healthcare settings where they have been objectified as a disease or a research subject, or have been treated as teaching material (Fein, 1982). These identities are carried

over to home care. The medical diagnosis, for example, is the key to qualifying for referral to home care, and it determines what division patients will be assigned to in the field. At Riverside, there was a cardiac team, a dementia team, a comfort care team, an adult services division, and a maternal–child health division.

When the marketplace is added to the picture of patient care, patients are labeled another type of object. They are customers. And further, when home care is added, patients become "referrals" with a "pay source." It gets even worse. According to Medicare billing, patients are "skilled nursing visits" required to be "homebound." On the daily scheduling board, patients are "off-loaded" from one nurse to another. Patient care is documented on a form called a "single-visit flow sheet," as if one visit was disconnected from the other visits. Every 60 days patients become "recerts," when paperwork has to be updated for reimbursement.

In these examples, the language of the corporation displaces talk about persons and compassion. The language of human interactions in relationships is silenced to a point where it becomes nearly impossible to nurture a consciousness about caring for patients in healthcare. When business talk and data systems are emphasized, the institution's interests are reinforced. One executive at Riverside reflected about the power of the corporation to change views about patients and institutional life:

We never even used the word corporate at UniCare until the top executives moved into the corporate headquarters downtown. Once we had [offices at] 1250 Main Street we were corporate. We started saying things like "I have a meeting at corporate" and "You have a call from corporate." We were making decisions about services and consolidation, but the problem was nobody ever saw patients. When the offices were in the hospital we at least saw patients in the hallways and on stretchers. They kept you focused on the reason there is healthcare. At corporate, there were decisions without patients and not many people felt good about going there to work. The most telling evidence of distancing ourselves from patients was that the front door was locked for security reasons. Even if patients found their way downtown, they couldn't walk in the front door. They had to be buzzed in over an intercom. . . . One of the best moves we made was relocating the executive offices back to the hospital. Closing the corporate office sent the message that we were refocusing on patients.

2. Cost-control strategies. Cost control, a national theme in healthcare, is another business model that objectifies patients. It is currently the predominant health policy objective and at the core of most discussions in

healthcare (Caplan, 1996). When taken to this extreme, patient identity is co-opted, and patients can encounter poor quality of care and lack of attention to caregiving (Abramson, 1996). Nationally, cost cutting combined with a nursing shortage is limiting patients' access to nursing care.

The dominance of cost control reinforces an earlier claim: patients and nurses are so intertwined that a dilemma for one group significantly affects the other. For example, nurses at Riverside spent time copying and filing forms and tracking down medical records. At the same time nurses were doing clerical work, executives were considering replacing community health nurses with licensed practical nurses in the field. Using nurses for non-nursing work and substituting less qualified staff members for skilled community health nurses limits patients' access to nurses. Classic strategies for reducing salary expenses in the short term inherently treat patients as objects, as if they were separate from nurses and could be used as trade-offs for the bottom line.

3. Hierarchical authority. This third mechanism contributing to the objectification of patients is so deeply embedded in institutional life that the subtle and disturbing message being sent to nurses on the front line is that their value to healthcare increases the farther they move away from the bedside.[3] Nowhere was the devaluing of nurses' professional judgment more evident at Riverside than with the gatekeeping function of HMOs. Fran was angry about the relentless and mortifying challenges to her clinical judgment by the gatekeepers:

I hate begging for visits from HMOs. It makes me crazy. I'm the nurse; don't tell me how to do my job. They'll argue with you and sometimes the nurses are the worst ones. "Isn't there someone who can do that evening dressing?" or "Can't you teach so and so?" You have to fight with them and say, "No, that's not working." It's frustrating. I don't like the managed care patients because of that.

In the last line of the quotation, Fran did not distinguish the patient from the health plan, which shows that nurses' attitudes toward patients can get mixed up with the reputation and requirements of the health plan. When a patient is referred to as a Medicare patient, Medicaid patient, PCI patient, and so on, social attitudes and institutional failings associated with the health plan are transferred to the patient. Alternatively, patients' health plans and associated socioeconomic status can work in their favor; as one nurse commented, "I almost prefer to have the inner city [patients], because you know they are going to be poor, and I can get the stuff they need through [Medi]caid." Nurses' central concern is with patients, but these data show they are not immune to contributing to the objectification of patients. In no small measure, culture and social structures construct the language and worldviews of persons in everyday encounters (Fein, 1982).

4. Prescribed home care services. Patients also become objects in home care via the rigid criteria that define who is eligible for home care and what counts as home care. Two main groups of patients access home care services: post-hospital patients and disabled and chronically ill patients. The health plans mete out services for both groups, but here I focus on the latter group because of the growing demand for long-term, chronic-care services and a shrinking safety net of services to meet the demand (Himmelstein, Wollhandler, & Hellander, 2001; Mason & Leavitt, 1998).

Home care services are changeable, fragmented, and uncertain, which tips the scale of power toward the health plan. At Riverside, patients and families had a notable unease about how and when shifting policies, economics, and services would disrupt their lives. Mrs. E. described the uncertainty she faces over the home health service she relies upon for Jonathan, her disabled son:

MRS. E.: "The aide service is key to what I need, and I can understand there are problems with scheduling because of shortages, but I get a lot of them. I request to get the same aides, and I get mad because they send me aides right out of school. Jonathan is their first case. He scares them or they really don't want to work with disabled people. If they stay, once I get them trained they are good now, so they go on to someplace else. So I got to train somebody else."

T.O.: "How many aides has Jonathan had over 12 years in home care?"

MRS. E.: "Oh my God, I don't think I could count them all, I've had so many. I've had aides that have stayed a long time and then I've had aides for the shift. If she can't come in, then I don't get an aide. It makes me feel bad. I need help getting him into bed. If there is nobody around to help me, Jonathan ends up sleeping on the floor. Sometimes I just can't get him up. He is 31 now and he is getting a little bit heavy for me to lift."

T.O.: "How often is it that the aide doesn't come?"

MRS. E.: "I don't get aide service a lot. Today is Thursday. I haven't got aide service twice this week. Like right now it is 3:00 p.m. and I'm not sure whether I'm going to have an aide this afternoon. They used to guarantee me coverage, but now they tell me they can't guarantee me coverage. It puts me in such a predicament. It makes me wonder about the people that don't have anybody to care for them, that don't have a family to come in and do for them. I can say, okay, I am burned out or I am not feeling well enough to get him ready for the day program, but I can keep him home with me. I'm here with him, but there's people who don't have family to care for them. So I think the aide service should be much, much better than it is. And I think they should get paid for what they do."

Mrs. E.'s situation is consistent with the trend of family caregiving. Reemerging in the 1980s, family caregiving has grown even more common in the era of managed care and cost containment to the point where family caregivers provide 80% of all long-term care in the United States (Fagin, 2001; O'Brien & DeMarco, 1999; Wagner, 1997). The home, actually the family farm with several generations of caregivers, was the primary location for healthcare delivery prior to urbanization in the 19th century, but now one of the structural problems of institutions is that the role of family caregivers is still largely taken for granted as one that families are expected to undertake willingly and lovingly (Fisher, 1998). Mrs. E. wanted to care for her son at home, but she was weary from the ongoing 24-hour responsibility for caregiving and worried about a time when she might be sick or otherwise unable to care for her son.

When the caregiver is a child caring for a parent, the caregiver may end up quitting his or her job and struggling with the loss of income (O'Brien & DeMarco, 1999). Mrs. L. relied on her only daughter and nursing assistants for care at home. Her daughter was stressed trying to care for her mother and keep a job:

Basically, I am elected when my mom's aides don't come or are here too short of a time to get things done. . . . She's supposed to get 4 hours, but when they are short of aides they cut her down to 2. Basically an aide can't get everything done in 2 hours. They can't get her out of her bed, give her a bath, give her something to eat, and then take her back to the bathroom before she [aide] leaves all in 2 hours. They can't do it. Then I come home from work and I've got to pick up where they left off. I know it's my mother and in the past, yes, I was taking care of her, but I wasn't working at the time. Now I'm working, and they think I can just go ahead and do everything. It is basically like they are telling my mother, "You need to call your daughter at work to come home and take care of you because we don't have any aides," or it's 2:00 and I don't come home until 7:00 or

8:00 p.m. She's got to sit there, and if she ain't went to the bathroom since 2:00 in the afternoon she has to keep trying to maneuver herself so that she don't wet herself until I come home.

The changing needs of patients and family caregivers have also produced a situation where a prescribed list of unalterable home care benefits may not always match the services that patients need. Mrs. B. named this problem "The One Person Theory," in which she conceptualized home care as a book, constructed with ideal patients and ideal outcomes. Mrs. B. said she "did not fit the quotes of the book." Socially, physically, and economically vulnerable, she was an unemployed, single parent and matriarch for four generations of family members. Her voice of experience was illuminating:

They should see us as individuals with individual needs. But it's not so. The aides go in and do a structured routine; it's all the same for everyone. They don't look to see that if Mrs. Jones has minor children it's OK to cook a meal for her plus a little bit extra for the children. The aide can only cook for Mrs. Jones, but it's just as easy to cook for three than it is for one you know.

We're individuals in one sense because we might need a dressing, we might need decubitus care, or some might need to be turned in bed, but overall we are looked at the same when it comes to family. The individual's situation is overlooked because a certain service is provided. When it comes down to the aide service, I've progressed, I am doing better, but I have aide service because I am eligible for aide service. What I could use now is chore service.

I'm hoping you just don't keep this to yourself. I hope that this gets to somebody. We need more individual care. The nurse has a lot with treatments and drips and taking care of so many in the field. I understand that they're overwhelmed in that way. But part of the nurses' job is to cut services, so they are also telling you what you don't need. The business gets mixed up with what you count on them for. I would like it left outside when my nurses come into my home. I am not trying to get extra [chore] services, I am trying to find the tools to keep up the fight. So, when I get overlooked I push everybody away at the agency. I hold them out there because I don't trust the service anymore.

Mrs. B. pointed out that the typical home care benefit structure objectifies patients by focusing on medical problems, as if they were separate from the social context of patients' lives. As a subscriber of a health plan, the need for chore service is irrelevant when only aide service is covered. Mrs. B. also highlighted nurses' dual role of gatekeeper and professional, which raises questions about conflict of interest in relationships with patients.

Even a dying patient could not escape being objectified as a commodity by the prescribed package of home care services. April reflected about a situation that had troubled her for a long time:

Two years ago I had a patient on comfort care. She wanted to stay with UniCare, rather than transfer to a certified hospice, but the insurance company only allotted so many visits per year and she had used most of them. She wanted hydration, which in her eyes was comfort. She had a Foley in, so that takes visits, and she needed pain control, dressing changes, and monitoring the medi-port. We could have been out there three times a day. She had dressings like you would not believe. But it just wasn't meant to be and it broke my heart watching these people struggle. They couldn't just spend time with their mom, they had to be the nurse. They had to lift, tug, and turn her for positioning, the aide situation was horrible, and they could only have so many hours of aide service anyway. It was a nightmare.

I went every day, but of course, I couldn't charge every day because they would have run out of visits and they didn't have enough money to private pay. So for me, the ethical issue involved the policies of the agency and the government, and the insurance company. I only officially had enough visits for one visit a week, but I saw her once a day, sometimes twice a day. I was going on my weekends off to see her because the family was at their wits' end; there was nothing they could do. They were told plain and simple, "She can be admitted to the hospital or long-term care, or you can keep her at home and keep going like this." They didn't have any positive options. It was a very sad case and I was very emotionally involved.

I got a lot of support here from my supervisor, my fellow workers, and the behavioral health nurse. We met, we talked, and she made a couple of visits with me. The case sticks out in my mind. I almost quit home care because it was so draining. She got poor home care and I didn't like that. She wanted care that didn't fit into the category of comfort care or hospice. Nobody wanted her to go into the hospital and the hospice nurse said there really wasn't too much more they could offer. They don't cover everything and they don't take patients with IVs. Care shouldn't come down to having the right or wrong insurance. I just felt bad that I couldn't get her more support, but money was running the show. The question is how can we educate people about insurance and what is covered and not covered. Pay source, it is my biggest dilemma.

The institutional aspects of patient care dilemmas—home care as a business, productivity, regulatory paperwork, and the objectification of patients—reflect incremental change and chaos in home care that puts patients and nurses in the position of trying to figure out what to do in everyday situations. The quandaries showed up vividly in the nurses' questions, "Now what do I do?" (Fran), "When am I asking the patient to do too much?" (Chris), "Have we done everything we can do?" (Holly), "How do I justify using a cheaper version that might not work as well because Medicare pays but Medicaid doesn't?" (Eva). These are the types of questions responsible nurses ask when institutional structures have little to do with the world of patient care. In an effort to fulfill their obligations to patients, the nurses approached the dilemmas by wrestling with the marketplace.

Wrestling with the Marketplace

Wrestling is a metaphor that captures nurses' expressions of their moral agency in patient care. As a noun meaning *a struggle* and as a verb meaning *to throw or immobilize one's opponent* (American Heritage Dictionary of the English Language, 2000), the nurses' wrestling involved confronting institutional structures that did not respect their values and aims in patient care. A thoughtful, proactive form of resistance on behalf of patients, the nurses' wrestled to overcome barriers to what they viewed as their ineluctable obligation to care for patients. The opponents changed and the wrestling took different forms, but in grappling with the home care system, the nurses refused to submit unquestioningly to formal rules, regulations, and practices governing patient care. Representing the strength of the nurses' character, wrestling mitigated the intrusion of the corporation into patient care.

As a practical matter, wrestling was the only way to get the job done: "Rules need to be interpreted" (Sam), because nurses "go into different situations all the time" (Holly). "Not everything is neat and clean or black and white. In home care we live in the gray" (Brenda). "You have to work around and through things to get patients what they need" (Eva). And Esther explained:

The system drives you to break the rules, because it is so complex nothing is clear. You have to learn a loose way of working, to do what is best for the patients. It is not cut and dried, and it is a tremendous amount of responsibility because the boundaries are open and fluid and we need room to maneuver and be creative. The goal is patient care, but that goal gets lost in paperwork and regulations and time pressures. To the degree that the system works, it is because we are well-educated professionals and take our responsibility to try and do what is right for patients seriously.

When the bureaucracy threatened to get in the way of the nurses doing their job, wrestling was a way of creating a zone of control over barriers to effectiveness. Claire commented:

I love home care. It is important work, and I feel like I make a contribution to patients every day, but the work is like a rolling ball. You have to be conscious of not letting it roll over you. You have to keep kicking it back. Our basic goal is to assess patients' needs and then plan how to meet those needs. It requires basic nursing knowledge plus critical thinking skills. But to really make things happen you have to have expert networking skills. The idea is to find people who know ways to get in the back door and then learn what they know. If you don't, the work rolls over you and you can't overcome it.

Justifications for wrestling varied by nurse and by situation. Marian explained, "Home care is real life, so we keep going. There is always something else to try. We don't give up, otherwise there is no hope." Other nurses wrestled with the formal rules on the basis that they were putting patients ahead of a home care system concerned with cost cutting and protecting profits. At the level of the home care system, they wrestled as strong advocates:

When people trust me with their life story and their information, I have to do something. If I see a case that's got multiple needs not being addressed, I can't ignore them. (Marge)

For Jeanne, wrestling was morally responsible. She said, "I do it because I tell my patients I will be their best advocate. I take cues from them about what I should do for them as a nurse." Wrestling also preserved nursing as a caring profession:

I want to be the guy down here who breaks those rules and keeps the heart in nursing. We have to show that healthcare is given with the heart and the hands. It goes beyond oximeters and stitches, but the problem is you can't see it and insurance companies don't want to pay for it. (Fran)

Four strategies employed by the nurses in confronting the marketplace show the nurses' skillful approach to institutional dilemmas as they try to do what they judge to be the right thing for patients.

1. *Making the system see the patient in a different way* was one of Eva's strategies for meeting patients' needs. This strategy aimed at overcoming barriers to patients' access to home care services. The home care system works best for insured patients, who have a short-term, post-hospital acute-care illness and who have supportive family members or friends able to assist in caregiving. Nurses wrestle with the system when their patients fall outside of these criteria.

Following a stroke, one of Fran's patients experienced impaired judgment and lapses of memory. A woman in her fifties, classified as high risk, the patient was largely immobile and lived by herself. She was stranded at the bus station without a place to live, so the police called Riverside and Fran was assigned to be the woman's case manager.

Fran was diligent in trying to get her patient a doctor's appointment, but unwittingly the patient kept getting in the way of her own care. One morning, for example, the woman awoke around 4:00 a.m. It was snowing and she wondered why her home health aide, scheduled for 7:00 a.m., had not yet arrived. Concerned that she was not going to make her doctor's appointment on time, the patient cancelled the home health aide, the transportation service, and the appointment with the doctor. By the time Fran figured out what had happened in the morning, it was too late to undo the cancellations:

I got her an appointment at Marie Rossi Health Center, which is a bear to start with, and then I struggled all week to get her transportation because her Medicaid wasn't active yet. I made a couple calls to people higher up, pulling strings to get her transportation. Then I moved her aide service from her usual 9–11 to 7–9 so she would be ready for her doctor's appointment. And then, she cancelled everything. It's a problem because she needs to see the doctor to get her pills. She was self-dosing on HCTZ [blood pressure medication] and she has hypertension. It wasn't the first time she screwed up either, but I've got her number. We have learned to work together, but she does bully people and she can be really intimidating. So when you get a patient like this, the doctors write them off, the agency writes them off, and I have to keep defending her. When I say to people it is because of her stroke that she did this, she has memory lapses, sometimes they'll listen. So you know, the doctor scheduled another appointment, and I told the schedulers to put in the computer that when she calls in the future, not to cancel any aides until they check with the nurse first.

In this story, Fran wrestled with a home care system that did not see an uninsured patient. With a reputation for "screwing up," care providers, who did not know her, were inclined to be impatient with her. To make her patient visible, Fran called higher-ups, pulled strings, and defended her patient.

Kathleen's patient was missed when transfers and multiple physicians fragmented her care:

Emma Jacobs is a Medicare patient with a pericardial window, poorly medically managed. She went to rehab and the doctor [on the referral] was her rehab doctor. He refused to do anything about her medical problems and her primary physician didn't know her. When I called with a low heart rate, in the 50s, and the patient was having problems with nausea and vomiting, the office said we have never seen her, she is a new patient, you need to talk to her cardiologist.

Well, it turned out there was no cardiologist assigned to her, so I called the primary back the next morning and I said to the nurse, you can't mismanage this situation. We need to have something done for her. She's on Digoxin and Lopressor and her heart rate is low. I said, "She's not taking those two medications this morning and she is waiting to hear from you about coming in to be evaluated by the doctor or whatever we are going to do." They ended up seeing her right away and she was in heart block. She was dig toxic and [found] herself going to the hospital. They couldn't get her out of heart block, so she [found herself with] a pacer [pacemaker]. When she came out of the hospital she had a cardiologist.

Because Emma was repeatedly seen as another physician's patient, Kathleen acted to fill a crack in the physician referral and transfer process and pressed the nurse in the primary care physician's office to see her patient and to respond to a person requiring immediate medical attention.

One of Natalie's patients got completely lost by the home care system at the critical juncture between the hospital and the home care agency:

This is a lady who had endocarditis and became increasingly more confused with the Vanco [antibiotic] to the point where the doctor decreased the dosage. After talking to him that she was having mental status changes, she went to the hospital and then ended up actually having an anaphylactic reaction to it. When she came home it was a frustrating thing.

I had called the discharge coordinator to tell her that we weren't going to accept her back to home care [because she was not safe to be at home by herself]. She had a PICC line and I found her in the bathtub, and there was an episode where she had left the gas on in the house all night long on the stove. But she slipped out [of the hospital] by mistake and ended up coming home on a Saturday. I called the hospital Monday and they said she had been discharged but I didn't get a report from weekends. Nobody knew anything about her. So she went for two days at home without antibiotic therapy or a PICC line flush. The coordinator didn't follow up on her over the weekend.

Fran's, Kathleen's, and Natalie's stories are representative of the many times nurses advocated to help others see their patients. Patients, whether chronically ill or in need of acute care services, including patients who had insurance, were vulnerable to being bypassed precisely because they were getting care at home. They were not, as the nurses said, the "good patients" that could "move efficiently" through the home care system.

2. *Stretching services and supplies* is a form of wrestling used to fill the cracks between reimbursed services and services needed by patients. This strategy was nuanced and detailed and could only be used by experienced nurses who understood the home care system. Getting approval for visits is the best example of hypervigilant wrestling with HMOs. It was a process Eva likened to "pulling teeth from a chicken."

In some situations the need for visits was indisputable. The difficulty occurred when the case manager wanted visits that the HMO gatekeeper did not agree were needed. With a stunning scarcity of research in home care about the relationship of nursing care to patient outcomes, decision making about the right number of visits comes down to conflicts between case management nurses' clinical judgment and HMO gatekeepers' interests in denying visits to protect profits. This wrestling match occurred every day, time and time again.

Efforts to humanize healthcare with support and tender loving care led nurses to stretch visits as far as possible:

There have been times when I've stretched people out. It's like creative writing 101, you know, to make the patient appear sick enough so that you can justify visits. I mean, these are sick people, but I've added a little more flavor to it, the wording is a little different. . . . Maybe I give them six or seven weeks because they needed that little extra TLC to get a little stronger, a little more independent. (Esther)

When patients were on the borderline between skilled nursing care and supportive care, stretching visits was viewed as more cost effective than institutionalization:

I had a patient with colon cancer with mets to the liver who ended up getting a nasty, itchy, open eschar. She is independent with the dressing change, but if she gets a massive infection she goes back in the hospital for weeks and weeks. Wouldn't it be better to have a skilled assessment once a week to make sure the wound is doing well? So I try to tell them that my visits are saving a hospital admission, that it is more efficient. . . . You say, "Let's stay ahead of this to keep her out of trouble by going in once a week, then once every two weeks, and then finally discharge her." I mention she has COPD [chronic obstructive pulmonary disease]. You try to add things together. (Kathleen)

There were also appeals to the gatekeepers' own sense of doing the right thing by pointing out the absurdity of denying visits:

I had a patient with a 9-cm-deep wound on her abdomen. She was a very heavy woman, a diabetic. Her husband was legally blind and they wanted him to do the dressing. You sit there and you say, "Are you out of your mind? He's legally blind. How is he going to do the dressing? Feel around to find where it is? How would you feel about this if it was your mother?" (Eva)

When the nurses could not justify stretching visits for medical reasons, some resorted to unofficial patient visits, which are visits not recorded in the medical record or billed to insurance companies. The nurses also accumulated unused supplies from one patient to use with another. They turned to charitable community services and sometimes made modest purchases for patients, such as groceries, a special meal, or more rarely, medication when a patient did not have money to fill his prescriptions.

3. *Turning a blind eye and a deaf ear* to circumstances that might threaten patients' eligibility for home care services was a strategy that allowed the nurses to continue care when they judged it was needed. One of the nurses' strongest opponents in this wrestling match was the Medicare requirement that a patient be "confined to his home," or "homebound." Assessing a patient's homebound status is a moral morass, because the standards are confusing and have been challenged in the courts.

To meet the homebound test, a patient's trips outside the home must require the aid of another individual or an assist device. The second, and stricter, standard requires that the trips involve considerable and taxing effort, be infrequent and of short duration, and be for the purpose of medical treatment. A patient discharged from the hospital with abdominal drains and dressing changes, restricted by physician order from leaving the house, is indisputably homebound. Other situations are not so clear.

When a patient with Alzheimer's disease required nursing visits for new-onset diabetes, but wandered freely from her home, the nurses struggled with the possibility of denying Medicare visits that would help family members manage her diabetes. A patient with heart failure received daily help from a home health aide and stabilized to the point where he could leave home to go to the grocery store. No longer homebound, he lost the home health aide service that made it possible for him to leave the house in the first place. Even experienced nurses struggled with the homebound test, as Jackie explained:

Just recently, an experienced community health nurse had a difficult time with the homebound requirement. There's a patient on the cardiac team status post CABG [coronary artery bypass surgery]. He is not homebound, but he has a sternal wound that requires dressing changes. The nurse said to me, "The person really needs my services; there's no way that anybody else in the family could do it." Yet, the person wasn't homebound. We talked and I explained that there is no disputing nursing services are needed, but you can't bill Medicare because the patient isn't homebound. He is out and doing all kinds of things. He shouldn't be out with an open sternal wound, but that's beside the point. Functionally he was able to be out and about.

Turning a blind eye and a deaf ear to possible reasons for disqualification from home care was also a way of responding to patients' need for comfort and well-being:

When I was case managing, the thing that I always did turn a blind eye and a deaf ear to, by not documenting the conversation, was my little ole ladies going out to get their hair done and going out to visit a spouse in the cemetery. In both of those cases, 9 times out of 10 it was family or friend or somebody that was helping them to get out and I just always figured getting their hair done promoted more of a sense of well-being than going to any physician or health professional. So I never had any quandaries about sort of not documenting that they went out. (Deborah)

Chris and other nurses who used this strategy tended to adjust the homebound rule more readily at the beginning of a patient's admission to home care than at the end:

I feel strongly about the criteria set and that we need to follow it, but we need to mold and bend it. If the patient is questionably homebound and needs a couple of visits, is bending the rule deception? I will not do it six months down the road, and I make that clear in the beginning. Home care is acute, for two to three months. If you need more, we need to do something else. You have to set the table and make it clear that the preponderance of cases are short term. As nurses, we are softhearted, which is a good thing, but we can get into trouble because so much is subjective data. You have to see it for what it is. There is beauty in it, but it is also painful for the nurse to have to make judgments about level of services.

Chris's statement reveals the double-bind nature of the homebound rule, because in the moment there was no way out of his dilemma. He could not mold the homebound rule and adhere to it, so he used time and openness to balance conflicting forces.

4. *Teaching patients the problems with the rules* is a strategy by which nurses sought to empower patients to be their own advocates. Eva took a straightforward approach:

I've actually told my patients, if you are not getting what you need, you have to do something. It you are not getting the treatment you need you make a list of questions and stand in front of that door and don't let the doctor out till you get your questions answered. If you are not getting what you think you need from the HMO, you go to the president. You have to be your own advocate because nobody else is going to do it for you. It's pretty sad [but] I have patients say, you know I've got more information from you in three visits than I have from my doctor in my whole disease process.

Sam coached patients about the problem of homebound status:

There are people I have said to, fairly early, I need to tell you the rules for homebound according to Medicare. And you need to listen to me so that you can answer my questions appropriately. And they'll figure out what they can't say. I can't say, "I'm telling you how to lie," but I'll tell them things that will make them homebound. We all do that.

Mr. D., a patient, was aware that Ruth had adjusted the rules on his behalf:

I liked Ruth. She was funny, and we got along, so I don't want to get her in trouble. . . . If her supervisor finds out that she helped me with a problem other than my leg, she could get in trouble. . . . She wasn't supposed to mess with other things besides my leg, but I had a hernia about a year ago and it [incision] has never healed right. So, I said, "All you are doing is looking at it. It seems to me if you are here for something and something else is wrong, why don't you look at it before it gets really bad? It may save them money, don't you think?" They want to save money, but they don't want to save money. It is the stupidest thing I have ever seen. The nurses have to sneak around to help their patients. I said, "I won't tell anybody, you don't tell anybody."

Nurses wrestled with the marketplace to bypass formal institutional structures that prevented them from doing what they perceived was the right thing to do for patients. Their strategies struck me as responsible moral actions, which made it possible for them to care for patients and advocate for needed services. Wrestling with the marketplace is likewise responsible resistance, in which the nurses did what was possible to fill the cracks in a broken system that is failing to meet the needs of patients it was designed to serve.

Taking Personhood Seriously

Taking note of the nurses' experiences over four years at Riverside brings the institutional aspects of morality in home care into view. Changing values and institutional structures at Riverside transformed the nurses' standing as persons in the workplace and brought about accompanying moral problems. The nurses did not stand next to the workplace, nor did they stand as individual persons within it. Rather, their personhood was intimately defined and redefined by prevailing values, principles, priorities, and expectations of the institution and of the local healthcare culture.

Depersonalization was a disturbing feature of corporatization. The nurses' corporate persona was so distorted that they did not see it as consistent with their professional identity. Without recognized values, symbols, roles, and relationships, the nurses were abandoned in a workplace that refused to value them and nursing work.

The nurses at Riverside were thrice exploited. First, practicing in the shadow of the corporate ethos, nurses spent countless hours filling cracks in a fragmented, redundant, inefficient home care system. In these predictable and common instances, the institution exploited the expertise and altruistic capital that reside within nurses' personhood to meet the needs of patients. Second, nurses' work, beyond what was selectively recorded on payroll forms and insurance claims, was not acknowledged or accounted for in formal discussions and assessments of home care services. Third, nurses' knowledge and experience was not reimbursed and was left uncompensated.

For patients, the situation is worse morally because they are sick and vulnerable and they turn to the home care system for help. Treated as a routine according to the "One Person Theory," Mrs. B. was desperate to be recognized as a person in a confusing system she experienced as untrustworthy. Mrs. E. encountered reprehensible gaps in home health aide service. Once Mrs. L.'s daughter finally found a job, she risked losing it. These examples illustrate situations in which home care as a business is not good business. Services provided do not meet minimal standards for reliability, customization, and consistent quality. In an era of customer service, it is clear that home care is not patient driven (Kearney & Bandley, 1990).

The moral consequence of the home care system in terms of personhood is that the personhood of patients and nurses is treated with complete disregard, and worse, indifference. Patients are objectified as "referrals" with "a pay source." When nurses are not considered persons they are ineligible to be full participants in a dialogue about patient care and work practices. The nurses at Riverside refused to be passive automatons and fully integrate a corporate persona into their understanding of self, but at a time in healthcare when the priority is efficiency and cost control, it is unconscionable that nursing time and expertise is squandered on dysfunctional institutional systems.

To the extent that Mohr and Mahon (1996) are right in concluding that "ethics has become the stepchild to 'real research,' which is outcome and intervention oriented and geared to what can or cannot be funded in a competitive atmosphere" (p. 35), it would be a mistake to think that depersonalization is not a serious moral problem worthy of research. The loss of personhood in the marketplace warrants moral outrage and response in its own right. It also has implications for the larger healthcare system, as the same impersonal forces redefining nurses' personhood undergird the structures, processes, and outcomes in patient care, administration, research, and education.

Another mistake related to the first would be to think that the problems at Riverside could not occur in some frequency or form in other institutions being transformed by corporatization. Although the healthcare system is intended to be about respect for persons along with integrity, care, compassion, trust, and so on, evidence at Riverside and in other healthcare settings across the United States (Abramson, 1996; Adams, 2002; Aroskar, 1995; Baer, Fagin, & Gordon, 1996; Bingham, 2002;

David, 1999; Dombeck & Olsan, 2002; Fagin, 2001; Fein, 1982; Marck, 2000; SmithBattle, Diekemper, & Drake, 1999) indicates those values are being eclipsed by a business plan that does not include persons. Personhood is an abstract concept that can easily be ignored. Sadly, it is sometimes only appreciated once it is lost.

Thus, in order to assess the full impact of corporatization it is important to examine the relationships between health policy, institutions, and small acts of living in daily encounters in healthcare (Goffman, 1961). It is in these relationships that the often insidious disregard of personhood occurs. If we do not consider personhood in assessing changing values and structures in healthcare, then our only guides for organizational change will be business principles and organizational theories narrowly construed as efficiency, productivity, and segmentalism. What we learn from the nurses at Riverside is that relationships cannot be sustained without meaningful moral attachments, and certainly a humane healthcare system cannot exist if persons are not valued *as* persons.

Some nurses at Riverside told me their stories because they wanted to explain how changes imposed by the marketplace were affecting their practice. Some trusted that their experiences would matter to the people who read about them. Others wondered if their stories would be believed. Personally, I am optimistic that we can improve the home care system we have created if we attend to the findings and the questions that have emerged in this research.

First, this research was conducted during a time in healthcare when two competing paradigms framed assessments of healthcare reform—basic entitlements and commercialization. The tension between the two is not easily addressed, but unless institutional structures are infused with personhood and meaning, depersonalization and objectification will continue to wound and leave scars on nurses and put quality of patient care at risk. The pressing question is, Will key stakeholders commit to challenging the dominant paradigm of corporatization through ongoing processes of involvement to negotiate workable solutions to moral problems?

Second, it is uncommon to invite nurses from the rank and file into boardrooms and policy making arenas in healthcare, but that lack of invitation is a mistake. If workable, cost-effective models of care delivery are to be developed, it is essential that community health nurses, and other professions providing direct care to patients, be positioned to create policies. Rather than wrestling with the marketplace, nurses need to be part of setting the agenda for home care—and healthcare in general—in the present and future.

In a healthcare system oriented toward improving health outcomes and producing cost-effective care, leaving community health nurses out of discussions about quality and costs is deeply misguided. Nurses' expertise and experience are relevant to reform, especially since the new rules for redesigning healthcare proposed by the Institute of Medicine (2001) are consistent with the principles upon which public health nursing was established over 100 years ago. The key question is, will public health nursing principles and approaches to patient care continue to be ignored, or will they be embraced for restructuring care delivery systems and institutions in home care?

Third, the reliance on informal cultural systems as a corrective to impersonal formal institutional structures raises many questions. No rational system of care delivery would intentionally be designed to require moral agents to adjust rules and stretch the truth in order to do the right thing for patients. Rule adjustment and other forms of resistance comprise a fruitful area for further research in philosophy and the social sciences. Systematic flaws in the system generating the problem need to be identified and alternatives proposed. An important question is, in the current culture of blame in healthcare (Institute of Medicine, 2000), will we find a way to sensitively explore and elaborate the practice of wrestling with the marketplace that does not risk nurses' integrity, and more practically, their jobs?

Fourth, the home care system, as it appears in health policy analyses and government reports, misrepresents resources and services invested in patient care on the front line. Nursing work is most commonly operationalized and evaluated by home visits, but there is quite a difference between formal services that are allowed and what is actually provided. Rigorous analyses of the effects of reimbursement controls on patient care and nursing practice in home care are needed. Family caregiving in home care also needs to be examined to determine the scope, stressors, skill sets, and services needed by family members. One question worth pursuing is, Will investments be made in a more in-depth analysis of home care costs for redesigning benefit structures or will policies continue that exploit the altruistic work of nurses and the love of family members for the sake of the bottom line?

Finally, institutions raise complex issues about responsibility. Decision-making processes in healthcare have become so complex that it may not be unfair to say that often decisions are made by no one (Vladeck, 1993). The human costs of restructuring and corporatization, however, cannot be ignored if we want a healthcare system that embodies human good.

The imperative that emerged from Riverside calls for leaders to engage in serious self-reflection to understand their personal contexts for decision making and for acting in the workplace (Gross et al., 1993). The first order of business is to create work environments that appeal to social values and foster expressions of human dignity (Brodeur, 1997). An important question for every member of a work group is, What strategies can be employed to transcend segmentalist structures in institutions in order to meet the demands of the marketplace without sacrificing personhood?

Postscript

In the early 1990s, the contemporary wisdom was that home care would be a pivotal link in comprehensive healthcare reform (O'Donnell & Sampson, 1994). By 1997, an estimated 60% of acute hospital systems were affiliated with home care agencies (Meyer, 1997). But uncertainty about whether home care could actually reduce inpatient costs by earlier discharge, combined with declining Medicare reimbursement, led some IHSs to sell their home care affiliate and some other agencies to close. Since the federal Balanced Budget Act was passed in 1997, approximately 3,500 home care agencies have closed (National Association for Home Care, 2000).

Similarly, five years after a turbulent affiliation, UniCare sold Riverside to a large regional health insurance company. Riverside was subsequently dismantled and merged with another home care agency. These mergers represent the most dramatic cases of effaced personhood in the Riverside nurses' story. The official role of public health nurse was eliminated from the nurses themselves and from the patients they cared for at the county for almost a century. Following the sale of Riverside to the health insurance company, community health nurses likewise disappeared from the UniCare health system.

For over a century social and economic forces in the United States have pushed and pulled on home care, and also on nurses. At the start of this research I wondered if I would be able to find and interpret institutional forces in the nurses' stories. At the conclusion of this work, I have come to appreciate that institutions were part of nurses' stories all along, especially the stories of community health nurses. They expertly navigate blurred boundaries and work in multiple conflicting contexts simultaneously.

What is different from the past, however, is the authority of the marketplace in home care. It is at odds with nurses' ideals. It silences the voices and the changing needs of patients. In its current form, the market model does not respond to the requirements of caregiving. Embracing the market model as the sole paradigm for restructuring healthcare has put the humanness of nurses and patients on the endangered list.

In the midst of chaos, the incremental approach to reform will likely continue, at least for the short term. But we have learned from the nurses at Riverside that expressions of personhood can raise consciousness about changing contexts in healthcare and the significance of new institutional arrangements. The open question is, Will our response to the moral dilemmas created by healthcare institutions acknowledge the manifest urgency of the problems?

Notes

1. Community health nurse refers to nurses working in home care agencies and holding positions as managers, support staff, procedure nurses, and case management nurses. Case management nurses were the main participants in this research, and unless otherwise indicated, they are the nurses quoted in the text.

2. To protect the privacy of participants, organizations, and places in this study, fictitious names have been used in place of information that could identify the actual home care agency in this study. Details of circumstances and events have been changed when they did not alter the meaning of the nurses' experiences.

3. I am grateful to Rebecca Forbes, RN, for raising my consciousness of institutional attitudes and forces that push nurses away from direct patient care.

References

Abramson, H. S. (1996). A patient's view. In E. D. Baer, C. M. Fagin, & S. Gordon (Eds.), *Abandonment of the patient: The impact of profit-driven health care on the public* (pp. 25–30). New York: Springer.

Adams, B. (2002). Accountable but powerless. *Health Affairs, 21,* 218–223.

Allen, N. J. (1989). The category of the person: A reading of Mauss's last essay. In M. Carrithers, S. Collins, & S. Lukes (Eds.), *The category of the person: Anthropology, philosophy, history* (pp. 26–45). New York: Cambridge University Press.

American Heritage Dictionary of the English Language. (2000). *Wrestle.* Retrieved November 16, 2001, from http://www.bartleby.com

Aroskar, M. A. (1995). Managed care and nursing values: A reflection. *Trends in Health Care, Law, and Ethics, 10,* 83–86.

Ayto, J. (1990). *Dictionary of word origins.* New York: Arcade Publishing.

Baer, E. D., Fagin, C. M., & Gordon, S. (Eds.). (1996). *Abandonment of the patient: The impact of profit-driven health care on the public.* New York: Springer.

Bingham, R. (2002). High-intensity care. *Health Affairs, 21,* 212–217.

Bowers, B. J., Lauring, C., & Jacobson, N. (2001). How nurses manage time and work in long term care. *Journal of Advanced Nursing, 33,* 484–491.

Brodeur, D. (1997). Health care institutional ethics: Broader than clinical ethics. In J. F. Monagle & D. C. Thomasma (Eds.), *Health care ethics: Critical issues for the 21st century* (pp. 497–504). Gaithersburg, MD: Aspen.

Caplan, A. (1996). Do ethics and money mix? In E. D. Baer, C. M. Fagan, & S. Gordon (Eds.), *Abandonment of the patient: The impact of profit driven health care on the public* (pp. 87–99). New York: Springer.

Creswell, J. W. (1998). *Qualitative inquiry and research design: Choosing among five traditions.* Thousand Oaks, CA: Sage Publications.

David, B. A. (1999). Nurses' conflicting values in competitively managed health care. *Image: Journal of Nursing Scholarship, 31,* 188.

Dombeck, M. (1997). Professional personhood: Training, territoriality and tolerance. *Journal of Interprofessional Care, 11,* 9–21.

Dombeck, M., Markakis, K., Brachman, L., Dalal, B., & Olsan, T. (2002). Analysis of a biopsychosocial correspondence: Models, mentors, and meanings. In S. M. R. Frankel & T. Quill (Eds.), *The biopsychosocial approach: Past, present and future* (pp. 231–251). Rochester, NY: University of Rochester Press.

Dombeck, M. T., & Olsan, T. H. (2002). Ethics and managed care. *Journal of Interprofessional Care, 16,* 221–233.

Douglas, M. (1986). *How institutions think.* Syracuse, NY: Syracuse University Press.

Durkheim, E. (1947). *Elementary forms of religious life.* New York: Swain.

Emerson, R. M., Fretz, R. I., & Shaw, L. L. (1995). *Writing ethnographic fieldnotes.* Chicago: University of Chicago Press.

Fagin, C. (2001). *When care becomes a burden: Diminishing access to adequate nursing.* New York: Milbank Memorial Fund.

Fein, R. (1982). What is wrong with the language of medicine? *New England Journal of Medicine, 306,* 863–864.

Fisher, I. (1998, June 7). Families providing complex medical care, tubes and all. *New York Times,* pp. 1A, 30A.

Fortes, M. (1987). *Religion, morality, and the person: Essays on the Tallensi religion.* Cambridge, England: Cambridge University Press.

Goffman, E. (1961). *Asylums: Essays on the sociological situation of mental patients and other inmates.* New York: Doubleday.

Gross, T., Pascale, R., & Athos, A. (1993). The reinvention roller coaster: Risking the present for a powerful future. *Harvard Business Review, 72,* 97–108.

Hall, J. K. (1996). *Nursing ethics and law.* Philadelphia: W. B. Saunders.

Harris, G. G. (1989). Concepts of individual, self, and person in description and analysis. *American Anthropologist, 91,* 599–612.

Henry, J. (1973). *On sham, vulnerability and other forms of self-destruction.* London: Penguin Press.

Himmelstein, D., Wollhandler, S., & Hellander, I. (2001). *Bleeding the patient: The consequences of corporate health care.* Philadelphia: Common Courage Press.

HR107: Health Care Financing Administration paperwork burdens: Hearings before the Committee on Small Business, 107th Cong., 6 (2001).

Huberman, M., & Miles, M. (1994). Data management and analysis methods. In N. K. Denzin & Y. S. Lincoln (Eds.), *Handbook of qualitative research* (pp. 428–444). Thousand Oaks, CA: Sage Publications.

Institute of Medicine. (2000). *To err is human: Building a safer health system.* Washington, DC: National Academies Press.

Institute of Medicine. (2001). *Crossing the quality chasm: A new health system for the 21st century.* Washington, DC: National Academies Press.

Jameton, A. (1990). Culture, morality, and ethics: Twirling the spindle. *Critical Care Nursing Clinics of North America, 2,* 443–451.

Kayser-Jones, J. S. (1981). *Old, alone, and neglected: Care of the aged in the United States and Scotland.* Berkeley: University of California Press.

Kearney, E. I., & Bandley, M. J. (1990). *Customers run your company: They pay the bills.* Provo, UT: Community Press.

Little, W., Fowler, H. W., & Couslon, J. (Eds.). (1955). *The Oxford universal dictionary of historical principles* (3rd ed.). Oxford, England: Clarendon Press.

Marck, P. (2000). Nursing in a technological world: Searching for healing communities. *Advances in Nursing Science, 23,* 62–81.

Mason, D. J., & Leavitt, J. K. (1998). *Policy and politics in nursing and in health care* (3rd ed.). Philadelphia: W. B. Saunders.

Mauss, M. (1989). A category of the human mind: The notion of persons; the notion of self (W. D. Halls, Trans.). In M. Carrithers, S. Collins, & S. Lukes (Eds.), *The category of the person: Anthropology, philosophy, history* (pp. 1–25). New York: Cambridge University Press.

Meyer, H. (1997). Home care goes corporate. *Hospitals & Health Networks, 71*(9), 20–22, 24, 26.

Mohr, W. K., & Mahon, M. M. (1996). Dirty hands: The underside of marketplace health care. *Advances in Nursing Science, 19,* 28–37.

Morgan, G. (1997). *Images of organization* (2nd ed.). Thousands Oaks, CA: Sage.

National Association for Home Care. (2000). *Basic statistics about home care.* Retrieved from http://www.nahc.org/Consumer/hcstats.html

Neilson, W. A. (Ed.). (1947). *Webster's new international dictionary* (2nd ed.). Springfield, MA: G & C Merriam.

O'Brien, L., & DeMarco, R. (1999, April). *Transfer of home health care to lay caregivers: Economic and policy implications.* Paper presented at the meeting of the Eastern Nursing Research Society, New York.

O'Donnell, K. P., & Sampson, E. M. (1994). Home health care: The pivotal link in the creation of a new health care delivery system. *Journal of Health Care Finance, 21,* 74–86.

Peacock, J. L. (1986). *The anthropological lens: Harsh light, soft focus.* New York: Cambridge University Press.

Phillips, E. K., Cloonan, P., Irvine, A., & Fisher, M. E. (1990). Nonreimbursed home health care: Beyond the bills. *Public Health Nursing, 7,* 60–64.

Potter, R. L. (1999). On our way to integrated bioethics: Clinical/Organizational/Communal. *The Journal of Clinical Ethics, 10,* 171–177.

PricewaterhouseCoopers. (2001). *Patients or paperwork: The regulatory burden facing America's hospitals.* Retrieved March 23, 2002, from http://www.aha.org

Scott, K. S., Moore, K. S., & Miceli, M. P. (1997). An exploration of the meaning and consequences of workaholism. *Human Resources, 50,* 287–314.

Scott, P. A. (1995). Role, role enactment and the health care practitioner. *Journal of Advanced Nursing, 22,* 323–328.

SmithBattle, L., Diekemper, M., Drake, M. A. (1999). Articulating the culture and tradition of community health nursing. *Public Health Nursing, 16,* 215–222.

Steinfelds, P. (2001, December 29). How should time be lived? A professor (M. Cathleen Kaveny) sees a billable-hour culture, and religious antidotes. *New York Times,* p. A10.

Taylor, C. (1985). *Human agency and language: Philosophical papers 1.* Cambridge, England: Cambridge University Press.

Taylor, S. J., & Bogdan, R. (1984). Working with data. In S. J. Taylor & R. Bogdan (Eds.), *Introduction to qualitative research methods: The search for meanings* (2nd ed., pp. 123–145). New York: John Wiley & Sons.

Thompson, I. E., Melia, K. M., & Boyd, K. M. (2000). *Nursing ethics* (4th ed.). Edinburgh, Scotland: Churchill Livingstone.

Todd, J. M. (1999). The trouble with mergers. *Healthcare Business,* Sept/Oct, 92–101.

Turner, V. (1974). *Drama, fields, and metaphors: Symbolic action in human society.* Ithaca, NY: Cornell University Press.

Van Maanen, J. (1988). *Tales of the field.* Chicago: University of Chicago Press.

Vladeck, B. (1993). Editorial: Beliefs vs. behaviors in healthcare decision making. *American Journal of Public Health, 83,* 13–14.

Vladeck, B. C. (1996). The corporatization of American health care and why it is happening. In E. D. Baer, C. M. Fagin, & S. Gordon (Eds.), *Abandonment of the patient: The impact of profit-driven health care on the public* (pp. 9–19). New York: Springer Publishing.

Wagner, D. L. (1997). *Comparative analysis of caregiver data for caregivers to the elderly, 1987 and 1997.* Bethesda, MD: National Alliance for Caregiving.

Wolgast, E. (1992). *Ethics of an artificial person: Lost responsibility in professions and organizations.* Stanford, CA: Stanford University Press.

Out of the Danger, the Saving Power Grows

Olsan's study gives us the opportunity to hear stories from nurses and patients about the threat of depersonalization under corporatization. The patients find themselves thrown into a world that is chaotic and impersonal. The nurses find their workplace and profession transformed into something that marginalizes them and their patients, measures productivity in terms of an incompatible business model, and takes away their professional identity as nurses. With each negative consequence of the transition to UniCare, though, comes the possibility of recognizing what was important in the first place. Segmentalism can lead us to appreciate the importance of integrated thinking and seeing "the big picture." The closing down of the nurses' possibilities can help us recognize the importance of always holding open possibilities when we are able. Finally, the recognition that nurses and patients are becoming what Heidegger calls "standing reserve" for health care institutions can help us find the saving power that lies within the very danger of depersonalization.

Integration and the Big Picture

Olsan reports that when she approached the nurses and explained her study, they viewed her work as being about "the other stuff." The nurses saw the realities of their workplace—including "business principles, bureaucracies, formal rules, regulations, expectations, and work group relationships"—as distinct from caregiving and relationships with patients (p. 10). Their work world had become a segmented, nonintegrated dwelling place where connections between key components had been severed. Holly vividly expresses her frustration with this lack of

61

integration, saying "I'm not just caring for a leg" (p. 28). Holly struggles to maintain the holistic approach to patient care that she believes is morally required of her, but she does so in the context of a system that seems to destroy any chance at holistic treatment. It is a system that does not allow anyone to see the bigger picture. Ronald, a UniCare administrator, explains that

the ideal way would be that everybody who was creating this system would come together and say . . . this is the vision of the future and let's invest in it by starting a partnership. That wasn't the case at all. . . . Everything has got to stand on its own, not as a system, but as individual pieces. (p. 29)

This image of individual pieces that cannot find a way to fit or work together is also captured by Amy, a member of Riverside's support staff:

We are a system on paper, but integration has not occurred. It is every man for himself. I know I keep saying that, but it is true. We are all here but we are in separate cars, and it makes me feel ineffective. Some days it is like I am standing in the parking lot, surrounded by all these cars and watching things happen, but I am all alone. (p. 30)

These images are stark and disturbing, but the realization that "we are all here but we are in separate cars" can also point us toward a solution. Indeed, Olsan's own approach acknowledges that "we are all here," while trying to end the problem of being "in separate cars." As she explains, "the nurses' moral problems reveal structural features and relationships in institutions. Nurses' daily work provides an interpretive context for shedding light on the moral dimensions of changing values and structures in healthcare" (p. 19). By choosing to study healthcare institutions through the eyes of the persons—in this case nurses—within them, Olsan attempts to integrate what has become so segmentalized. By giving the nurses a voice, and by acknowledging that they can see things about the whole that others cannot, Olsan begins to make connections between the voices "crying in the wilderness" (p. 27) and the institutional problems that left them in the wilderness in the first place.

The understanding that we must look through human eyes and listen to human stories in order to understand the structures in which we live is in fact an ancient one. The Greek philosopher Protagoras, a contemporary of Socrates, was best known for his claim that "A human being is the measure of all things, of the things that are, that (how) they are, and of the things that are not, that (how) they are not" (1996, p. 98). Protagoras believed that truth and morality have no meaning outside of human understanding. Centuries later, in Germany, Heidegger picks up a similar thread:

"There is" truth only insofar as Da-sein is and as long as it is. Beings are discovered only *when* Da-sein *is,* and only *as long as* Da-sein *is* are they disclosed. . . . Before there was any Da-sein, there was no truth; nor will there be any after Da-sein is no more. For in such a case truth as disclosedness, dis-covering, and discoveredness *cannot* be. (1996, p. 208)

Here, Heidegger argues that the very nature of truth is dis-covering, an act that can only be performed by human beings. Thus, without looking through the eyes of nurses when we attempt to understand the institutions of healthcare, we can find no way for the truth to be un-covered or disclosed.

Olsan further advances a solution to segmentalism and lack of integration in her call for a change in the way decisions are made about the future of healthcare and healthcare institutions. As she says,

it is uncommon to invite nurses from the rank and file into boardrooms and policy-making arenas in healthcare, but that lack of invitation is a mistake. If workable, cost-effective models of care delivery are to be developed, it is essential that community health nurses, and other professions providing direct care to patients, be positioned to create policies. (p. 54)

Olsan insists that policy makers listen to the voices that have been left crying in the wilderness too long. Her presentation of this argument implies that a difference of goals may not even be the primary problem, that instead it is the lack of integration. Nurses may be able to help institutions achieve their goals of profit and efficiency while also keeping healthcare safe and effective for patients:

In a healthcare system oriented toward improving health outcomes and producing cost-effective care, leaving community health nurses out of discussions about quality and costs is deeply misguided. Nurses' expertise and experience are relevant to reform, especially since the new rules for redesigning healthcare proposed by the Institute of Medicine are consistent with the principles upon which public health nursing was established over 100 years ago. (p. 55)

If nurses have wisdom dating back over 100 years on matters of utmost importance in the 21st century, then clearly the problem, and thus the solution, lies with giving these nurses a voice and integrating them into the policy-making system.

Holding Open Possibilities

The nurses at Riverside told Olsan, "We can't be nurses anymore." As Olsan says, this is "a disturbing phrase signaling a loss of personhood" (p. 23). In addition, the phrase signals a loss of possibility. The nurses find that their possible ways of caring for their patients—their possible ways of being-with and being-there-for their patients—have been severely limited or even in some cases eliminated. At the same time, the nurses find their "professional and personal lives . . . gradually eclipsed by their economic purpose for Riverside" (p. 23). They are losing possibilities as nurses, as family members, as friends. Their economic purpose for Riverside is limiting their possibilities in many or all of their different modes of being-in-the-world.

Institutions such as Riverside close down possibilities in another way: through language. Olsan notes that at Riverside, "the language of the corporation displaces talk about persons and compassion. The language of human interactions in relationships is silenced to a point where it becomes nearly impossible to nurture a consciousness about caring for patients in healthcare" (p. 38). Silencing certain types of language is tantamount to silencing types of thinking, for as human beings, we dwell in language. Language creates, sustains, and enriches the world we share. Therefore, without proper language, not only can we not communicate our thoughts to one another, we cannot easily *think* those thoughts in the first place.

Heidegger raises a similar concern when he reflects upon a favorite poem by Stefan George called "The Word":

> Wonder or dream from distant land
> I carried to my country strand
>
> And waited till the twilit norn
> Had found the name within her bourn–
>
> Then I could grasp it close and strong
> It blooms and shines now the front along . . .

Once I returned from happy sail,
I had a prize so rich and frail,

She sought for long and tidings told:
"No like of this these depths enfold."

And straight it vanished from my hand,
The treasure never graced by land . . .

So I renounced and sadly see:
Where word breaks off no thing may be.

(1971, p. 60)

As Heidegger interprets it, the poem tells us that when the word or name is lacking, no thing may be present for us, because "the being of anything that is resides in the word. Therefore this statement holds true: Language is the house of Being" (1971, p. 63). Only when we have a word or a name for something or someone can that something or someone appear as what it is and be present for us (1971, p. 65). Therefore, as the language at Riverside shifts to marketplace terms that refer to patients by diagnoses or visit codes, the nurses' own ability to think of their patients as individual human beings to be cared for is hampered.

The realization of the mechanisms involved in closing down possibilities can lead us to reopening those possibilities and even seeking new realms of possibilities. Knowledge that part of the nurses' loss of personhood is caused by the restriction of professional and personal possibilities should guide policy makers and institution executives to pay particular attention to the possibilities the nurses could have, particularly since many of those possibilities might lead to a better functioning and morally healthier institution. Likewise, knowledge that the language of the marketplace restricts possibilities of nurse–patient relationships should lead administrators and nurses alike to seek out both the language that was lost and new possibilities for language. Should Mrs. B. be considered a "patient," a "client," or is there some other word that would better respect and maintain her personhood? Should the group of nurses interviewed at Riverside be called "case managers," or is there a term that better captures the complexities and possibilities of their role within the institution? Once nurses and administrators heighten their awareness of language and its importance, the possibilities are many indeed.

Standing Reserve and the Saving Power

Heidegger is well aware of the dangers of the age in which we live, and he expresses concern that the way we treat each other and the way we treat our world may cause us to view the earth, the animals, other human beings, and even ourselves as "standing reserve" (1993, p. 322). People and things become standing reserve when "everywhere everything is ordered to stand by, to be immediately on hand, indeed to stand there just so that it may be on call for a further ordering" (1993, p. 322). It is alarming how well these words describe the place of the nurses in the institution of Riverside. They are a resource to be exploited to maximum capacity; they exist to stand by and do the job that is assigned them, rather than the job their own morality or professional integrity would lead them to do. Olsan reports that "the nurses were viewed as identical and interchangeable" (p. 24) and that productivity was "used to measure nurses' contribution to the bottom line" (p. 32). Furthermore, she underlines a problem she says is new to healthcare as of this age:

The authority of the marketplace in home care . . . is at odds with nurses' ideals. It silences the voices and the changing needs of patients. In its current form, the market model does not respond to the requirements of caregiving. Embracing the market model as the sole paradigm for restructuring healthcare has put the humanness of nurses and patients on the endangered list. (p. 57)

Olsan's own description here is a vivid illustration of how nurses and patients are becoming standing reserve in the modern healthcare institution.

When people become standing reserve, they may also lose their ties to their world and to their own being, which they experience as a loss of rootedness. Heidegger laments:

The loss of rootedness is caused not merely by circumstance and fortune, nor does it stem only from the negligence and the superficiality of man's way of life. The loss of autochthony springs from the spirit of the age into which all of us were born. . . . Will everything now fall into the clutches of planning and calculation, of organization and automation? (1966, pp. 48–49)

The nurses at Riverside, as they become standing reserve for the institution, find themselves losing ties with each other, their profession, their patients, and even the institution. The nurses are uprooted from their own professional world as they find their educational qualifications and their professional judgment ignored.

While the transformation of people into standing reserve is a frightening and dangerous thing, Heidegger finds hope in the words of the poet, Hölderlin: "But where danger is, grows / The saving power also" (1993, p. 333). When danger is at its most extreme, that is when we can catch a glimpse of what might save us. Such is the case here. Faced with the fact that institutions such as Riverside under UniCare may be here to stay, at least in some form, we must look for a way to preserve personhood in that context; we must find a way to avoid treating nurses and patients as standing reserve while being realistic about the constraints of the current healthcare system.

One possibility lies in the approach Heidegger offers for our relationship to technology: *Gelassenheit.* Just as healthcare ethicists and policy makers must find a way to preserve personhood without rejecting the current healthcare system outright, Heidegger suggests a way to preserve personhood without rejecting technology:

We can use technical devices as they ought to be used, and also let them alone as something which does not affect our inner and real core. We can affirm the unavoidable use of technical devices, and also deny them the right to dominate us, and so to warp, confuse and lay waste our nature. . . . I would call this comportment toward technology which expresses "yes" and at the same time "no," by an old word, *releasement [Gelassenheit] toward things.* (1966, p. 54)

Nurses, patients, administrators, and physicians can likewise find a comportment toward institutional care that expresses "yes" and at the same time "no." They can "affirm the unavoidable" restrictions placed on healthcare by the need for efficiency, but also deny those restrictions the right to dominate them "and so to warp, confuse and lay waste" their nature. This task is not easily accomplished, of course, but it is important to note that this approach avoids tilting at windmills. If the system is here to stay, in some form like its current one, then it is pointless to rail against that system or to ignore the requirements and needs of that system. Instead, we can look for creative ways to alter the system from within, preserving efficiency and productivity as much as possible while placing equal priority on preserving personhood and professional integrity.

Another saving power surely grows in Olsan's very study, and in other studies that may follow a similar path. Olsan's work lets us hear the stories that reveal the truth about what is happening in healthcare today. These stories are told by persons, as persons, not by social security numbers and productivity ratings. As such, these stories hold a saving power of their own: the power to invite us to listen to voices that might otherwise have been unheard whispers in the margins of modern healthcare.

References

Heidegger, M. (1966). *Discourse on thinking* (J. M. Anderson and E. H. Freund, Trans.). New York: Harper & Row.

Heidegger, M. (1971). *On the way to language* (P. Hertz, Trans.). San Francisco: Harper & Row.

Heidegger, M. (1993). The question concerning technology (W. Lovitt, Trans.). In D. F. Krell (Ed.), *Martin Heidegger: Basic writings*. San Francisco: Harper Collins.

Heidegger, M. (1996). *Being and time* (J. Stambaugh, Trans.). Albany: State University of New York.

Protagoras. (1996). Fragments (R. D. McKirahan, Jr., Trans.). In P. Curd (Ed.), *A presocratics reader: Selected fragments and testimonia*. Indianapolis: Hackett.

3

Ethics of Articulation

Constituting Organizational Identity in a Catholic Hospital System

SIMON J. CRADDOCK LEE

Introduction

The religious morality underpinning Catholic healthcare informs the ethical motivation to provide care for the poor and the sick in the modern world. The challenge posed by the world is how to sustain an organizational identity that is at once the descendant of the formal Catholic Church and yet a distinctive response to the demands of the pluralistic environment of contemporary healthcare. This chapter documents and analyzes the pragmatic dimension of ethics at work in a Catholic hospital system through the daily work of women religious (sisters) and their lay colleagues.[1] In describing the ethico-political constitution of Catholic Pacific Healthsystem (CPH),[2] this chapter demonstrates how the practice of ethics extends beyond sets of rules and guidelines to a way of thinking, of self-fashioning, not only of individuals but also of a new *catholicity*—a model that engages religious legacy and community values, navigating the increasing social pluralization of contemporary society, to reflect truly cultural dimensions of ethical praxis.

First, I will define my terms and briefly describe the research methodology. Then, I will provide the context of anthropological research in Catholic healthcare ministry and preface my analysis of CPH with the particular historical setting of contemporary California that has helped shape American assumptions about, and expectations of, Catholic hospitals. My analysis will show the relation of faith and agency in the CPH

69

system and makes a case for the ethical effects of values articulation through a juxtaposition of the anthropology of organizations with a Catholic ethics of discourse. Explicit examples of exteriorizing processes, programmatic devices, and language intervention reinforce mission, creating an ethico-political culture to which business practices should conform. The implementation of an ethical decision-making process tracks this ethical culture in practice. My analysis concludes with the problem of translation that attends such organizational processes at the intersection of healthcare, religion, and modern pluralization.

Terms and Methodology

In Catholic terminology, "women religious" is the generic term for those who have taken vows of religious life; this story concerns "sisters," who are active in public ministry, rather than "nuns" of contemplative orders (cloistered or not). For ease of analysis, I use the label "secular community hospitals" to describe facilities that are traditionally not-Catholic, to distinguish them from the traditionally Catholic-identified hospitals. But as my informants reminded me, Catholic facilities are arguably also community hospitals; CPH generally refers to their secular partners as simply "community hospitals."

A sponsoring congregation is the official group of sisters (e.g., Sisters of Charity of the Incarnate Word) who founded a hospital as one of their works. "Sister-sponsors" may be employed across the system according to their individual training as nurses, lab techs, or administrators, yet because they are both employees and sisters, they occupy a unique social role and are perceived as conduits to CPH leadership. "Mission" is a ubiquitous term in not-for-profit healthcare now, but in Catholic hospitals, it refers to the religious purpose of caring for the poor and the sick through the core values, especially of particular congregations. CPH core values are dignity, collaboration, justice, stewardship, and excellence. "Mission Integration" refers to the division charged with fostering that sense of purpose in every aspect of the organization's daily operations, literally ensuring that mission is integral to each function.

Fieldwork Methods and Analysis

This chapter is drawn from a larger study based on 18 months of sustained ethnographic fieldwork capping a six-year critical engagement with one of the largest hospital systems in the United States (Lee, 2003). In my fieldwork, I chose individual hospital sites that have a history of community and partnership interaction, focusing especially on secular facilities now operated by this Catholic system. I conducted daily participant observation at a charity clinic arm of a Catholic hospital, the system office, and two regional offices. I spent one month per facility among: three nonreligious community hospitals in southern, central, and northern California as well as a Catholic hospital sponsored by a different order (Saint Catherine-by-Sea) than the hospital where I had earlier conducted an additional six months of comparative fieldwork in chaplaincy and spiritual care (Incarnation Hospital). I attended administrative and executive meetings, including strategy, planning, operations, mission integration, and governance with management, medical staff, and sisters. Finally, I conducted more than 20 modified life history interviews with men and women religious and lay Catholics as well as other key individuals whose career or vocation entails involved participation in Catholic healthcare operations and policy across the CPH system.

Most ethnographic material for this chapter is drawn from participant observation in hospital and system administration. I had engaged with key actors in system leadership for over four years prior to fieldwork, building trust and rapport that facilitated the transition to full-time participant observation. I shadowed key actors in each location as well as at off-site retreats and system summits (Coffey & Atkinson, 1996; Miles & Huberman, 1994). Topics like community benefit, care management, finance, and revenue all provided entrée into how value frameworks operate in the provision of healthcare. I tracked how indigent cases were handled and how new staff hires were oriented, listening for moral judgments in both the language of providers and experienced staff. I listened for comments about Catholic facilities and other services available in the various service areas to explore if these providers conceptualize differences between religiously sponsored and "secular" healthcare. I did not observe direct medical procedures but monitored provider offices and clinic rooms as providers discussed patients and went about their daily routines. I observed daily life in the common areas, the waiting rooms, cafeteria, and hallways. I also socialized with physicians, hospital staff, and board members at CPH functions.

The interviews used in this chapter focus on those key actors engaged in Mission Integration activities at various levels throughout the system. Each interview was fully transcribed and the resulting text checked repeatedly against its recording. They were structured, one-on-one inter-actions, private conversations held in closed rooms on hospital grounds or system offices, and all save one informant allowed me to tape-record the sessions. The conversations were modeled on abbreviated life history interviews, using a common template of generic questions provided in advance, further tailored to particular groups (current and former sisters, lay administrators, men religious and/or priests, and chaplains) and par-ticular geographic site locations (Kvale, 1996; Silverman, 1993). I asked about changes in subjects' lifetimes, and what drew them to service, and the focus of their occupation or vocation. The interviews lent perspective on institutional history and social change to provide context and comple-ment the insights gained from participant observation. In some cases, in-dividual perspectives provide contrast or counterpoint to the collective or official stances, and these comments are reported precisely to demon-strate the texture and complexity of this organization and the lives of the people who constitute it. Actual questions differed depending on the informant, and many emerged out of earlier field observation. Many in-formants expounded at length, sharing their opinions about values, the state of healthcare, or hospital operations. This flexibility allowed me to pursue individual conceptions of values tied to self-identity and greater collectivities or group function (Stewart & Strathern, 2000, p. 21).

Documents can be regarded as part of social life itself, the "elements that enable or prevent or subvert social events" (Asad, 1993, p. 8). In ad-dition to their immediate content, documents provided a point of entry to further discussion that elicited informants' own terms and labels, as well as priorities and challenges. I had free access to current undertak-ings, meeting minutes, and other internal memos in addition to my own notes taken each day. Since May 1997, I had collected written material in the form of memos, newsletters, official publications, press releases, and procedures related to operations across the system. I continued to moni-tor both the Catholic and secular healthcare industry press in California as well as the activities and policy positions of the U.S. Catholic bishops and the Vatican. Reports concerning the Roman Catholic Church and child abuse appeared regularly in national and local media, simultane-ously facilitating and complicating the ease of talking about social values, ethics, religion, and the care of others.

Field notes were reread daily while in the field to track initial themes and map new directions for the next day. Field notes, interviews, and many documents were later coded using qualitative analysis software (Nvivo 2.0) in an iterative process that generated core categories and thematic hierarchies. The simultaneous development of analytic memos was critical to the process, particularly in the cyclic analysis that moved from interview to field note to interview and back. Repeated reanalysis revealed implications for theory building, variations on themes, and linkages in and among codes (Coffey & Atkinson, 1996).

Anthropological Context

This chapter provides an anthropological "ethnographic account," a description in the sense of Weber and Wittgenstein, to describe in order that the material stand out in the context of normative liberal assumptions about identity and religiosity. Embedded ethnographic elements weave a sustained argument about values frameworks in the face of pluralization that also attend to the coherent and consistent thread of Catholic-ness within the lived experience of this hospital system, even as the agents that constitute it work out their own accommodations with contemporary life-in-the-world. Fieldwork also engaged an implicit comparison—for to consider Catholic healthcare necessarily undertakes the question of other forms of healthcare. Why is such a distinction necessary? What is "not-Catholic healthcare"? Further, what is meant by religious- or faith-based healthcare? What do those terms mean, and who mobilizes those meanings? How do these understandings play out in the larger field of not-for-profit hospital management and healthcare services delivery? Each of these questions frame the organizational life of Catholic Pacific Healthsystem.

Ideas and constructs about what Catholic healthcare ministry is or should be, reminiscent of what Weber called "ideal types," circulate, but may not fully reflect practical arrangements and their attendant characteristics. Anthropological fieldwork grounds the historically documented distortions that are part and parcel of lived experience and engages the principle of coexistence that lies at the heart of contemporary pluralism, for informants here are not exotic, distant Others. They inhabit the same Real Time as the researcher and the reader, and yet this anthropology is about what makes them different and distinct as well as similar. It is about identity, and its politics—their external manifestation in the world we share. But it is also about an ethics of individuals—the internal, the self-formation linked to *caritas,* caring for others—the sense of work and purpose, that is, of *mission* broadly writ. These are the forms of life that anthropologist Talal Asad gestures to, and acknowledging his reading of Foucault, that he asserts are the substance of anthropological analysis. In this sense, my conception of ethics differs from other operating definitions of ethics in medicine and healthcare (e.g., Kleinman, 1995).

There are socially constructed spheres of for-profit and not-for-profit, where health is a vague notion only gestured at but health services are quantified and allocated monetary value. Those valuations in turn fuel a discourse on commodity acquisition, social position, and resources that dictate whether healthcare is something an individual can or cannot get, though an abstract "health" remains a common good. Social rhetoric, social organization, the law, and government programs follow from the assumptions that accrue to these constellations. And thus, healthcare in the United States is an experiment in morality.

Study of local effects of this mainstream religion in health and medicine is a key task for a modern anthropology of pluralism. The historical demands of philosophy and politics have concerned moral universalities—for example, what is the good life? But, "the consistent brotherly ethic of salvation religions has come into an equally sharp tension with the *political* orders of the world" (Weber, 1958a, p. 333). Foucault maintained that the modern state took as its object the statistical, normative model of *healthy man* and created "public health" (Foucault, 1994, p. 34). This might lead one to construct the problem as one of the state as theological object. However, the mission of Catholic hospitals entails what Weber would recognize as the appropriation of health as practiced by a religiously identified institution, not the state. Thus, this research inquiry concerns a new *problematization* produced by the extreme situations of changing fields of knowledge and the exigencies of extra-Church religiosity. Weber linked charismatic authority to leadership (Weber, 1958b); women religious cite the "charism" within their sponsoring congregations as the vehicle of social values in Catholic healthcare (Kennelly, 1989). Thus, Catholic hospital administrators are contemporary theological subjects amidst the technical rationalism of healthcare delivery, representing a redefinition of the Roman Catholic Church-in-the-world through various articulations of the Catholic healing mission by its own professional enterprises in healthcare (Cheney, 1990; McCormick, 1984; Walsh, 2000).

Not-for-profit organizations dominate the hospital industry throughout the United States, despite an ongoing debate about their value, distinctive contributions, and efficiency (Schlesinger, Gray, & Bradley, 1996; Young & Desai, 1999). In the words of the late Cardinal Bernardin, nonprofit hospitals are "mediating institutions": they stand between the individual and the state and "mediate against the rougher edges of capitalism's inclination toward excessive individualism" (1999, p. 91). Historically, the Catholic Church has been a primary source of moral values and a pragmatic engagement with healthcare as a common societal good (Redican, 1981; Risse, 1999; Rosner, 1987). The Catholic magisterium has repeatedly critiqued American society for failing to articulate an adequate conception of the common good and human purpose (Byrnes, 1991; Douglass, Mara, & Richardson, 1990; Gaillardetz, 1997).

The ethics and social values of Catholic healthcare, then, are not about the number of hospitalizations or surgical procedures that go without reimbursement and constitute charity care in the sense deployed by the state of California for its nonprofit bookkeeping. My fieldwork takes as its object an even broader "community benefit" picture. It is about corporate citizenship, not in the sense of a hospital as a business entity, but corporate in the sense of a collective subject acting in the social world. Many social formations and dissolutions happen around notions of "the good." Catholics in their mission of healthcare negotiate many of the same concerns that others in a pluralist society do; Catholics just do it in a visible and organized way that reflects their particular history as a formal religious institution. This analysis would ask, is Catholic healthcare practice distinctive, how, and to whom? Is religious or values language used to make accommodations palatable or do they signal true difference?

There is a prevailing rhetoric about inhumane, capitalist economics that labor unions and consumer groups use to batter hospital systems like the one examined here, which they perceive as impersonal corporations acting in spite of their not-for-profit designation and, in the case of Catholic Pacific Healthsystem, their religious healthcare ministry. But the righteous stance of this chastisement itself derives its social weight by invoking an underlying cultural rhetoric suggesting that all spiritual endeavors in the temporal realm are somehow imbued with moral superiority. That is, it indicates an expectation that religious hospitals should, by definition, be held to a higher standard than their secular counterparts. Studies of nonprofit healthcare abound that recount finance and policy, but they do not explain how faith shapes ethical practice in people's lives (K. R. White, 2000). If we are to understand the philanthropic impetus to care for our neighbors more broadly, we must understand how contemporary Catholic hospital administrators navigate the constraints of maintaining a religious identity while collaborating with secular partners to implement their commitment to healthcare provision for the poor. Further, we might consider the cultural meanings that adhere to the not-for-profit designation, and the distinctions between faith-based organizations and their supposedly secular counterparts.

Considerations and Constraints

Despite an espoused American secularity, religious perspectives continue to inform and influence health and medical policy. To designate something or someone as "religious" often seems to evoke a cultural cachet that connotes moral propriety. As Asad has noted, religion is used to unite and divide (Asad, 1992). The charged atmosphere of the United States persistently reduces the analysis of the Catholic engagement with healthcare to the political conflict (in the policy sense) over reproductive health services, namely abortion provision or its prohibition. In the United States today, access to reproductive healthcare remains at risk, often represented as in crisis (Baumgardner, 1999; Bucar, 1998; Dinsmore, 1998; Uttley & Pawelko, 2002). Many people continue to oppose the presence of Catholic hospitals in their communities because those hospitals are unable to provide particular reproductive services, despite their dedication to serving other local needs. These issues remain critical concerns in people's lives and sites for advocacy and action. They also mark fault lines for successful pluralization in the world, as well as for any anthropological inquiry that takes ethics and politics as its objects. That said, this chapter neither defends nor attacks the values and "choices" of my informants, nor Catholicism more broadly, on this policy issue. Studies in the anthropology of reproduction, bioethics, and feminist anthropologies have already extensively engaged many of the controversial elements (Dillon, 1995; Ginsburg, 1998; Heriot, 1996; Lazarus, 1994; Martin, 1987; Mensch & Freeman, 1993; Purdy, 1996; Whitbeck, 1983). Though those particular dynamics are important, I set them aside here in order to take up the larger domain of Catholic healthcare to demonstrate what I refer to as the ethics of articulation, namely, the effects on forming and sustaining organizational identity of explicitly articulating through social processes. My research argues that CPH manifests as an onto-political entity through the ethics of articulation.[3]

Distinctiveness is real. It is also true that identity politics at the individual level can be driven by ego, an insistence on difference that can itself challenge pluralization (Brown, 1992). However, though calling something "Catholic" makes it distinct from something that is called other than "Catholic," or "not Catholic" (a distinction often taken as a priori), a true anthropology requires moving beyond the taken-for-granted to determine what that difference actually looks like to those who understand it to be so. Identity is multidimensional; it extends beyond Action X to the rationale driving that action. Within a collective of persons, this raises the additional question of collaboration, an identified founding principle of CPH. Different identities exist under the single label of "Catholic." This is true of both individuals, even sisters, and the different organizations and social groups operating within the tradition of the Mother Church. The members of an organization, individually and collectively, together engage in an ethos or worldview, what Geertz writes is the "tone, character, and quality of their life, its moral and aesthetic style and mood; it is the underlying attitude toward themselves and their world that life reflects. Their world view is their picture of the way things in sheer actuality are [*and should be*], their concept of nature, of self, of society" (Geertz, 2000, p. 127). My emphasis reflects the ethical projection—the prophetic witness—that Catholic healthcare is called to and that is the touchstone for many of the women religious and their colleagues of Catholic Pacific Healthsystem.

Historical Context

The sisters, their role, and social location are central to any anthropological account of Catholic healthcare. The presence of women religious, both historical and contemporary, is an obvious characteristic that sets Catholic hospitals apart from their "secular" not-for-profit cousins and investor-owned facilities. This easy observation bears greater elaboration, for it sets the scene for the ethnographic account of ethical practices that follows.

The story of Catholic healthcare in the United States reflects the history of migration across the country. It follows the efforts of Roman Catholic sisters who sought to minister amidst the poverty and disease that attended new frontier settlements and emerged in the streets and shelters of new cities, like San Francisco. For example, in 1854, already struggling to care for the burgeoning poor trampled in the gold rush of 1849, the Daughters of Charity welcomed Mary Baptist Russell and seven other Sisters of Mercy to the Bay area. One hundred and fifty years later, both orders of women religious remain involved in extensive healthcare ministry throughout the state of California and the United States.

The sociopolitical history of the United States, especially in the latter half of the 20th century, is one of great change. Those forces affected both the climate in which Catholic healthcare is practiced and those who practice it. Though convened abroad in 1963, perhaps the most central event for American Roman Catholics was the 21st Ecumenical Council (Vatican II) that was held to usher in a new era in the life of the Church throughout the world (Abbott, 1963; Lernoux, 1989; Varacalli, 1983). The American Catholic hierarchy worked to understand its role in national civic life as well as in the lives of the faithful (Byrnes, 1991; National Conference of Catholic Bishops, 1983, 1986). As Darryl Caterine has emphasized, the council was called just as the first Catholic was elected to the office of President of the United States, in part by

minimizing the difference between Roman Catholic and Protestant American identity. . . . Ecclesiastically, the council triggered profound critiques of hierarchical structures in the name of that most hallowed of all American institutions, democracy, while ecumenically the church's claim as defender of the exclusive faith gave way to dialogue with other churches as well as with traditions outside the Christian and even Judeo-Christian faith. (Caterine, 2001, p. xv)

No Catholic group took the Council's efforts to heart more than Catholic women religious in the United States (Quiñonez & Turner, 1992; Ranke-Heinemann, 1990; Wittberg, 1994). Trained research sociologists and themselves Catholic women religious, Quiñonez and Turner in particular provide an excellent review of the emergence of the Leadership Conference of Women Religious of the United States of America (LCWR), which ultimately became the national association of chief governing officers of religious communities involved in active ministry (that is, not cloistered groups). Changes in language like the decision to refer to themselves as "women in the Church" rather than the traditional "daughters of the Church" illustrate the larger constitutional changes the women took on, encouraged by what many sisters perceived as a new spirit of openness embodied in Vatican II. The seriousness with which sisters redesigned the process of formation and embraced formal advanced education as a vehicle for social change within their ranks is pivotal to understanding modern women religious. In one CPH hospital, over 95% of the sisters, average age well over 60, have two master's degrees. Moreover, openly American civic values in the language of LCWR demonstrate the inextricable cultural identification that marked what Rome had always belittled as Americanism. The spirit of renewal through which American women religious understood Vatican II marks a turning point in the sociopolitical history of vowed life in the United States. The Vatican, and even the American arm of the magisterium, were taken aback by these transformations and undertook several steps to reassert Vatican authority over religious life. It is crucial to the analysis of CPH to understand the ethos of independent thought that took hold among American women religious. I cannot do justice to the breadth of this transformation here but present some examples to signal the import of this period in their social history.

One of the most significant acts to reflect this development came as a result of the first Women's Ordination Conference, held in 1975. The Vatican ordered the LCWR "to dissociate itself completely from the conference's proceedings and goals," but the LCWR board unanimously refused. Then in 1979, when the new pope visited the United States, Sister Theresa Kane, a Sister of Mercy and president of the LCWR that year, "greeted John Paul II before a national television audience by telling him that the Church 'must respond' to its own call for affirming the dignity of all persons by allowing women to become ordained. The pope visibly registered his disapproval of such audacity" (Wittberg, p. 218; cf. Quiñonez & Turner, p. 157). Tension flared throughout the ranks of women religious and reactions were mixed. The outcome, however, was an affirmation of a new sense of engagement with Rome, together with a commitment to self-determination grounded in the Church's own teachings.

Moreover, American women in general were part of other social movements and cultural attitudes that created new possibilities for women in the world. As one sister remembered:

It is true, when many of us entered the congregation, a lot of professions probably did not welcome women. There's always exceptions. But today, women have just unlimited opportunities for all kinds of—all kinds of careers. And it's just a different time.

In addition to civil rights and three waves of feminism, the spirit of the Peace Corps, Head Start, Model Cities, and war resistance all radically altered visions of life and work for women of faith. Extensively documented, the cumulative effect has been a steady decrease in the number of women entering vowed religious life, coupled with the steady aging of the professed. Nationally, the average age in 1990 was 65 among an estimated 94,000 religious sisters; less than 1% of them were recent recruits to vowed life (Wittberg, 1994, pp. 1–2). Today the estimate is 65,000 and the average age is 69 (Fialka, 2003).

For the ministries of Catholic women religious, the impact over time was enormous, especially in the central missions of healthcare and teaching. The transformation of American medicine into the dominant professional industry in the country, the intense level of regulation, and the attention to cost-containment measures and other business practices brought substantial organizational repercussions. Staffing shortages among sisters in the hospitals were increasingly a problem as the number of institutions grew. But, as a landmark study of Catholic philanthropy documents, the demands for professionalization in social work and financial management also pressured the sisterhoods, and many dioceses changed how institutions were managed in what one scholar terms the "Catholic charity consolidation movement" (Oates, 1995, pp. 86–90).

By the 1980s, the end of fee-for-service compensation and the emergence of managed care were accompanied by the rise of for-profit and investor-owned hospital players. Together, the challenges of competition struck hard at the backbone of not-for-profit healthcare in the United States—the Catholic hospitals sponsored by regional communities of women religious, like the Sisters of Mercy or the Daughters of Charity. This competition conspired with the demographic trends of women religious to increase the growing laicization of Catholic hospital ministry throughout the United States (Risse, 1999, pp. 513–568). Medical facilities that had once been managed, operated, and staffed by Catholic sisters, both in nursing and hospital administration itself, are now almost entirely run by professional lay administrators. And like healthcare administration in general, most senior administrators were male and, even in religious facilities, increasingly not Catholic. Today, some sisters remain active in the philanthropic arm of the hospital foundation or in particular positions that reflect their professional training. For the most part, however, in almost all Catholic hospitals, sisters retreated to positions of governance rather than operations, the sister-administrator replaced by a lay hospital president.

The need for increasing means to care for the poor and the sick arose in a healthcare economy marked by aggressive growth and competition in a decade of radical change in the healthcare services industry. California has been at the forefront of the health maintenance organization (HMO) expansion over the past 25 years and is considered a bellwether state in the nation for managed care trends (Wilkerson, Devers, & Given, 1996). Such managed care dominance has also made California's healthcare marketplace one of the nation's most competitive, or the "proving ground for managed competition" (Luft, 1996, p. 23). Managed care, in turn, drove changes in hospital organization and financial arrangements as hospitals were bought and sold and even multiple facility systems further integrated. From 1994 to 1997, 198 hospitals in the United States changed ownership, the majority of which occurred among investor-owned organizations (California Office of Statewide Health Planning and Development, 1999). The incorporation of CPH reflected the determination of the Catholic women religious that sponsor their hospitals to resist the incursion of for-profit hospital systems, like Columbia-HCA, and maintain an aggressive not-for-profit voice in the healthcare industry wilderness.

The CPH was a leading example of the business growth model applied in the not-for-profit sector. During that same period, in the years preceding my fieldwork, more than 24 different hospitals chose to affiliate with CPH. Some were county or district hospitals pounded by state and federal social welfare cutbacks, others were community-sponsored, not-for-profit facilities pressured by managed care or demographic change that shifted the burden of care for working people with insurance to increasingly partial or uninsured populations. By the beginning of my fieldwork, CPH had grown to more than 35 hospitals across a huge demographic and geographic swath of the western United States. By 2001, the level of secular affiliation was unprecedented in Catholic healthcare and remains a distinguishing characteristic of CPH.

For-profit healthcare companies can make, and are rewarded for making, growth decisions based solely on future revenue. Not-for-profit hospitals, especially those directed by their governing philosophy to commit resources to sustain a not-for-profit presence in healthcare, cannot. At CPH, the drive to sustain not-for-profit, hospital-based healthcare in local communities of need significantly shaped the network's growth until the late 1990s. This formative agenda has had real repercussions on Catholic Pacific Healthsystem as an ethico-political organization balanced between the realities of margin and demands of mission—that is, the need to maintain revenue for operations and the effort to sustain not-for-profit healthcare provision for the poor and underserved.

Catholic Healthcare Ministry in the United States

The United States has repeatedly been unable to enact comprehensive healthcare coverage at the national level. Social safety net measures are enacted and repealed in accord with the vacillations of the economy and electoral politics. Incremental change is espoused as the only effective political strategy. Ironically, in a nation premised on rhetoric of the separation of church and state, the Roman Catholic Church remains the largest institutional provider of healthcare services, second only to the federal government.

Catholic ministry hospitals constitute the largest single group of the nation's not-for-profit hospitals, more than 11% of the nation's total nonfederal hospitals, 15.2% of the nation's total nonfederal acute care hospital beds, and 15.8% of all nonfederal U.S. hospital admissions (American Hospital Association Annual Survey, 2002). To give some perspective on the position of Catholic healthcare providers in the United States as of September 1999,[4] the Catholic Health Association had a national membership comprised of 63 healthcare systems, 683 hospitals (of which 619 are Catholic facilities and 64 are non-Catholic members of Catholic systems), 354 long-term-care nursing facilities, 342 Catholic facilities, 12 non-Catholic members of Catholic systems, 76 home health agencies, 18 hospice organizations, 253 other services along the care continuum (e.g., adult day care, assisted living, senior housing, physician groups, and outpatient services), and 284 health-related organizations (e.g., HMOs, community-based services, and foundations). Finally, more than 774,000 employees worked full-time or part-time in Catholic hospitals. The staffs of Catholic hospitals cared for more than 85 million inpatients and outpatients in 2000. Catholic healthcare systems often span multiple states and sponsor regional healthcare networks. They range in size from a few to more than 100 facilities. Catholic hospitals and agencies minister through shelters, food programs, and hundreds of other community outreach efforts to people in need, regardless of creed.

The Roman Catholic Church provides healthcare services through a range of nonprofit hospitals and clinics that serve very disparate communities throughout the country. Increasing economic pressure to consolidate healthcare service providers encouraged religiously sponsored systems to acquire struggling secular community facilities, lending greater economies of scale. Currently, 10 of the 20 largest healthcare systems in the United States are affiliated with the Roman Catholic Church (Catholics for a Free Choice, 2002).

The provision of healthcare constitutes a foundational element of the mission of the Catholic Church in the United States. From an applied perspective, a richer understanding of the motivations and rationale behind this private sector approach to a public concern is valuable, if only to clarify the utility of this major partner in a social good. In an era of federal devolution of the social welfare and health services that has seen block grants shift these responsibilities to individual states, the Church's contributions to the social safety net has implications for the future direction of American health policy. The rhetoric of federal devolution is one of decreased government bureaucracy in favor of increased local control and an appeal to individual philanthropy over mandated societal structures. However, this private sector player operates within strict limitations that are central to its religious identity. The expansion of Catholic systems restricts the provision of particular services, while the religious identity of the institutions themselves challenges public distinctions in the separation of church and state. Community and other "secular" partnerships, project planning, and development are sites of reflection about the role of the church or state, "local control," "individual responsibility," or "philanthropy"—situations that call into question the nature of Catholic organizational identity.

Generally, Catholic identity is conferred on an institution by the bishop in whose diocese a facility is located. A Catholic facility is required to abide by the *Religious and Ethical Directives for Catholic Healthcare Institutions* and is periodically examined by representatives of the local diocese. Catholic hospitals differ from other religiously sponsored hospitals in that they are historically operated by men or women religious, rather than lay people or the more congregational, community-founded model typical of the Protestant or Jewish traditions (see, for example,

Rosner, 1987). In the CPH system, senior management and the sponsoring congregations of women religious are accountable to the local bishop for the operations of their facilities in so far as they impact the public identity of the Catholic presence in the community.[5]

The Catholic Church assumes a stance of action-in-the-world shaped by the perspective of the poor; specifically, the Church is called to voice a prophetic critique of society in fidelity to Jesus's option for the poor. Catholic hospitals must balance the commitment to their religious identity and values with the commitment to caring for people whose beliefs and practices may not conform to those of the hospitals (Kauffman, 1997). Catholic hospitals regularly find that ethics and values conflicts can directly impact the provision of services to vulnerable populations: the sick and those who are poor, especially women of color. Many of these hospitals are intentionally located in diverse communities with a disproportionate share of Medicare and Medicaid-supported populations. CPH is aggressively engaged with community projects caring for these populations, reporting $422 million in unsponsored community benefit, or nearly 9% of total operating expenses, in 2003. In addition to a direct grants program that funded 111 grants at $1.7 million, the hospital system works with community not-for-profits to increase access to jobs, housing, education, social services, and healthcare for people in low-income and minority communities (McKnight, 1994). Within the hospital system itself, these demands create organizational tension between the business-minded departments like finance or risk management and the staff more directly concerned with services like care management or community benefit services.

Catholic Pacific Healthsystem

Catholic Pacific Healthsystem is a leading network of hospitals with facilities in several states of the western United States; in 2001, it was one of the five largest systems and one of the largest religious-affiliated, non-profit healthcare corporations in the country. Due to its size and scope (in terms of patient volume), its hundreds of affiliated physicians, and its thousands of employees, CPH is a major player in regional healthcare. As a nonprofit hospital system, it occupies a significant niche in the state social welfare system and community benefit dynamics of the western United States.

CPH was founded in 1986 by the nonprofit incorporation of the hospitals of multiple congregations of women religious. This made CPH unique in Catholic healthcare. The Roman Catholic Church only recognizes canonical sponsorship of a hospital by one congregation of sisters. In effect, CPH had initiated a new form of religious sponsorship and a key site of pluralism even within Catholic healthcare (Francis, 1964; Quiñonez & Turner, 1992; Wittberg, 1994). This has had implications for both the politics of identity of the aggregate organization and the operations of the system and its member facilities in local service areas—particularly as the system grew to incorporate the secular community hospitals, as above. Finally, these transformations occurred in one of the most multicultural parts of the country. Even with its dynamic demography, California is considered the most secular state in the union: 9% of residents reportedly have no religious affiliation (Gallup & Castelli, 1989)—in a nation where a civic separation of church and state colors all activities in the public sphere.

These Catholic hospital administrators must balance the official Church teachings, bishops' public policies, and the implications of the Second Vatican Council while conforming to local, state, and federal regulations that qualify their facilities for public funds. Simultaneously, their facilities are buffeted by the healthcare marketplace, particularly the stiff competition from secular nonprofits and investor-owned hospitals (Buchmueller & Feldstein, 1996; MacStravic, 1987; McClellan, 1997; Young & Desai, 1999). To successfully enact its mission, this Catholic system must offer "standard of care" services to maintain patient volume to compete with neighboring medical facilities; the mediating value lies in the Catholic principle of stewardship (National Conference of Catholic Bishops, 1986).

Having set the stage, the sections that follow explore the relationship of faith to agency, the articulation of values, and ethical praxis in constituting organizational identity in the CPH system. I make the case for understanding the ethico-political constitution of CPH by interweaving social ethics and political theory into the ethnographic account of the practices of the hospital organization and its actors.

Faith in Agency

Academic research in the United States, supposedly a site of impartial, objective intellectual evaluation and innovation, is itself subject to the vagaries of culture. As a product of modern social structures, academia more often than not suffers from a conceptual blind spot, namely that secularization is a universal phenomenon, which therefore renders the religious faithful social anomalies or holdouts from modernity that need to be explained. Consequently, many academic researchers often proceed from a questionable presumption that religious knowledge as a means to organizing daily life and political action in a liberal society is obsolete or inappropriate. Political theorist William Connolly, as we shall see, suggests that this "conceit of secularism" is a basic challenge of social pluralism (Connolly, 1999, pp. 19–46). Sociologist Peter Berger asserts that the far better project may be to explain why the professional knowledge industry is *not* theistic (Berger, 1992). Indeed, the "culture wars" may reflect the challenge that such an unexamined stance can present. For many people that presumption of irrelevancy would be overreaching. For the Catholic faithful, diocesan programs in many states seek to affirm the place of Catholic faith in the practices of modern life. By practices, I mean the forms of "socially established cooperative human activity through which goods internal to that form of activity are realized in the course of trying to achieve those standards of excellence which are appropriate to . . . that activity . . . with the result that . . . human conceptions of ends and goods are systematically extended" (MacIntyre, 1984, p. 187).

San Francisco is one of the most politically significant archdioceses in the United States because of its historic Catholic roots as well as the ethnic and cultural diversity of the Catholic demographic that draws on both eastern and western European and Asian Catholic communities. The weekly Catholic newspaper there reports on the events and activities within the archdiocese, focusing on parochial schools and universities, but carrying news from Rome and the Catholic diaspora worldwide. It also carries editorials and opinion columns applying Catholic morality to daily life with commentary on current events, the family, and spirituality. Film reviews, often a staple of local papers, are a syndicated series from the Office of Film and Broadcasting of the U.S. Conference of Catholic Bishops, and each review ends with a moral rating system paired with the U.S. Motion Picture of America (MPAA) rating.

A critical reading of the newspaper demonstrates a distinct difference in understanding the role of religion in social life than academic discourse would suggest. It represents a religious ethic wherein being Catholic involves *acting* Catholic; *catholicity* is made manifest in the way one lives and structures daily life. Religion is reflected in the choices one makes and in the acts or works one undertakes, either alone or as part of a collective. The vowed life of Catholic women religious necessarily formalizes that premise.

Mother Catherine McAuley, founder of the Sisters of Mercy (c. 1830), established the unity of prayer as the basis for an *active* apostolate for her order. McAuley argued that "love of God (and) love of neighbor . . . are as cause and effect, . . . *for the proof of love is deed*" (Bolster, 1990, p. 75). Mother McAuley's spirituality was original in its "novel synthesis of contemplation and action, a preferential option for the poor in whom she found Christ and in which she anticipated . . . the encyclical *Populorum Progressio* which stressed a social mission which is at the same time profoundly religious that it permits those who practice it 'to be present to their brothers and sisters in a deeper way in the charity of Christ'" (Bolster, p. 104). Healthcare provision is an explicit ministry and Catholic hospitals are both the symbolic and pragmatic instantiation of the mission to be-Catholic-in-the-world. The particular positionality of women religious, and by extension, of former women religious, is a force of both power and influence that differs from any other group of players in CPH, and their presence adds a layer of complexity to any treatment of ethical leadership in the hospital system.

A substantial countercultural element of religious life involves the valuation of virtues, like humility and modesty, that are no longer appreciated in the same way by secular society. In the modern world of postfeminist activism, such traditional virtues are often associated with passivity and inaction. This association works only if the analytic reference point is an emancipatory agenda framed by the "flat narrative of succumbing to or resisting relations of domination" (Mahmood, 2001). But there are other frames through which to view these virtues that are more applicable to the situation of the women religious of CPH, frames that I have gestured to in my treatment of the changing history of Catholic sisters after Vatican II.

In her writing on the women involved in the Egyptian Islamic revival, anthropologist Saba Mahmood posits a definition of agency "not as a synonym for resistance to relations of domination, but as a capacity for action that historically specific relations of subordination enable and create" (Mahmood, 2001, p. 203). This supposition is provocative within feminist discourse because, as Mahmood writes, feminism maintains a dual character that is both an *analytical* and *politically prescriptive* project

(p. 206). Such analyses, then, are largely built on a foundation of liberal assumptions about emancipatory frameworks; agency is understood "as the capacity to realize one's own interests against the weight of custom, tradition, transcendental will, or other obstacles (whether individual or collective)" (p. 206). Beyond Mahmood's effort to parochialize the normative feminist subject, the significance of her scholarship lies in the move to account for contemporary women who explicitly constitute themselves as ethical subjects in and through the very structures of religiosity, supposedly oppressive, from which liberal theory would ostensibly seek to free them.

A theme in my work is the heterogeneous character of what it means to be "Catholic" in contradistinction to what is often an unexamined presumption of uniformity. Such presumption is understandable given the voice the Church often deploys, the historical and publicly visible individual Holy Father and his magisterium, independent of the theological implications of the apostolic authority of the "one, holy, catholic, and apostolic Church." However, the diversity of peoples who call themselves Catholic, as well as the countries and nation-states that identify themselves as Catholic, demonstrate that cultural manifestations of what such an identity and faith in practice may mean to lived experience are worthy of anthropological analysis (Anderson & Friend, 1995). Just as Mahmood's ethnographic analysis of contemporary Egyptian women demonstrates, analytical and political distinctions are easily erased and forms of life and self-fashioning are flattened out, obviating the significance and meaning such efforts hold in people's lives.

A character of late Western modernity is a growing acknowledgment that the dominant conversations have often been carried out with a false, universalist self-understanding (S. K. White, 2000). Catholicity, or Catholic-ness, may play out as an identity theme that is diverse and variable, but the Church always mounts a universality within its hegemonic claims; certainly, the history of the Church in early Europe engaged a constitutive cultural hegemony. Today, the Church proper still represents one of those dominant conversations, a historic "strong ontology" emerging from a doctrine of a singular truth in the one true church and invested with that particular history of Church as sovereign nation-state. But the nature of identity within the push–pull dynamic of power and resistance is such that there are niches or margins, even, within such a universal claim, and a consequent diversity and variability with regard to what the lived experience of Catholic-ness might be. It is useful to recall Foucault here because the genealogical method draws attention "to the way dominant conversations might contain hegemonic silences or may be drawn into certain paths rather than others simply through the subtle force of dominant discursive formations" (S. K. White, 2000, p. 57). It is my contention that we can understand the sisters' identity/ethical articulation as happening in such a space, neither directly within hegemonic silences nor on those certain paths, but rather in between. It is from that space in between that the sisters and their organization come into being.

The sisters act in their capacity as ethical agents whose spiritual convictions give them an official role within a religious identity and institution, not from within a framework of oppression or domination. It would be a mistake to characterize the experience of women religious as marginalized or peripheral. Such descriptors are referential and always demand, peripheral to what? In their own mission and ethical constitution, women religious are the actors and the center. Certainly, there are historically situated structural constraints to how that role has been constituted, drawn in the context of the Church's masculinist theology, along lines of biological sex, then articulated in terms of ecclesiology. Since only men are eligible for ordination to the priesthood, Catholic women who wish to undertake a life of service to the Church are restricted to other ministries, notably education and healthcare. But as Mahmood (2001) has argued, any analytic that reduces these experiences to a simple narrative of religious oppression or false consciousness and then narrates "moments of disruption of, and articulation of points of opposition to, male authority" does violence to the ethical reality of the women religious (p. 206).

When you speak to sisters about their healthcare facilities, they clearly refer to them as "our hospitals." Moreover, the tenure of their ministries in many locales signifies their moral commitments to the healing mission of the Church, quite distinct from local churches, missions, or new cathedrals. Indeed, in the course of years of interaction with Catholic Pacific Healthsystem, the sisters and their colleagues rarely if ever made reference to the works of their religious brothers (fathers?) in the Church. A description of ethico-politics of the hospital system hinges on the varying dynamics of power and influence of sister-sponsors and the independence with which they articulate their own ministries within the tradition of the Church. As Gene Burns has written, "American sisters with a quite different set of priorities than the bishops, are an excellent example of the power of the powerless to turn their exclusion into an asset of autonomy" (Burns, 1992, p. 5). Some sisters have bluntly drawn distinctions between what they call the women's Church and the men's Church. Consequently, when the sister-sponsors speak of the "Mother Church," they are invoking a very different political and theological entity than that which the magisterium imagines when it uses that term.

Scholar Wendy Brown, who has written extensively on the interstices of political theory and feminism, argues cogently to the limitations of what she calls "injured states" (1992). Her analysis points up the challenge of advancing a political analysis on the basis of a perceived identity based on having been wronged. In her thesis, speaking from a concretized identity of oppression can never be liberatory because the terms of one's very ethical constitution are fixed, bonded to those lacunae. The sister-sponsors and their healthcare ministries in CPH do not proceed from such concretized identities. They have distinct and explicit faith in their agency.

Philosopher Charles Scott engages the implications of the tendency of ethics and politics to drift toward claims of universalization and a consequent tribalism (1996). In this respect, his work echoes William Connolly and others I have engaged elsewhere (Connolly, 1995, 2002). I want to be mindful of my informants within CPH who try to walk that line with care, both maintaining the historical tradition of an originating organization (the Church, their sponsoring congregations) that asserts a transcendental notion of the good and the lived reality of the indeterminacy of normative claims when they extend beyond communal standards and habits (as in sponsoring a community hospital or serving a non-Catholic population through a religious hospital). It is a challenge to sustain such an affirmative ethical identity, cognizant of fears for the loss or erosion of ethico-political sensibility, while remaining open to the possibilities that pluralization may bring to even stronger reconfigurations. As one corporate member insisted, "We will not become catholic-lite."

Ethical Effects of Articulation

I turn now to the daily and programmatic interventions of Mission Integration in the operations of Catholic Pacific Healthsystem. The examples I use will document the tactics of mission agents, both sister-sponsors and lay people, in a strategy I have labeled the ethics of articulation. First, I will consider the work of Mary Douglas and George Cheney within an anthropology of organizations to set the stage for a discussion of identity and group dynamics. Then, I will examine a Catholic perspective on the ethics of discourse through the work of theologian John Courtney Murray that contributes to an analytic frame for the social life of CPH. Framing this analysis in terms of an ethics of articulation, I set my analysis against a background of the work of Charles Taylor and others, marking the discourse that emphasizes the role of qualitative distinctions in defining identity and the role of narrative in literally making sense of human lives.

The terms in/through which people live their lives cannot be separated from the explication of ethico-moral choices, particularly in regard to what makes a social "good" as well as "moral sources" for such goods (Taylor, 1990, p. 63). One might consider the CPH mission to care for the sick and those who are poor as an echo of what Taylor calls a "hyper-good." These are higher order goods, "which not only are incomparably more important than others but provide the standpoint from which these must be weighed, judged, decided about" (Taylor, p. 63). Taylor's argument works through the problem of naturalism that results from the embeddedness of values wherein we perceive existing valuations as objective. Naturalism obscures the possibility of value pluralism and tends toward an ethic of inarticulacy that Taylor dismantles (pp. 67–72). An ethic of articulacy, then, develops from a range of ethical views that see reason, in the sense of the logos—the linguistic articulacy—as part of the telos of human beings. That *anthropos,* what Kant called humanity and Foucault called *l'homme,* reflects a being with the capacity to be moral through his rational faculties, the conceptual apparatus necessary for ethical reflection (Rabinow, 2003). The language of that moral becoming, or *logos,* informs what I am calling an "ethic of articulation." This then is *anthropology* and clearly resonates with the theological anthropology (the nature of being human in relation to God) within the Catholic tradition. Such an ethical view suggests people are "not fully human beings until we can say what moves us, what our lives are built around" (Taylor, p. 92).

In the context of my ethnographic account of CPH, the suggestion of a hyper-good is not one of the broader society in which the system operates, but one of the collective ethico-moral constitution of Catholic Pacific Healthsystem, understood as crucial to the formation of organizational identity precisely for the ability of such an orientation to provide a distinctive qualitative dimension to the *catholicity* or Catholic-ness of the hospital network. It is just this articulation of those values that supports a common understanding of the good *for* CPH, *as* CPH. Further, as I will later demonstrate, the means by which that good is articulated, as a deliberative and collective process, enables Catholic Pacific Healthsystem to engage its diverse inspirational constituencies in such a way that accommodates an ethos of pluralization—in working with non-Catholic partners and the public—and incorporates that ethos as means to a common end, namely, a sustained witness of not-for-profit healthcare.

Modes of Engagement

The challenge of identity always lies in its communication. For an individual, how identity is recognized and affirmed within herself, as well as how it is made manifest to others, is a dialogic process; similarly for an organization, how identity is constituted and shared within the group and manifestly demonstrated for those who interact with it involves a social dialectic, stages of production both deliberative and less so. What this means in the context of Catholic Pacific Healthsystem is a move to recognize that values work, first, a recognition of self and, what follows, the recognition of the Other. I am thinking in this sense of Hegel and Gadamer—what Charles Taylor synthesizes as recognizing "Verstehen is a Seinsmodus"—namely, recognizing the action of conversation and dialogue within which interpretations of ourselves and of others come together (S. K. White, 2000, p. 53). At CPH, one might tally up the constituent groups as the sister-sponsors, lay colleagues (including the secular community hospital partners), agents of mission and margin, and of course the communities they all serve. "Intercultural" conversations have some unifying *telos:* in articulation and conversation lies possibility for connection, reconciliation between what seems initially to be irredeemably incommensurable (Bayley, 1995).

For our purposes, the significance of Taylor's argument in *Sources of the Self* lies in the assertion that in the space of late modern conversation there is no single trump card with regard to moral sources. The utility of foundational arguments—like Taylor's ontological constellations that vie to underpin some concordance over "life goods" (1990, pp. 50–51)—is not their specific truth value but their contribution to a motivation to care for conversational engagement between ontological constellations and the dedication to interpretive work that engagement requires. The ideal, as political theorist Stephen K. White points out, is not the guarantee of progress but the motivation to try (2000). As subsequent details will illustrate, CPH is an entity that takes this effort seriously. In some cases, the effort falls short, but the commitment of the organization to such an orientation toward *becoming* is grounded in its very identity.

White argues that having knowledge of one's values is equivalent to the claim that one has an explicit understanding "about one's form of life, moral source, and so on sufficient to know its precise boundaries" (S. K. White, 2000, p. 55). Thus, he suggests, to declare irreconcilability with others is to fail to recognize "that the very activity of articulating those things that are morally and spiritually crucial to one's form of life unavoidably puts one in a position of seeing/feeling them in new contexts and with new possibilities" (2000, p. 55). That is to say, conceptualizing values requires that one also conceptualize what is external to those values. Acknowledging this conceptualization of internal/external bounds of values, the "what is/is not" resonates with Adorno's *negative dialectic* and it reveals the narrative artifice of the margin/mission binary that peppers not-for-profit healthcare experience. In essence, White's argument is that since self-understanding is a linguistic act—of articulation to the self—that very determination is transactional and carries with it the potential for reconciliation by shifting the bounds within the conceptualization.

To the extent that the ethico-moral conundrum of modernity lies in the realization that "underneath the agreement on moral standards lies uncertainty and division concerning constitutive goods" (Taylor, p. 498), strong ontologies that insist on any particular fundamentalisms about self, other, and the world are contestable. However, such foundations lie at the heart of a reflective and ethical life. We are inclined, then, to consider what White calls "weak ontologies" that reflect fully the processual aspects of self-cultivation marked by the small narratives *(petits recits)* that Lyotard asserts mark our postmodern times (S. K. White, 2000, p. 12). To the extent that it is possible, I want to look to the common deliberations that mark CPH's daily operations as something that approaches *phronesis*. To recall Aristotelian ethics, this engages both complete excellence of practical intellect (comprising a true conception of the good life) and the deliberative excellence necessary to realize that conception in practice via choice (which Aristotle contrasts with *sophia*, operating in the theoretical sphere *(thewria)* in the context of the notion of well-being and man as both ethical and political animal). Common, everyday deliberations in CPH are the goods of social interchange that contribute to the rational life of the ethico-moral collective embodied in the hospital organization. As Mary Douglas has argued, institutions do not have minds of their own, but they do confer identity (Douglas, 1986).

Anthropology of Organizations

In the 1985 Abrams lectures, anthropologist Mary Douglas sought to push through the Durkheimian inheritance of suprapersonal cognitive systems constitutive of institutions and social groups. She has maintained that a theory of institutions is needed to "amend the current unsociological [*sic*] view of human cognition" (1986), while a theory of cognition is needed "to supplement the weaknesses of institutional analysis" (Gregg, 1999, p. 31). In her introduction, Douglas reminds readers that the theory of rational behavior presumes that each thinker is a sovereign individual. Rational choice seems at odds with the idea of true cooperation and solidarity that, arguing from Durkheim and Ludwig Fleck, Douglas claims would require that individuals share the categories of their thought (Douglas, p. 8). The Abrams lectures, How Institutions Think, are intended to bring rational choice and solidarity to a theoretical rapprochement. Douglas seeks to construct a better functionalist argument, while addressing the objection that rational choice undermines any collective action that causes an individual to act against her self-interest.

Douglas builds outward from a foundation in Durkheim's division of labor. If, as he argued, the increasing division of labor breaks down the shared symbolic universe on which solidarity was based in primitive society, then in industrial society, sacredness is "transferred to the individual" and solidarity shifts to become "dependent on the workings of the market" (Douglas, p. 13). Fleck's treatment of organizational structure, the gradations from thought collective (more bound) to thought community (looser constraints but still retaining membership), works for Douglas to provide a positivistic counterbalance for Durkheim's apparent invocation of a "mysterious, super-organic group mind" that Douglas is wary of affirming. Douglas chides Durkheim for using "religion" as the escape system to answer the problem of the collective acting against individual self-interest. As Douglas reminds us, Fleck understood a system of knowledge itself to be a public good, thus religion cannot be the exception that Durkheim claims it to be.

Juxtapose to Douglas's anthropological treatment George Cheney's analysis of corporate rhetoric in which an organization is understood as a system of communication that involves the persuasion of individuals and groups (Cheney, 1990). His case study revolves around the creation of the 1983 pastoral letter, *The Challenge of Peace,* by American Catholic bishops. At the center of his analysis is the question of how an organization maintains a traditional identity yet adapts to external change without risking the loss of internal authority and legitimacy. Citing sociologist Kenneth Burke, Cheney proposes to understand organizational rhetoric, literally persuasion, as the management of multiple identities as it relates to intended audience and organizational message. Though undertheorized from an anthropological perspective, Cheney recognizes identity as a focal point in contemporary social theory and emphasizes its role in the symbolic representation of perceived shared interests. Thus, Cheney addresses a lacuna in Douglas's theorizing—how to make the move to observed phenomena in the contemporary world. His answer is to examine the development of position statements and other "corporate" documents of the organizational body, though he runs the risk of treating an organization as individual writ large. He considers individual principal actors as directional influences in the broader management of multiple identities but concurs with Douglas that the effect of organizations is to embody, read incorporate, decisions for individuals, setting categories for thought and fixing identity (Cheney, p. 164). They proceed from different frameworks; where Douglas uses Durkheim and Fleck, Cheney deploys Weber and Burke.

I introduce Douglas and Cheney to point to a consistent problem in anthropological inquiry that these authors begin to address. We can identify an organization as an entity, but it is not solely reducible to a group of individuals, for it bears a collective identity. And in the case of a religion or faith group, there is an appeal to that collective, suprapersonal construction. But how does such an entity act, evaluate and prioritize, and then sustain those processes against the arrival and departure of individual actors within it? Religion and religious practice are necessarily concerned with the metaphysics of human experience. Those concerns, however, are acted out in the social realm and take on social forms. The following analysis of documents and bureaucratic processes within the hospital system is set against participant observation of individual actors and agent groups in hopes of filling in that analytic gap within this anthropological inquiry and demonstrating the ethico-political nature of the hospital system.

Ethics of Discourse

A similar emphasis on the possibility inherent in discourse underlies the critical contributions to contemporary Catholic social politics of John Courtney Murray. Murray was a key contributor, if not central voice, of *Dignitatis Humanae Personae*, the Declaration on Religious Liberty that emerged from Vatican II. The Declaration expresses three doctrinal elements: an ethical doctrine of religious freedom as an individual human right, the political doctrine on limits and functions of government in matters religious, and the theological doctrine of the freedom of the Church as the basis for relations between the sociopolitical order and the Church itself (Murray writing in Abbott, 1963, p. 673). It is the third aspect that concerns us here.

Murray's broader works concerned the mode of Christian engagement with public life, asserting particularly a reliance on persuasion rather than historically sanctioned coercion or manipulation (Hooper, 1986, pp. 187–189). Importantly, Murray's effort to broaden the lines of dialogue were based on an authorization principle that recognized the active, ethical agency of the people in contrast to the hierarchical model of Church authority (Hooper, pp. 82–120). The actual argumentation is complex, bringing in both historical observation and philosophical treatise, but the central theme advocates an openness through which not only the teachings of the Church but the Church itself as a sociohistorical entity continues to experience moral growth. To fulfill its own mission, and to behave responsibly within the actual environment of the larger social world, requires ethical conversation—public theological discourse for the Church means open discussion of Church doctrine, interpretation, and application creating ethical relations between the magisterium and the faithful, as well as public sociopolitical engagement that is open to the possibility of moral, and even religious, insights which might arise outside of the Church and to which the Church should nonetheless attend. It is these precepts for ethical discourse that affirms for the Church the secular value of religious liberty (S. K. White, 2000, p. 169). Indeed, to return to Vatican II, the Declaration itself not only acknowledges non-Catholics and non-Christians but also directly addresses them. The Response to the Declaration points out that the assertion of religious freedom begun as work among the faithful is "completed in the reshaping of the created order" by explicitly engaging these non-Catholics as audience and partner in social life (Abbott, 1963, p. 700). That engagement with non-Catholics as audience and partner illustrates how Vatican II is representative of what White calls a "weak ontology." An ontology is inherently foundational and, as such, tends toward reification and naturalization. To accommodate an ethos of pluralization, a weak ontology instead exhibits the capacity to fold back on itself, such that contestability can be enacted and not simply announced (S. K. White, p. 8).

Understanding CPH as an ethico-moral project hinges on the fact that my informants actively engage in reflection and articulation of the purpose of their work and relate it to a larger teleology of social engagement. Their conscious efforts to link their actions to social and religio-spiritual values only begins with the superficial work of linking operations to the espoused "core values" of the hospital corporation: dignity, collaboration, justice, stewardship, and excellence. It is most significantly manifest in the small disciplinary techniques of individuals, mainly in mission services, sisters and former sisters, who alone and together, conceive and shape an organizational culture that is more than just the action plan of organizational development in the Human Resources department. Rather, the explicit goals and objectives of the organizational development staff result from the tactical maneuvers of agents from Mission Services, later deliberately renamed Mission Integration.

Explicit Processes: Exteriorizing Interiors

In the sections that follow, I document how various disciplinary techniques and tactical maneuvers of several key actors work to make values an integral part of daily operations at CPH and thus shape the organization's culture. Though I have called this an ethics of articulation, it also connotes a reconceptualization of ethical practice. Rather than relying on internal virtues of Catholic sisters, for example, the ethics of articulation acts to externalize values into the lived experience of everyday hospital operations. As the lead ethicist in the system, Marie sees that part of her role as she understands it is to make things explicit. She says of herself:

Understanding how those functions work, then I can make the connections. . . . And one way to be effective is to learn more about other people's work. And then show them, by not doing anything basically, how they're already doing what they think I do. They're already doing it. Giving it a name, giving it a language, giving it a legitimacy for conversation [that's my task].

The idea of being explicit—of articulating an ethics—invokes concepts of authenticity and sincerity. Further, the intention that underlies naming—which is the process of legitimizing that Marie's comment points to—obliges us to recognize that a form of linguistic ideology is at work. Language use, in this sense, makes an interior state transparent through articulation. Sincerity reflects the idea that thoughts and words constitute a parallel discourse that correspond to each other; though thought precedes the spoken word and shapes it, the two match. To wit, religious conversion would require authenticity and sincerity to be real and true (Keane, 2002, pp. 74–75). In CPH, the Mission Integration team has as its charge the articulation of an ethics of *catholicity,* particular to this collectivity of Catholic and secular community hospitals working in partnership. Marie's role, as she herself reports, is to engage CPH employees, physicians, and other professional staff and assist them to see "how they're already doing what they think I do [as the nominal ethicist]" in their own work. That is, her efforts help her colleagues to be reflexive about their work in healthcare, undertaking ethical decision making, and then ultimately, constituting CPH as an ethical collective entity. With this guidance, they are able to make *conscious,* to make explicit, the values underlying actions and thereby to extend into new spheres a *signifying practice.* Another sister put it this way:

It's the conversation that keeps—tries to keep people on that thin line of integrity. And the fact that there's conversation around it probably is a very healthy sign. . . . .You know. If there's no conversation around it, that might be a very dangerous thing, too, that everybody should think it's all hunky dory.

The simple refrain "no margin, no mission," often heard amongst financial staff, is a real reminder of both the pragmatics of healthcare services and the easy social risks of insincerity, of mere lip service to values that do not, in actuality, reflect an internal state. We only ever have incomplete access to motivations; however, we also need to acknowledge that one's form of life is tied to the language that interprets the larger lifeworld within that such a form manifests. Like etiquette, using religious language in the CPH context may merely be a matter of observing social forms.

Both Taylor (1990) and Asad (1993) have developed the idea that an individual's interiority is the main site that can elude political coercion. It is unclear how such a view may reflect a broader "protestantization" that itself could be an element of secularization: the Calvinist view that actions and behaviors are external manifestations of an always-and-already elect is very different from the Catholic conception of spiritual practices wherein particular behaviors repeated can lead to correct internal states—parallel but distinct from any conception of *habitus* and the cultivation of virtues. Here, I want to think about the connection to Foucault's genealogy of ethical discipline that he argues emerges from the Christian conception of the pastorate, particularly, the idea that it is possible to know what is in people's minds (Dreyfus & Rabinow, 1983, p. 214). Taylor argues that the concept of having responsibility for one's desires and motives is distinctively modern. Foucault's work defines modern forms of subjectification through which the subject is "tied to his own identity by conscience or self-knowledge"—a necessary element to the functioning of pastoral power (Dreyfus & Rabinow, 1983, p. 212). If his typologies hold as marked characteristics of modern subjectivity, life at CPH also suggests that there is a Catholic dimension to that subjectivity that carries threads of older forms through into the contemporary. The catholicity here is a subjectivity constituted through pastoral care that creates a collective that undertakes to consciously care for the Other. *Communitas,* then, is both the collective that is CPH-as-organization, which mobilizes external agents in society to care *(caritas),* as well as the group of Others for whom the hospital cares, or the social body from which the cared-for are drawn—what the hospital literature repeatedly refers to as the "community," as in community outreach, community services, community needs, or community assessment.

The Mission Integration structure, its functions, and its members are a social intermediary that is key to pastoral power in the Catholic sense. Protestant conceptions understand power to be internalized in the individual, obviating the need for an intermediary agent. The Mission Integration structure echoes, too, the denominational contrast between the notion of assigning holiness to a particular sanctified "priestly" group, which we may recognize in the power and influence of sister-sponsors, over the more democratic ideal of a "priesthood of all believers." This has

important implications for the future of Catholic healthcare as the number of active sisters continues to decline. The Mission Integration team
occupies a "middle ground as social technicians articulating a normative
or middling modernism" for the hospital system (Rabinow, 1989, p. 13).
In CPH, the application of social technologies, like the mission standards
I discuss below, are deployed to cultivate norms and forms of caring and
community, emergent values motivated by a religious orientation.

It is difficult to imagine a Catholic hospital without some form of mission agent. It is precisely the fact that ethical reflection and organizational self-fashioning is an articulated role tied to actual budget items and
full-time equivalents in personnel that distinguishes this Catholic system
from its non-Catholic secular counterparts. Other systems and facilities
may have organizational development staff within a larger human resources department, but at CPH, mission and values extend well beyond
organizational development because of the ontological legacy embedded
in a religious history of identity. It remains to be seen the extent to which
the mediation of the Mission Integration staff may be a transitional medium from the previous era of Catholic hospitals, replete with sisters, to
new and emerging forms yet to be called into being. I am diagnosing a
context that may be part of a larger transition, though that context constitutes a distinct ethico-moral moment in fieldwork. Another way to conceptualize this development is to consider how mission integration might
be different if it took place in a Protestant hospital. That is, might it be
helpful to imagine this account as a sort of protestantization of Catholic
healthcare: the diffusion of the values from religious specialists (the
sister-sponsors) to the broader group (the priesthood of all believers) that
in this sense follows a "secular rationalization" model suggested by some
sociologists of religion.

Mission Integration standards are itemized tenets of practice designed to tie CPH core values to concrete actions across the spectrum of
operations at every level of the hospital system. The approach of Mission
Integration standards resembles a "theology of inculturation," a Catholic
pastoral strategy that revalorizes indigenous cultural forms and culturally
specific expressions of universally translatable Christian values and
themes. The "theology of inculturation" represents a reformulation of liberation theology, ascendant in Latin America in the 1970s and early 1980s
but resisted and arguably co-opted by the Roman magisterium. Originally,
liberation theology espoused a dissident pastoral approach articulating a

class-based rhetoric for structural change grounded in Christian values; the theology of inculturation is a discourse of ethnic solidarity and identity politics. The reformulation is understood by some to be a conscious and conscientious project of the Roman magisterium to recoup the revolutionary theological doctrine of priests and bishops of whom Rome had become wary, particularly in the overtly political context of developing countries.

At CPH, the Mission Integration philosophy seeks to routinize local appreciation of posited parallels between indigenous sensibilities and the values of the Christian founders in collaboration with the historical commitments of the secular, not-for-profit hospitals. For example, orientation for new hires at Incarnation Hospital is a program that is largely led by Sister Josephine. Standing in front of the assembly hall, in her lavender blazer and cream skirt suit, a dove and cross pinned to her lapel, Josephine is a living example of the religious origins of the hospital's sociopolitical legacy, and she repeatedly uses the history of her congregation to explain what employees at all levels are contributing in their new role within Incarnation.

Down the road, at City Physicians' Hospital, the same new hire orientation program is led by Marsha Cooper, a registered nurse who has worked at City Physicians' for nearly 20 years. Beginning as a staff nurse, she has risen through management to become the vice president for patient care services and chief nurse executive. Instead of setting out work at City Physicians' in terms of the larger religious history of Catholic Pacific Healthsystem, she begins with the story of a small group of physicians and their decision to build a hospital to serve the city and the demographic changes that have shaped the facility's commitment to serving the needs of the immigrant poor, for the hospital sits between an established, wealthy neighborhood and a transient low-income area near the downtown area. Marsha explicitly positions her narrative at the level of her secular community facility that "is not a Catholic hospital," but which had rather sought out CPH as a parent system in order to sustain its not-for-profit commitment to the needs of the local populace.

As an original site of the Catholic system, Incarnation sets its identity firmly within that religious legacy. In contrast, City Physicians' spokespeople are wary of losing their secular history and make conscious efforts to distinguish themselves as community partners, even as their operations are increasingly regulated and standardized according to the dictates of the parent system that sustains their local not-for-profit identity and objectives. CPH promotes the localization of core values to match the on-site traditions, both reinforcing indigenous sensibilities and forging links across the system as an ethico-political entity.

Mission Integration standards build on the impetus of rationalization in care management and other operational functions, adapting by casting themselves as simply another development process compatible with the locally accepted trends already underway toward greater quantification and reporting, vital to competitive healthcare. Mission integration agents capitalize on that trend, but they see themselves as something other than another bureaucratic process; they perceive a purpose in their interventions that lends an additional dimension to their work. In the realm of faith and belief, "spirituality in the workplace" is something more than a vehicle for making the office more pleasant. Some see the Mission Integration department as the soul of the system; others are uncomfortable with such a designation, arguing that it reifies the perception of precisely the "priestliness" they are trying to dismantle in the diffusion of values and mission amongst all CPH employees and partners.

Our Patients, Our People, Our Future

In 2001, a strategic plan produced by a broad swath of the various constituencies and guided by key actors in the CPH system office brought new attention to organizational development and the focus on the system as a "learning organization." Indeed, when I first began participant observation at the system office, I was welcomed in under the auspices of the Mission Integration department because its senior leadership perceived my presence at CPH—the outsider perspective—and the discussions that might ensue as contributing to that "learning organization." The strategic planning process itself was met with enthusiasm in Mission Integration because discussion of employee recruitment and retention began to focus on ideas of continuing education and training that could allow for succession planning. Furthermore, the planning process represented an opportunity to integrate the mission and values perspectives across the spectrum of CPH's action plan for all operations. Even the title, *Our Patients, Our People, Our Future,* suggested a trajectory, and this resonated strongly with the mission agents who were thinking over ideas to adapt religious formation as a model for organizational development in CPH.

The religious sponsorship of CPH and its Catholic hospitals, especially incarnated in the social vision of sister-sponsors, stands out as a distinguishing characteristic that sets CPH apart from other not-for-profit hospitals. Evocations of Catholic identity may rub off on other Catholic healthcare players in California, but as the dominant Catholic system, CPH does not risk much in its geographic markets. In the face of economic crisis, the system strategists in Strategic Planning and Corporate Communications converged on the religious history as a marketing message. That convergence indicates how the charisma of the past as an inalienable possession—"our unique history of ministry"—can itself be used as a commodity. Thus, the media specialists in CPH Corporate Communications became unexpected collaborators with the Mission Integration department. Consultations were scheduled and people across the system worked to market the history of the hospitals, especially capitalizing on lay perceptions of women religious. This collaboration saw a resurgence in the language of healing and caring (as opposed to scientific or technical vocabularies) in system and hospital publications, especially caring for the whole person through spiritual care, continuity of care and discharge planning, palliative care, and birthing suites that recognized the familial needs of obstetrical patients. Telling those stories in CPH ad campaigns, Web site narratives, and internal newsletters and recounting the redesign of wards and service lines as indicators of the historical religious orientation that underlay CPH also articulated how the system operations reflected mission and values. A cynic would see savvy approaches to niche marketing; a romantic, ministry ideals. In truth, both things converged.

Mary Douglas's characterization of Ludwig Fleck evokes Ian Hacking in arguing that "the development of knowledge depends on how the knowledge is expected to intervene in practical life. Thinking has more to do with intervening than with representing" (Douglas, 1986, p. 50; Hacking, 1983). In contrast, Arendt would assert that thinking makes things visible: through speech, thought objects are made "an appearance" (Arendt, 1981). My analysis suggests both understandings are applicable here.

Expression, or articulation, is an aesthetic process. In articulating what we find within us, Taylor argues, we also make something manifest and bring something of fundamental human nature into expression

(1990, p. 374). Two distinct qualities characterize this act. First, that which is brought to expression is "not something that was already fully formulated beforehand; rather, its very character is partially constituted by the expression." Second, this "curious quality of creating and/or discovering" has to do both with being engaged in articulation and the wider world (S. K. White, 2000, p. 59). In this sense, anthropological fieldwork, too, has a hermeneutic effect; during interviews and hallway conversations, my inquiries become part of the social processes through which articulation occurs. During the time I was part of their daily work lives, my participant observation was interpolated in discourse and reflection around my informants' ethical stances and other aspects of their worldview, particularly in the sense that experience is "écrit aprés coup" [written after the fact] (Jay, 1998, pp. 62–78). Similarly, what is repeatedly constituted as "operations" within a hospital system, in fact, means people collectively engaged in a series of practices; "management" happens as a social exchange between people, not in paper trails as such, though documents may be the medium through which that exchange takes place. Thus, there is validity to attending meetings, strategy sessions, and Mission department activities as a participant-observer that converges with the overall argument for the ethics of articulation: articulation has ethical effects derived from the possibility of reconciliation and collaboration. For better or for worse, there are aspects of being a participant-observer that echo some of the more effective characteristics of a management consultant; indeed, anthropology has engaged this under the rubric of "complicity" (Marcus, 1998, pp. 105–131).

As I read Taylor and S. K. White, then, the fundamental ontological center of gravity in moral life is the process of articulating moral sources and even perhaps, as Taylor has argued elsewhere, contributing to a refocusing on the good of a flourishing culture in ethical–political terms. When such an ethic is articulated, it is done in the language of an organization and its members. Syntax and semantics are fundamental elements of rhetoric. In this sense, they are political tools of persuasion. Language choice represents an aspect of how values are set; it is through language that mission is made explicit and how practices driven by CPH core values are set as an expectation or a quarterly target. Language is thus a representation of a way of being, and as we know, representations are social facts (Rabinow, 1986).

Language Marking Culture

In a meeting of the system vice presidents for group operations, one executive was so determined to ensure that the system's financial turnaround continue that he proclaimed he would not hire any new people unless they had extensive for-profit experience and "came from *that world.*" This emphatic assertion met with no objections, no comments to the contrary, or even furrowed brows, but rather nods of agreement. This comment percolated through to other venues, for I heard it reported back to the Mission Integration team as a whole in a department meeting one day. There it was met with some consternation and taken as partial proof of the need to aggressively orient new leadership to CPH mission and core values.

Anthropologist Stacey Leigh Pigg writes of the incommensurability of language and the social production of commensurability (Pigg, 2001). I want to suggest that this may be a useful way to think about the efforts of Mission Integration to intervene in the perceived cultural ascendancy of the margin oriented—the finance and accounting managers across the hospital system. In her work on international public health interventions in Nepal, Pigg muses on how language can be used for political expediency (p. 508). She turns to linguistic anthropologist Michael Silverstein's treatment of code switching to illustrate how language practices can reflect tensions created by social difference and stratification. Pigg goes on to argue that language can be a tool to reconfigure social position. Mission agents encourage colleagues to change the terms they use to align with what the sisters want to hear; in effect, colleagues switch the code of business for one of mission. Linguistic anthropologists call the strategy of altering one's terms to match a particular social context "code switching."

Similarly, I want to suggest that the values language of faith, mission, and values in CPH is used to soften otherwise blatant business language–marked concepts. "Languages and their locally recognized variants become emblems (iconically essentialized indexes) of their users' positions in a shifting field of identities" (Silverstein, 1998, p. 411). Thus, at CPH, the core value of stewardship can also be appropriated as the gloss for corporate rightsizing, itself a recoded term that began as downsizing. Code switching as a social practice "must be seen as the socioculturally meaningful creation and transformation of interactional context through the use of entextualized forms" (Silverstein, p. 413). In her work on the problem of disease prevention in developing countries, Pigg uses this explanation to explain how AIDS education sessions are particular entextualized forms that are, in practice, communicative events that actually *aim* to transform interactional contexts by creating new forms of awareness. As Pigg's analysis points out, greater social complexities underlie any word choice. At CPH, a strategic intervention by sister-sponsors or their allies in Mission Integration carries a similar transformative hope: they want to routinely recategorize business practices as extensions of mission and core values.

I was present for a number of conversations among various managers, directors, and senior management about the use of the label "corporate" for internal descriptions of the CPH system. One manager maintained that ever since some senior executives had used the word, the sense of familiarity among people had changed. Another disagreed, blaming the changes on both rapid growth and significant staff turnover in the former regions and divisions of CPH. When sister-sponsors heard this during their lunch before a governance meeting, there were discussions among staff and sisters about whether "company" had a softer tone to it, as in the name of their sister-colleagues to the south, the Little Company of Mary. The political stance in the United States that considers corporations as individuals with constitutional rights of free speech and other protections may resonate here. A staffperson at Saint-Catherine-by-Sea shared the following explantion:

a legal "corpus," a body, [of] an organization that allows it to assume debt and make covenants that exist beyond the physical life of the people who created the company. Some . . . might observe that the problem with many modern corporations is they are . . . legal bodies that are without any spirit or soul. They are alive legally, but dead when it comes to having feelings that link the souls and spirits of those who are part of the corporation.

At lunch that day, someone pointed out that corporation really echoed "corpus" and liked the idea of the system as part of the body of Christ. This initiated a larger debate, and some executives scoffed that this kind of semantics had little bearing on reality. When the sister-sponsors later convened by themselves, they discussed their discomfort with what seemed like the language of a colder, for-profit world, particularly given the CPH stance on access to healthcare as a fundamental human right. While they regretted the permeating effects of market capitalism, they were quite outspoken about stemming the flow of military language into common parlance. One of the sisters reported that she had overheard a discussion among strategy department staff about efforts by the state hospital association to "kill" legislation tying community benefit to a percentage of net revenue. Another sister suggested we could find a better way to communicate itemized lists than "bullet points," and "hitting targets." She expressed her disgust at recent news coverage reporting the U.S. State Department's and Pentagon's use of "collateral damage" to refer to unintended violence done to noncombatants, civilian buildings, etc.

The sister-sponsors asked Catherine, the senior vice president who served as the liaison to system governance, to communicate their concerns to senior management, encouraging them to endeavor to seek alternatives. "Our documents, our strategic plans, should reflect who we are and what we stand for, just as much as our mission statement and our investment practices," Sister Mary Frances told me. Returning to the notion of the corporation as an individual, the sisters recognize their corporate documents as speech acts of a legally constituted person. This is why the choice of language is important. Policy and procedure are the means by which the public identity of the organization is presented and language constructs that representation.

Language is an issue, but one with multiple meanings for different people. The sister-sponsors adopted the stance that even minor slippage could create an inappropriate familiarity with terms that otherwise connote violence and other aspects of culture that they did not want their organization to foster. One politically active sister very much involved in daily operations of a CPH hospital's information systems shared this perspective:

PARTICIPANT: You know, with so many different professions [in healthcare]—so many people come from different strands of professional education, and they bring with it that language. . . . [Y]ou bring in people, let's say, in terms of management or finance, they bring with it a management/finance language. Right? . . . whereas, if you bring in somebody from the clinical side, they're gonna bring in a clinical language. So that—we almost have like a cacophony of sounds coming out from different traditions.

I remember back in the '80s, . . . in strategic planning now, you were supposed to identify your cash cows and the dogs. I love that. I can't imagine going to the faculty and telling them that their Medieval Latin was a dog and not a cash cow. . . . Those words and that whole concept of strategic planning came out of an engineering tradition, or military tradition. . . . Not—probably people wouldn't enjoy that, but . . . words are created out of certain disciplines . . . then they're borrowed by other disciplines, and they adapt, because everybody's adapting, trying to get the best ideas in order to function. But we bring in these words, like cash cow and dog [laughs]. . . . I sure wouldn't want to tell anybody that they were dogs, but obviously, they were the ones that we're losing money on, you know. But you know, to an engineer, that would just roll off the tongue—they'd roll that out without any sense, right? Now, in the sense of ministry, you're more concerned about the feelings—can you imagine using that language? . . .

The concept made sense . . . the context was fine, but the language was way off. [In some of our schools] the faculty would be horrified if we were talking about strategic planning, because they thought it was just so—I mean, out of our culture. Well, of course it was a way of saying, look, we've gotta be realistic about what we're doing here, right? . . . Anyway when you get into a system, where you're trying to bring in people with a variety of skills—financial, legal, clinical, whatever, clinical, ministerial, right, the chaplains are . . . gonna be horrified with some of this language. So—and I hear some of our people, occasionally I've heard people say, oh, you know, the language at corporate office is so—harsh and military. Well, I'm wondering if . . . there's a good possibility that they were attracted to the system and what it stood for and its values, but the language that they speak hasn't quite caught up with it. . . . .

I think we are great imitators. We pick up words unconsciously and find ourselves repeating something, if we're associated with people who . . . use a phrase we hadn't heard before, and it fits, and we find ourselves borrowing it. So there's a lot of imitation in language. And [the hospital's senior vice president] would probably say, "She's off the wall." But—so I don't know if—if we can say that the system is headed for—is headed for bad times, or that we're getting off course with our values system because we have all these mixed expressions that are there. I think more important is what we do. You know, how—people can talk about having values, but when you look at your budget, and what do you spend, does it reflect your values. That to me is what's real. That's where it's right, whether I'm coming from an engineering school or a military school or medical school or theological school, it seems to me, the values are really reflected in the decisions. . . . It's the decision-making mode, to me, that's the heart of the matter.

As anthropologist Stacey Leigh Pigg suggests, there is a power element at work in the substitution of language by Mission Integration. Language choice (framing a decision in terms of "stewardship") reintroduces the hierarchical structure of the organization (Pigg, 2001). Even the sister-sponsor quoted above uses terms of an economic/financial origin, like "cash cows"; the language of capitalism is ubiquitous. In CPH, users are cognizant of where particular language choice comes from, and why it is being deployed. Those lay staff members who dismiss language terms as insignificant nonetheless change the terms they use in speech and organizational documents. The power and influence of the sponsors may be the cause, and lay staff may retain their skepticism about the actual effects of such semantic juggling, but the result is that values are made evident in the products. Transformative ethical effects take place, becoming habit, and such practices repeated result in new internal states at the organizational level. Some might argue this is also true for individuals; certainly, the Church based its emphasis on transformative spiritual practices on such an idea of habituation.

Code switching does enable entrée into particular levels of social legitimacy: medical in the case of Pigg's Nepal, and in the conference rooms of CPH, religious. Just as mentioning "charism" marked me as a mission ally for sister-sponsors and former sisters, because I can "speak Catholic theology," it mattered to my field informants in operations and administration that I could toss about the language of managed care contracting and the economics of physician reimbursement and banter about "DRG creep" and the significance of Medicare waivers. Though my label as an anthropology researcher made people uncertain of my position, my former graduate student status allowed me to be categorized as a subordinate, and my use of coded terms from the business of healthcare further made me something of an insider. I am trained in the modalities of public health and healthcare administration, and I care about the practices of this organization in the social world. Though it is analogous to the work of Mission Integration in CPH, it also suggests the complexity of complicity that may be inherent to anthropological inquiry.

To import yet another insight from Pigg's concept of the social production of commensurability, in the healthcare environment of a hospital system, two dominant epistemologies of medicine and business together organize arenas of life and social interaction. Both demand recognition and, as the sister quoted above points out, invite emulation. Catholic healthcare ministry, as a configuration of both not-for-profit and religio-spiritual values, continually seeks to resist the dominant epistemologies, at once trying to engage them as vehicles for its own ends while avoiding co-optation within those efforts. The task of mission integration is to fa-cilitate engagement without being marginalized as simple window dress-ing. While it may be that the margin makes the mission possible, the mis-sion makes the margin necessary. As the last quote of the sister above emphasizes, the concern of ethical practice does not end in language use and speech acts. Action—"what we do"—is important because talk is cheap; budgets and spending reflect real values. Later discussion of an explicit "process for ethical decision making" will link these two sites of concern.

It is the practice throughout CPH for an individual participant, as-signed in advance on a rotating basis, to read a "reflection" before any meeting, both large and small. This represents a mapping of morality into each operational session at CPH; no matter the agenda or area of con-cern, the participants and guests are obliged to observe a moment of re-flection that calls people to the task at hand in the context of an organiza-tion founded on religious values that bear directly on their mission in healthcare that day. The practice that began with the sister-sponsors was codified into corporate systemwide policy in the mid-1990s and has since been reaffirmed in the mission standards created in 2002:

Mission Standard 9: CPH promotes spirituality in the lives of its co-workers and in the work(s) of the organization, (d) All gatherings and meetings begin with prayer/inspirational reflection.

Because each person who "does the reflection" is free to choose their own selection, the practice allows for the diversity of the employee body while still creating an ethical space that derives from the religious heri-tage of its sponsors. This seems to be a type of moral mapping more com-monly recognized in explicitly religious ritual (Muelebach, 2001). Conse-quently, there is general acceptance of this practice in the system office and many of the hospitals, especially the traditionally Catholic facilities. At Denomination North Hospital, however, the management meetings over a three-month period rarely ever began with a reflection, except for the new staff orientation session. There, the reflection provided an easy entrée into a discussion of the hospital's culture and what it meant to be a part of Catholic Pacific Healthsystem.

Senior management at Denomination North happily trotted out the obligatory reflection for conference calls with the system office, but its reading would elicit smiles and twinkling eyes from the on-site staff. Denomination North holds on tightly to its secular community identity, exacerbated by its competitive history in a local geography dominated by the ancestral group of hospitals that cofounded CPH. The resistance to reflections is allowed by the hospital president as a gesture of indulgence for a management staff that has been struggling to keep the hospital successful, particularly because he feels that his facility is a leading example of a mission-driven hospital even as its operations suffer from rapidly changing demographics. This hospital serves a largely indigent population on insufficient Medicaid reimbursements, and a new competing specialty center down the road that provides outpatient surgery and obstetrics is a significant challenge to patient flow as well as a dilution of Denomination North's marketing efforts. Run by the other leading not-for-profit hospital chain, the new center seems to skim the self-insured patients from the community pool. Nonetheless, Denomination North manages to do well and is quite respected within the CPH system.

Interestingly, even finance and business management staff have adapted to the organizational expectation of an opening reflection; one vice president of finance at a southern hospital read from Adam Smith at a revenue stream meeting. Most people exert themselves to find poems, literary references, inspirational anecdotes, or new stories, often combing the Internet or soliciting their friends and family for good "reflections" that in many cases seek to address the task at hand. Some staff people find it easy to read selections from a range of faith traditions that are overtly religious; others reach for quotes from Gandhi, Thoreau, or Faulkner. After September 11, and throughout the earlier Gulf War, many selections were culled from translations of the Qur'an or quoted from leading Arab intellectuals with the specific goal of consciousness-raising during a difficult time. Many executives keep a file of ideas for reflections. There is a thriving CPH intranet barter trade in reflections shared between coworkers across the system, and people recommend colleagues' selections to others in different departments over lunch and coffee breaks. I have even heard people introduce an out-of-town colleague with: "Oh, you'll remember Sheila; she read that great reflection on homelessness for the video conference last fall."

At a system board meeting later in the year, the board member who earlier had been assigned to lead the opening reflection was absent due to illness. The board chair appealed to a sister-sponsor and asked her to fill in. Putting aside her breakfast orange juice and smartly pulling her chair up to the table, the sister said: "I knew it, I knew it. We have to change the culture so that it isn't just Sister who can *offer* a reflection." She responded with good humor, but her point was not lost on the group, some of whom looked sheepish at having dodged the appeal to lead. The practice of reading a reflection represents a commitment to catholic—in the universal rather than sectarian sense—pluralism that nonetheless resonates with a Catholic tradition of mission, understood here as workplace spirituality. The intent is to systematize an explicit articulation that reflects an organizational identity through ritual practice. Conformity is expected, but how one conforms is individualized and demonstrates an accommodation of intragroup diversity across the CPH system.

In his examination of international health interventions, P. Stanley Yoder posits that operative intervention models treat culture "as a set of beliefs, values and individual goals that pattern behavior. . . . Individuals are constrained by their image of normative action as they seek to conform to the values of their society" (Yoder, 1997, p. 135). At CPH, Mission Integration uses language as a tactical tool within a broader strategy to set the organizational expectation of an articulated mission and values to which business practices, and other social behaviors, are expected to conform.

A Problem of Distinctions

Bene docet qui bene distinguit

Learning lies in drawing careful distinctions. We assume that calling a facility "Catholic" means that it is different from those facilities we do not call "Catholic." But is such a distinction in language and labels *real?* Both Talal Asad and Charles Taylor have made the suggestion that language differences can, in fact, be used to mask the absence of true difference. Asad notes:

Some ways in which symbolization (discourse) can *disguise lack of distinctiveness* are well brought out in MacIntyre's trenchant critique of contemporary Christian writers, where he argues that "Christians behave like everyone else but use a different vocabulary in characterizing their behaviour, and also to conceal their lack of distinctiveness" (MacIntyre 1971, 24). (Asad 1993, p. 33)

What then is real? How does a group constitute a cultural mode of allegiance to particular linguistic forms? As the example of the sister who decried "collateral damage" suggests, dramatic differences in metaphor that play themselves out in language are representative of larger issues. Ruth Shalit, writing in the *New Republic,* raised a parallel question for the emergent industry of bioethics consultants (1997). Shalit asked: "Just who [are] the ethicists really serving? A swelling corps of HMO utilitarians are cashing in on their ethical expertise, marketing their services to managed care executives eager to dress up cost-cutting decisions in Latinate labels and lofty principles" (1997, p. 25). But does such labeling only signify a politically expedient strategy in the CPH setting, or are other dynamics at work? One researcher uses the phrase "the language of reflexive spirituality" to describe the way in which people seek to relate to religious meaning (Besecke, 2001). That approach asserts that language use acts as a cultural resource that enables my informants to reground modern life with a shared transcendent quality of a concept or experience, without necessarily agreeing on the content or meaning that emerges from it. What is useful here is the emphasis on religiosity's cultural, communicative dimension. It reflects modern expressivism, post-appeals to nature or reason, post-Schopenhauer, post-Nietzsche, "our sense of the certainty or problematicity of God is relative to our sense of moral sources" (Taylor, 1990, p. 312). As S. K. White maintains, this means that God as a moral source is functionally related to subjective articulation (2000), or as Taylor would argue, "theology is indexed to the languages of personal resonance" (Taylor, 1990, p. 512). The ethos of CPH is one that recognizes these dimensions and seeks to foster them within the bureaucratic processes of corporate operations, and amidst increasing pluralization.

Sisters in governance and Mission Integration staff have consistently encouraged language awareness, most particularly in strategic planning–related meetings. Marking language choice as culturally significant at the governance level initiates a policing effect in management. And as language choice and term sensitivity become an explicit expectation, Mission Integration opens a space for further discussion of motivation and the values that should drive decision making according to the precepts of this (C)atholic organization. This parenthetical *C* in (C)atholic draws attention to the emergence of a particular identity label at CPH that I am arguing draws on both the formal Roman Catholic Church identity and the catholic-as-universal. Together, in the context of the pluralistic demands of the contemporary healthcare environment, the ethos of CPH is neither purely Catholic nor catholic, but (C)atholic. Operations practices are endowed with explicit mission/values dimensions by marking risk management and resource/supply chain management as functions of stewardship as well as the more obvious management of investments. When the vice president presents her quarterly report at the board meeting, it is the "Stewardship Report" that she reads, detailing the state of revenue and expenses from operations and investments.

The struggle for CPH is to resist the tendency for operations managers to simply dress up decision-making processes in the language of Catholic ministry or social teachings. This is a challenge because administrators want to make their projects and decisions appealing to governance— board members who want to be ethically sensitive as well as the sister-sponsors who hold the final say. For example, at an executive meeting, the topic at hand was how to hold executive attention to system dictates, and particularly, whether a traveling in-system, best-practices consulting team would ever be utilized by local facility presidents. Here is an excerpt of the dialogue around the table:

A: What would it look like? How to pay or reward, down at the granular level? Who is our audience?

B: Processwise, yes, but what about the goal? We are "stymied."

C: I question what is appropriate to establish the driver of leadership attention; I want to see 25% of the time, not 5% of time for each president.

D: On the 27th, give the message to the hospital presidents, articulate the expectation. Make it part of the fabric of operations, to make them decide if they need outside help.

B: It's about internalization, yes. So how do we do this?

A: Make the mission–values connection, I say. Frame it as dignity, that'll sell better than the economic perspective.

E: Yes, I agree. Push the connection between HR and mission/values integration.

There is an explicit appeal to mission language as something that allows another goal to be cast in different objectives. Economic motivations are perceived as somehow less palatable than changes set forth as mission values. It is a risk that the language will simply be appropriated without the possibility of achieving actual values inculturation. It bears saying that not all values-driven decisions are easy or painless, just as religion or spirituality in healing is not limited to the warm and joyful dimensions of human experience.

Mission Integration stakeholders hope to ensure that they are engaged in the processes from the ground up, to truly integrate ethics and values into processes well before administrators begin to consider how to market plans to their governing boards. This is where the Mission Integration department as staff is crucial to an ethics of articulation, because they are a part of the daily meetings and routine functions of the system and the hospitals. This is why a chief objective of the Mission standards was to set the expectation for mission leaders to be part of senior management in each facility, and why a new job description and competencies for those positions were circulated to presidents as part of the new standards to which they would be held accountable.

Earlier I suggested that equating corporate rightsizing with an enactment of the core value of stewardship is problematic and unresolved. Some system ethicists would argue that such an equating in fact becomes something else and assert that such executives forget that mission is the original justification for operations and that everything must be interpreted in that light (Panicola, 2002). In CPH, the equation is still heatedly debated at capital allocation meetings and other discussions of the system portfolio. There, a vigorous argument is made that without successful operations, there is no surplus for charity and other mission endeavors. Consequently, facilities that cannot be made revenue positive should be sold. The role of mission integration lies in a process to support the ethical decision making that the system has developed to work through these concerns in an explicit way. Once the decision to sell is made, for example, how will it proceed and what considerations must be made to ensure that the needs of that geography continue to be served?

As the system ethicist for CPH, Marie was a key actor in designing a document that came to be called the CPH "Process for Ethical Decision-making." The Process flowed from "The CPH Statement of Common

Values," which was part of the legal architecture that explicated the relationship of secular community hospitals, providing a nonreligious basis of collaboration to parallel the canonical directives that govern the Catholic hospitals. The Process guidelines offer "a way to explicitly review options in the light of [our Core Values]," asserting, "some decisions clearly touch the heart of what we are about, affect many people and shape our future because of the critical choices that are being considered. In these instances we want to be as clear as possible about our values, our multiple responsibilities and our Mission." The Process clearly invokes a tradition of ethical reflection with a Catholic syntax: "We witness to Mercy and Truth when we pursue integrity of word and action in our life and in our decision-making." It details the pragmatics of a six-step process and timeline for implementation. These elaborate the social hermeneutic of discussion/reflection/discussion to be undertaken by representative parties and delineate how the Process itself may require a series of cycles of implementation before, during, and after decision making is called for. Furthermore, it elaborates on the CPH core values (dignity, collaboration, justice, stewardship, excellence), asking a series of questions concerning how a decision affects quality of care, response to community need, recognition of dignity, rights of all to healthcare, and advocacy of the poor and those with special needs. The document attends to how core values may conflict, which are affirmed, and which denied. Various ethical principles are laid out in the form of illustrative questions to guide rationale and reasoning. The Process explicitly allows for reflective silence, "during which group members can bring all these factors into the light of their religious beliefs, traditions and personal convictions," and then invites individual participants to state their concerns, without discussion, before everyone addresses articulated options as a group.

The guidelines were never intended as a guarantee of an ethical decision; rather, they articulate a procedure designed to elicit a social process of convening, reflection, and discussion among multiple stakeholders from across the system, or hospital, with the explicit intention of bringing system core values directly to bear on a problem facing CPH. The guidelines expressly recognize that such a social process could require multiple cycles to move participants forward. Those stakeholders in the problem, not all senior executives, prepare a summary explanation for review by the senior management team, again at the system or hospital level, as the situation dictates. An example will illustrate how the mission-oriented dimension of the process for ethical decision making aligned with the concerns of operations executives for a centralized system strategy for CPH.

During my fieldwork, healthcare organizations across the state of California were beginning to engage with state and national projections that indicated an enormous shortfall in the nursing workforce needed to provide care into the 21st century (Health Care Advisory Board, 2001). Several hospitals in the CPH system had initiated efforts to address their individual needs, and at least one hospital had already planned to recruit nurses from developing countries for relocation to their service areas.

In February 2002 the system office recognized that individual member hospitals were moving ahead without a systemwide plan; somewhat belatedly, they convened a Foreign Nurse Recruitment Summit. In this forum, consultants reported information from other hospital systems around the country, showing very mixed results, and a team from regional division of CPH showcased its experiences as "lessons learned." Unfortunately, it was clear that go-it-alone initiatives were not consistently successful and the duplication of preparatory work was not cost-efficient. Moreover, as 2002 progressed, several nurse executives expressed concerns voiced by their staffs around the system, raising questions about the ethics of a foreign recruitment strategy (Prystay, 2002). The new relationships with healthcare worker unions contributed to the complexity of the issue for CPH, and the sister-sponsors, particularly those from congregations with histories of Irish nursing in the United States, had made it clear that governance was interested that nursing staffing solutions be in keeping with the system's mission and core values.

Many stakeholders were uncertain about the implications of such a foreign nurse recruitment strategy. They feared that CPH would be ignoring local education needs and job creation opportunities in the United States, encouraging "brain drain" in developing nations, and risking ethnic and racial prejudice, challenges of acculturation, significant financial investment, and perhaps overlooking long-term goals for short-term objectives. In a different vein, system senior management wanted to ensure that CPH would be able to adopt a uniform plan that would best leverage the system's resources as a whole. The sister-sponsors in governance and the system CEO imposed a systemwide freeze on new recruitment efforts abroad. A leadership group of chief nurse executives and business development and strategic planning staff approached Marie for guidance, and the group decided to implement the Process for Ethical

Decision-making to work through their concerns in an ordered and engaged way.

The guidelines and practices that Marie and her colleagues developed go beyond the policing of language that I earlier documented to actually foster social practices of group reflection. Identifying the project as an "ethical" undertaking within the organization seems also to diminish the gatekeeping normally exhibited by functional areas and staff wary of surrendering control over an initiative's direction. In this case, business development, care management, and senior nursing leadership were positioned as coequal collaborators (a CPH core value), where their respective competencies were called on to deliberate over the ethics of a proposed project. Under the cover of "an ethical problem," stakeholders were more disposed to take in broad considerations of the proposed strategy, rather than blindly championing their disciplinary perspective and the needs of their departments. Moreover, during the deliberations that Marie led, the participants were visibly determined to think through the issues and were earnestly conscientious about giving each other time to sit with an objection as well as to raise new angles.

In its ultimate effect, casting the problem as an ethical issue also allowed the system to centralize control of foreign nurse recruitment planning. The usual asides and grumblings of local facility management that "corporate was taking over again" and "no one understands that our local issues are unique" were noticeably absent. In fact, several participants commented informally that they felt the system leadership was taking their fears seriously in providing a forum for a sustained treatment of the issue among colleagues from distant geographies within CPH. The final recommendations to system senior management called for CPH to approach a foreign government directly and to seek formal permission to recruit nurses with the goal of avoiding the exploitation of developing countries. The recommendations also insisted that CPH commit resources to local service area training programs in community colleges to facilitate job creation and longer-term career tracking within the United States.

It seems that people perceive an "ethics problem" to involve determining the good and right action from the wrong. Further, while everyone wants to "be good" and "do the right thing," only Marie is a recognized "expert." As a result, there is little jockeying for control of the process by participants; rather, casting it as an "ethics problem" sets it in a different light, which participants approach differently. The process for ethical decision making creates a space for group process to go beyond the particular goals of an individual department or function to enable multiple facilities to work together as an actual unified system. Ironically, in contrast to their apprehension about reifying a "priestly elite," Mission Integration objectives in the form of the Process of Ethical Decision-making seem to benefit from the "otherness" associated with framing an issue as an "ethics problem."

After my fieldwork had ended, I learned from another staff person of an internal quandary within CPH about advocating against increased development of specialty hospitals with one state legislature, while simultaneously seeking to open one such CPH hospital in another state service area. The ethical decision-making process was again implemented, this time at a higher level of management, highlighting ethical dilemmas between maximizing reimbursement and providing better services for more seriously ill patients. Participants floated a justification about not-for-profit cost shifting that allocated revenue from one source to cover expenses, like charity care or other services oriented toward the poor and the uninsured. The discussion extended beyond the particulars of new services to consider CPH in its larger social role.

Perhaps the most fraught context for engaging seriously with explicit mission and values criteria in system decision making lay in the work of the Capital Allocation Committee. Catherine's involvement with the system office's senior operations team led to the incorporation of particular mission criteria, like service demographics and other annual targets for established levels of charity care and community benefit activities, in the evaluation matrix that the committee used to determine if a hospital would be successful in petitioning the system for access to capital in each quarterly cycle. For the first time, mission criteria formed a formal and necessary condition along with financial performance targets and utilization reviews. Again, as with foreign nurse recruitment, casting a possible operational change as a concern for mission and values enabled system leadership to bring local facilities into line with a centralized plan or strategy, while using a transparent process to allow individual factions and disparate stakeholders to make their case and express their local perspectives.

As the system moved through its operational reforms and management restructuring, system management also began to consider an internal assessment of all forty-plus hospitals. Acknowledging the historical problems of such rapid organizational growth and hospital acquisition strategy, the system management team began to quietly collect data in order to assess the individual hospitals that might be "weak or low performing assets." This internal assessment, alternately called a "portfolio review," had to be carefully presented, not only to allay rumors that would travel across the system generally, but also, specifically, to temper the reaction of sister-sponsors who might respond viscerally to the idea of abandoning a ministry in a particular area (owing to the emotional commitment to a facility that a group of sisters might have managed for over a century, not to mention concerns about the potential unmet needs of the community served by the hospital in question). Underperforming assets more often than not meant exactly those hospitals in depressed areas that lacked an insured, employed population but with plenty of poor and working-poor families who relied on community facilities, both religious and secular, for their healthcare needs.

The application of the process for ethical decision making here suggests what could happen were such a process not explicit within operations. In a national environment predicated on healthcare as commodity acquisition within a framework of for-profit capitalism, it would be easy for the priorities of margin to eclipse mission. Instead, all management decisions that might result in reductions or closures of service lines, never mind whole facilities, must be reviewed against criteria of purpose to ensure that operational decisions are not merely business expedient. It is important to emphasize that the process does not guarantee that the resulting action will not be an identical end, but that the means to that end are consistent with the greater mission and core-values context of the organization. Further, mission and values provide a more neutral ground over which to convene and unify disparate perspectives (the local facilities or functional groups within hospitals) in a way that facilitates central system leadership and oversight. Through these examples, the organizational behavior of CPH demonstrates how margin and mission can be mutually constitutive when Mission Integration Department perspective is engaged with operations.

Translation

In *Writing Culture,* Talal Asad maintains that the "process of cultural translation is inevitably enmeshed in conditions of power" (Asad, 1986,

p. 163). The faith-based hospital organization nonetheless speaks from within a national industry premised on a capitalist, for-profit worldview, no matter how values driven it may be. Within CPH, the role of sister-sponsors in governance—the sister-sponsors who sit above the CEO *and* the board of directors—is to deploy those power relations to set expectations, even if it is countercultural to the rhetoric of the free-market economy in the United States.

Translation is transformation, following Walter Benjamin (Benjamin 1978, p. 325). There is no one-to-one correspondence; the hybrid forms that emerge from translation are subject to reigning dynamics of power, and of inequality. The continuing presence of sister-sponsors in the CPH system complicate the power relations in the simple opposition of margin to mission. Sister-sponsors occupy the highest position of official authority. As one colleague wryly observed of the sister-sponsors, "if there is a buck at CPH, it stops there." CPH had become an operating company undertaking significant steps to centralize control. Consequently, the system that had been nominally Catholic but was, in reality, a diffuse assemblage of different kinds of hospitals sheltering under a Catholic umbrella now finds itself a Catholic hospital system in ways it had not been before. Mission standards reflect a rationalization, but rationalization also confers greater centralization to a system navigating shifting forces of (C)atholic governance.

As Asad suggests, using Christian language has meanings and effects, though they may be indirect or other than intended. For some staff in community hospitals, and even their presidents, Catholic language is threatening. Allegories, allusions, evocative descriptors that would go unremarked upon in a facility with a tradition of religious sponsorship can make people in a secular community facility nervous. I have suggested elsewhere the significance of language labels in the context of hospital facilities with differing histories and identities with regard to chaplaincy versus spiritual care services (Lee, 2002, p. 343). At the traditionally religious Incarnation Hospital, clinical pastoral education is provided through the Chaplaincy Department, while in the traditionally secular community City Physicians' Hospital, clinical pastoral education is based in the new department of Spiritual Care Services. "Chaplaincy" has a specific connotation in the Catholic context. I draw attention to that correlation because my observations occurred at the particular moment when pastoral care provision was extended to a new community partner in a religiously sponsored system. The administrators planning that extension of service were sensitive to cultural nuance and sought to dispel any anxiety at City Physicians' Hospital that "the Catholics were taking over." Consequently, while the clinical pastoral education programs were identical in the services they were to provide at each facility, the distinction in labels revolved around the perceived difference between "religion" as a social organization of belief and practice within a particular faith community (e.g., Roman Catholic, Methodist) and "spirituality," understood here as "the experiential integration of one's life in terms of one's ultimate values and meaning" without the institutional element connoted by "religion" (Lee, p. 343).

Using a theological or religious lexicon is not evangelism or proselytization in the sense of an effort to convert people to allegiance to a doctrinal institution. Rather, that language choice constitutes an explicit attempt to win over a business orientation to an organizational culture that has a particular sense about how people speak and behave, grounded in the belief that daily hospital operations or system office practices should articulate with the collective ethics of the organization, its mission, and its core values. In light of CPH's religious heritage, one might ask whether what I have documented here describes competing values systems or competing truth claims about the world.

How groups, as well as individuals, construct meaning and create relevance in their world, out of a range of life experiences is a central task of critical social analysis (Beckford, 1989, pp. 87–107). Rather than following Parsons's appeal to normative functionalism and systematicity, my analytic method has engaged symbolic processes and social interaction. As sociologist Peter Berger understands it, the creation of meaning ties intentionality to individual action, what he calls externalization, that is, cemented in community through objectivation (sic) in the forms of belief systems, institutions, ideologies, moral codes (Berger, 1967, pp. 8, 11). These social facts come back to the individual via internalization, as standards for discourse, acceptable behavior, and credible explanations of reality (S. K. White, 2000, p. 15). Only the organization of these meanings (as knowledge) and their symbolic counterparts provide "structure," and even then only through intersubjective, collective participation in those symbols (Wuthnow, Hunter, Bergeson, & Kurzweil, 1984, p. 25). Berger avoids the simple structural–functional tautology by always returning to the individual as the site of legitimation. The challenge remains to discern how legitimization for the individual transfers to the organizational level. Documenting the ethico-political constitution of CPH is an attempt to contribute to that analytic challenge within an anthropology of ethical pluralization.

Conclusion

The ethical effect of articulation is an emphasis on the formation of an organizational identity in explicit relation to its origins, social history, and contemporary context. The awareness of the system's Catholic legacy of its founders and governors, and the hospitals they brought to the system, enables CPH to sustain itself as a deliberately ethico-political entity because articulation of those values opens a space for reflection and expectation. There are significant operational implications for such an ethic in light of additional competing values from the non-Catholic worldviews of its secular community partner hospitals and the actual communities that make up the service areas of CPH hospitals. These contributing elements constitute an ethos of pluralization that CPH and its agents navigate to create a living *catholicity* that the sister-sponsors brought into being when CPH moved to incorporate secular community hospitals as full and equal members within a nominally Catholic hospital system. In doing so, CPH transformed traditional doctrinal sponsorship in the course of ethical praxis.

Given the particularity of this hospital system, this analysis has embedded its treatment of ethics and social values in the Catholic context. Mine is not a work of Catholic moral theology. The flexibility of lived experience, which anthropology takes as its object, lies in the fact that there is less need to structure human understanding to the tight logic required of philosophical treatises. Rather, the challenge lies in managing the contingent decisions of daily life. The relevance of the pragmatics of such organizational self-fashioning transcends the limits of what is nominally "religious." A critical engagement with these social actors is crucial to advancing interpretive scholarship of a possibly (post)modern healthcare. Parallel challenges exist in myriad contexts from mapping disease etiology to emerging medical technologies and the perennial demons of rationing and redistribution. Following Wendy Brown and others, static pluralisms—or retreats behind claims of a concretized "culture"—reduce us to petty games of identity politics, whereas dynamic pluralization could instead enrich the ontological dimensions that adhere to lived experience. If the goals of healthcare and medicine are not only epistemic but also aim to address human suffering, then the social practice of ethics is inherently political. As MacIntyre would suggest, *after virtue,* the rethinking of ethics requires incorporating the individual within the collective and its community. Ethical articulation is one such path.

Notes

1. Research was made possible by the Social Science Research Council's Program in Philanthropy and the Non-Profit Sector, with additional support of the National Science Foundation (SDEST #0114083). Writing and analysis of the larger study was made possible by a grant from the Agency for Healthcare Research and Quality (R03 HS11311–01).

2. CPH is a pseudonym. The names of individuals and facilities where research was conducted have been changed to protect those who provide and seek medical care on their premises. Where identifying elements are significant to the analysis, efforts have been made to retain plausibility in the narrative while still protecting individuals and the institutions where they work, per Institutional Review Board (IRB) human subjects protections for qualitative research.

3. I contend that this is a worthwhile move not solely to recognize the emic context but also the etic; the larger work from which this chapter is adapted makes this positioning more explicit. I am grateful for the willingness of my informants to suffer my presence among them and their trust that my analysis was neither apologetics nor diatribe. I recognize, however, that depending on the subject position of the reader, there may be temptation to read this account in such a vein.

4. The following data are adapted from Catholic Health Association Web site, www .chausa.org, reflecting the state of the ministry as reported at the time of fieldwork.

5. There are exceptions to this accountability: one Seattle-based system exists as a public juridical person under canon law and thus reports directly to Rome rather than to any of the dioceses in which its hospitals operate (Bridget Carney, personal communication, 2001, PeaceHealth).

References

Abbott, W. M. (Ed.). (1963). *Documents of Vatican II.* Vatican City, Italy: The America Press.

American Hospital Association Annual Survey. (2002). Retrieved January 2005, from http://www.chausa.org/ABOUTCHA/FACTSHEET.PDF

Anderson, J. W., & Friend, W. B. (Eds.). (1995). *The culture of Bible Belt Catholics.* New York: Paulist Press.

Arendt, H. (1981). *The life of the mind* (One-volume ed.). New York: Harvest/HBJ.

Asad, T. (1986) The concept of cultural translation in British social anthropology In J. Clifford & G. Marcus (Eds.), *Writing culture* (pp. 141–164). Berkeley: University of California Press.

Asad, T. (1992). Religion and politics: An introduction. *Social Research, 59*(2), 3–16.

Asad, T. (1993). *Genealogies of religion.* Baltimore: Johns Hopkins University Press.

Baumgardner, J. (1999, January 25). Immaculate contraception. *The Nation,* 11–15.

Bayley, C. (1995). Our world views (may be) incommensurable: Now what? *Journal of Medicine and Philosophy, 20,* 271–284.

Beckford, J. A. (1989). *Religion and advanced industrial society* (Vol. 23). London: Unwin Hyman.

Benjamin, W. (1978) *Reflections: Essays, aphorisms, autobiographical writings* (E. Jephcott, Trans.) New York: Schocken Books.

Berger, P. L. (1967). *The sacred canopy: Elements of a sociological theory of religion.* Garden City, NY: Doubleday.

Berger, P. L. (1992). Sociology: A disinvitation. *Society, 30*(1), 12–18.

Bernardin, J. C. (1999). *Celebrating the ministry of healing: Joseph Cardinal Bernardin's reflections on healthcare.* St. Louis, MO: Catholic Health Association.

Besecke, K. (2001). Speaking of meaning in modernity: Reflexive spirituality as a cultural resource. *Sociology of Religion, 62*(3), 365–381.

Bolster, M. A. (1990). *Catherine McAuley: Venerable for mercy.* Dublin: Dominican Publishers.

Brown, W. (1992). *States of injury: Power and freedom in late modernity.* Princeton, NJ: Princeton University Press.

Bucar, L. (1998). *When Catholic and non-Catholic hospitals merge: Reproductive health compromised.* Washington, DC: Catholics for a Free Choice.

Buchmueller, T., & Feldstein, P. (1996). Hospital community benefits other than charity care: Implications for tax exemption and public policy. *Hospital and health services administration, 41*(4), 461–471.

Burns, G. (1992). *The frontiers of Catholicism: The politics of ideology in a liberal world* (Vol. 3). Berkeley: University of California Press.

Byrnes, T. A. (1991). *Catholic bishops in American politics.* Princeton, NJ: Princeton University Press.

California Office of Statewide Health Planning and Development. (1999). *Hospital ownership change: Fiscal year 1993–1997.* Sacramento: State of California.

Caterine, D. V. (2001). *Conservative Catholicism and the Carmelites: Identity, ethnicity, and tradition in the modern Church* (Vol. 30). Bloomington: Indiana University Press.

Catholics for a Free Choice. *Catholic healthcare: An introduction to the issues.* Retrieved December 2002, from http://www.catholicsforchoice.org/healthissues.htm

Cheney, G. (1990). *Rhetoric in an organizational society: Managing multiple identities.* Columbia: University of South Carolina Press.

Coffey, A., & Atkinson, P. (1996). *Making sense of qualitative data: Complementary research strategies.* Thousand Oaks, CA: Sage.

Connolly, W. E. (1995). *Ethos of pluralization.* Minneapolis: University of Minnesota Press.

Connolly, W. E. (1999). *Why I am not a secularist.* Minneapolis: University of Minnesota Press.

Connolly, W. E. (2002). *Identity/difference: Democratic negotiations of political paradox* (Expanded ed.). Minneapolis: University of Minnesota Press. (Original work published 1991)

Dillon, M. (1995). Institutional legitimation and abortion: Monitoring the Catholic Church's discourse. *Journal for the Scientific Study of Religion, 34*(2), 141–151.

Dinsmore, C. (1998, July/August). Women's health: A casualty of hospital merger mania. *Ms.,* 17–22.

Douglas, M. (1986). *How institutions think.* Syracuse, NY: Syracuse University Press.

Douglass, R. B., Mara, G. R., & Richardson, H. S. (1990). *Liberalism and the good.* New York: Routledge.

Dreyfus, H., & Rabinow, P. (1983). *Michel Foucault: Beyond structuralism and hermeneutics* (2nd ed.). Chicago: University of Chicago Press.

Fialka, J. J. (2003). *Sisters: Catholic nuns and the making of America.* New York: St. Martin's Press.

Foucault, M. (1994). *The birth of the clinic: An archaeology of medical perception* (A. M. Sheridan Smith, Trans.). New York: Vintage Books. (Original work published 1973)

Francis, E. K. (1964). Toward a typology of religious orders. In L. Schneider (Ed.), *Religion, culture, society: A reader in the sociology of religion* (pp. 517–531). New York: Wiley and Sons.

Gaillardetz, R. (1997). *Teaching with authority: A theology of the magisterium in the Church.* Collegeville, MN: Liturgical Press.

Gallup, G., Jr., & Castelli, J. (1989). *The people's religion: American faith in the nineties.* New York: Macmillan.

Geertz, C. (2000). *The interpretation of cultures.* New York: Basic Books.

Ginsburg, F. D. (1998). *Contested lives: The abortion debate in an American community.* Berkeley: University of California Press.

Gregg, S. (1999). *Challenging the modern world: Karol Wojtyla/John Paul II and the development of Catholic social teaching.* Lanham, MD: Lexington Books.

Hacking, I. (1983). *Representing and intervening: Introductory topics in the philosophy of natural science.* Cambridge, England: Cambridge University Press.

Health Care Advisory Board. (2001). *Competing for talent: Recovering America's hospital workforce.* Washington, DC: The Advisory Board Company.

Heriot, M. J. (1996). Fetal rights vs. the female body: Contested domains. *Medical Anthropology Quarterly, 2*(2), 176–194.

Hooper, J. L. (1986). *The ethics of discourse: The social philosophy of John Courtney Murray.* Washington, DC: Georgetown University Press.

Jay, M. (1998). *Cultural semantics: Keywords of our time.* Amherst: University of Massachusetts Press.

Kauffman, C. (1997). *Ministry and meaning: A religious history of Catholic health care.* New York, NY: Crossroad.

Keane, W. (2002). Sincerity, "modernity," and the Protestants. *Cultural Anthropology, 17*(1), 65–92.

Kennelly, K. (Ed.). (1989). *American Catholic women: A historical explanation.* New York, NY: MacMillan.

Kleinman, A. (1995). *Writing at the margin: Discourse between anthropology and medicine.* Berkeley: University of California Press.

Kvale, S. (1996). *InterViews: An introduction to qualitative research interviewing.* Thousand Oaks, CA: Sage.

Lazarus, E. (1994). What do women want?: Issues of choice, control and class in pregnancy and childbirth. *Medical Anthropology Quarterly, 8*(1), 25–46.

Lee, S. J. C. (2002). In a secular spirit: Strategies of clinical pastoral education. *Health Care Analysis, 10*(4), 339–356.

Lee, S. J. F. C. (2003). *Caritas et communitas: An ethnographic account of the ethics and social values of Catholic healthcare in contemporary California.* Unpublished doctoral dissertation, University of California, San Francisco, with University of California, Berkeley.

Lernoux, P. (1989). *People of God: The struggle for world Catholicism.* New York: Viking.

Luft, H. (1996). Modifying managed competition to address cost and quality. *Health Affairs, 15*(1), 23–38.

MacIntyre, A. (1971). *Against the self-images of the age* (2nd ed.). London: Duckworth.

MacIntyre, A. (1984). *After virtue: A study in moral theory* (2nd ed.). Notre Dame, IN: University of Notre Dame Press.

MacStravic, R. S. (1987). *Marketing religious heath care.* St. Louis, MO: Catholic Health Association.

Mahmood, S. (2001). Feminist theory, embodiment, and the docile agent: Some reflections on the Egyptian Islamic revival. *Cultural Anthropology, 16*(2), 202–236.

Marcus, G. (1998). *Ethnography through thick and thin.* Princeton, NJ: Princeton University Press.

Martin, E. (1987). *The Woman in the body: A cultural analysis of reproduction.* Boston: Beacon Press.

McClellan, M. (1997). Hospital reimbursement incentives: An empirical analysis. *Journal of Economics and Management Strategy, 6*(1), 91–128.

McCormick, R. A. (1984). *Health and medicine in the Catholic tradition: Tradition in transition.* New York: Crossroad.

McKnight, J. L. (1994, January 5). Hospitals and the health of their communities. *Hospitals & Health Networks, 68,* 40–42.

Mensch, E., & Freeman, A. (1993). *The politics of virtue: Is abortion debatable?* Durham, NC: Duke University Press.

Miles, M. B., & Huberman, A. M. (1994). *Qualitative data analysis* (2nd ed.). Newbury Park, CA: Sage.

Muelebach, A. (2001). Making place at the United Nations: Indigenous cultural politics at the UN Working Group on Indigenous Populations. *Cultural Anthropology, 16*(3), 415–448.

National Conference of Catholic Bishops. (1983). *The challenge of peace: God's promise and our response—A pastoral letter on war and peace.* Washington, DC: United States Catholic Conference.

National Conference of Catholic Bishops. (1986). *Economic justice for all: A pastoral letter on Catholic social teaching and the U.S. economy.* Washington, DC: United States Catholic Conference.

Oates, M. J. (1995). *The Catholic philanthropic tradition in America.* Bloomington: Indiana University Press.

Panicola, M. R. (2002, April 29). A cautionary tale: Can Catholic health care maintain its identity and integrity while meeting the challenges of the marketplace? *America: The National Catholic Weekly, 186*(14): 13–15.

Pigg, S. L. (2001). Languages of sex and AIDS in Nepal: Notes on the social production of commensurability. *Cultural Anthropology, 16*(4), 481–541.

Prystay, C. (2002, July 18). U.S. solution is Philippine dilemma as recruiters snap up more nurses, hospitals in Manila are scrambling." *Wall Street Journal.*

Purdy, L. (1996). *Reproducing persons: Issues in feminist bioethics.* Ithaca, NY: Cornell University Press.

Quiñonez, L. A., & Turner, M. D. (1992). *The transformation of American Catholic sisters.* Philadelphia: Temple University Press.

Rabinow, P. (1986). Representations are social facts. In J. Clifford & G. Marcus (Eds.), *Writing culture* (pp. 234–261). Berkeley: University of California Press.

Rabinow, P. (1989). *French modern.* Chicago: University of Chicago Press.

Rabinow, P. (2003). *Anthropos today: Reflections on modern equipment.* Princeton, NJ: Princeton University Press.

Ranke-Heinemann, U. (1990). *Eunuchs for the kingdom of heaven: Women, sexuality, and the Catholic Church* (P. Heinegg, Trans., paperback ed.). New York: Bantam Doubleday.

Redican, G. (1981). *Catholic hospitals: History, development and policy implications.* Unpublished master's thesis, University of Texas at Austin.

Risse, G. (1999). *Mending bodies, saving souls.* Oxford, England: Oxford University Press.

Rosner, D. (1987). *A once charitable enterprise: Hospitals and health care in Brooklyn and New York, 1885–1915* (Paperback ed.). Princeton, NJ: Princeton University Press.

Schlesinger, M., Gray, B., & Bradley, E. (1996). Charity and community: The role of nonprofit ownership in a managed health care system. *Journal of Health Politics, Policy and Law, 21*(4), 697–751.

Scott, C. E. (1996). *On the advantages and disadvantages of ethics and politics.* Bloomington: Indiana University Press.

Shalit, R. (1997, April 28). When we were philosopher kings. *The New Republic, 216,* 24–28.

Silverman, D. (1993). *Interpreting qualitative data: Methods for analysing talk, text, and interaction.* London: Sage.

Silverstein, M. J. (1998). Contemporary transformations of linguistic communities. *Annual Review of Anthropology, 27,* 401–426.

Stewart, P. J., & Strathern, A. (Eds.). (2000). *Identity work: Constructing Pacific lives.* Pittsburgh: University of Pittsburgh Press.

Taylor, C. (1990). *Sources of the self: The making of modern identity.* Cambridge, MA: Harvard University Press.

Uttley, L., & Pawelko, R. (2002). *No strings attached: Public funding of religiously sponsored hospitals in the United States.* New York, NY: MergerWatch

Varacalli, J. A. (1983). *Toward the establishment of liberal Catholicism in America.* Washington, DC: University Press of America.

Walsh, A. D. (2000). *Religion, economics, and public policy: Ironies, tragedies, and absurdities of the contemporary culture wars.* Westport, CT: Praeger.

Weber, M. (1958a). Religious rejections of the world and their directions. In H. H. Gerth & C. W. Mills (Eds.), *From Max Weber: Essays in sociology* (Paperback ed., pp. 323–359). New York: Oxford University Press.

Weber, M. (1958b). The sociology of charismatic authority. In H. H. Gerth & C. W. Mills (Eds.), *From Max Weber: Essays in sociology* (paper ed., pp. 245–252). New York: Oxford University Press.

Whitbeck, C. (1983). Moral implications of recognizing women as people. In W. B. Bondeson, H. T. Engelhardt, S. F. Specker, & D. Windship (Eds.), *Abortion and the state of the fetus.* Dordrecht, Netherlands: Reidel.

White, K. R. (2000). Hospitals sponsored by the Roman Catholic Church: Separate, equal, and distinct? *Milbank Quarterly, 78*(2), 213–239.

White, S. K. (2000). *Sustaining affirmation: The strengths of weak ontology in political theory.* Princeton, NJ: Princeton University Press.

Wilkerson, J., Devers, K., & Given, R. (1996). The emerging competitive managed care marketplace. In J. Wilkerson, K. Devers, & R. Given (Eds.), *Competitive managed care* (pp. 7–10). San Francisco: Jossey-Bass.

Wittberg, P. (1994). *The rise and fall of Catholic religious orders: A social movement perspective.* Albany: State University of New York Press.

Wuthnow, R., Hunter, J. D., Bergeson, A., & Kurzweil, E. (1984). *Cultural analysis: The work of Peter L. Berger, Mary Douglas, Michel Foucault, and Jürgen Habermas.* Boston: Routledge & Kegan Paul.

Yoder, P. S. (1997). Negotiating relevance: Belief, knowledge, and practice in international health projects. *Medical Anthropology Quarterly, 11*(2), 131–146.

Young, G. J., & Desai, K. R. (1999). Nonprofit hospital conversions and community benefits: New evidence from three states. *Health Affairs, 18*(5), 146–155.

Creating Ethical Spaces Within Healthcare Organizations

Lee's study demonstrates how the practice of ethics extends beyond rules and regulations to a way of thinking and acting, not only of individuals, but collaboratively within and between organizations to establish what he refers to as "a new *catholicity*—a model that engages religious legacy and community values, navigating the increasing social pluralization of contemporary society, to reflect truly cultural dimensions of ethical praxis" (p. 69). He points out that this ethical praxis creates a space for ethical decision making to go beyond the particular goals of an individual or an isolated department to enable multiple entities in an organization to work together to support common values. Creating ethical spaces within an organization is essential in order to articulate the organization's values and provide opportunities for reflection and discussion about implementation of these values throughout the organization.

Most research in healthcare ethics has focused on individuals who provide care and the difficult choices they face in providing that care for patients (McCurdy, 2001; Silva, 1998; Taylor, 1999). It is only recently that the focus has turned to ethical concerns that organizations themselves should address, and most of this has been concentrated in healthcare organizations that focus on patients, not educational institutions that prepare healthcare professionals. Thus, it seems appropriate to discuss the characteristics of an ethical organization within the framework of an educational organization such as a school of nursing. It is interesting to consider how preparation of nurses might focus on the value of their work on interdisciplinary care teams as a sort of mission integration agent among other healthcare providers. This is the role chaplains sometimes assume. In the case of nursing, it need not be about extending a religious ethic or a not-for-profit ethic, but a humanistic nursing ethic to other provider disciplines in the common care of patients and the creation of an ethical organization, just like the mission agents in Catholic Pacific Healthsystem sought to enact in their hospitals, foster in their secular partners, and encourage among the business margin–minded.

To prepare future nurses to work effectively and ethically within the complexity of the healthcare system, it seems apparent that nursing education organizations need to consider what constitutes an ethical organization. The following is a true case, with specific information changed to protect confidentiality:

Nancy, a top administrator in a large school of nursing, described a problem she perceived within her organization. Several of the secretarial staff, who were ethnic minorities, had complained that they felt discrimination from nursing faculty. They felt that this involved racial bias and also that they were not treated with respect because of the lower status of their work roles. Nancy carried out some preliminary inquiries to determine the extent of the perceived discrimination and established that the complaints were directed at more than a few faculty members. She consulted with the University Human Resources Department and then brought the problem to light at the next faculty meeting, suggesting that the school might plan a session for staff and faculty to meet together with a facilitator for discussion and planning to address the problem.

After the faculty meeting, several faculty members came to Nancy individually to tell her that they were upset that she brought this problem up at a faculty meeting, especially since there were two students present at the meeting, who they felt should not have heard about the problem. Also, they felt that a joint meeting of faculty and staff would be detrimental and would only escalate the problem. Their advice was for Nancy to meet individually with the "one or two" staff members who had complained. When told that there were significantly more than one or two staff members who had complained, the faculty members expressed disbelief. It was evident to Nancy that she was almost alone among the faculty in the belief that the perceived discrimination was a problem that should be addressed as an organizational issue. This was shocking to her, since she had always believed that her faculty comprised a caring and ethical community of learning.

This true case causes us to consider: How many of us are working in ethical organizations? What is an ethical organization and how do employees build and maintain an ethical organization?

What Is an Ethical Organization?

What does it mean for an organization, as opposed to an individual, to be ethical? We may assume that employees only need to follow the rules and regulations set by the organization, or to act according to their own core values, but this doesn't mean that the organization itself is ethical (McCurdy, 2001). An ethical organization has a philosophy based on a value system that can be articulated to its employees. It strives to balance diverse needs of all employees, is committed to learning, fairness, and equity, supports morally courageous leadership, and communicates and models its core values. The organization fosters mutual trust and respect among members and maintains these values in interactions with other organizations.

It is important to recognize that although organizations reflect the values of society, they have unique cultures of their own that guide the activities of the organization and its members. Organizations consist of highly interdependent relationships in which not only individuals, but also groups influence each other in many ways (McCurdy, 2001). Creation of an ethical culture must provide for open communication systems among both individuals and groups to ensure a forum for open discussion of "gray areas" that relate to ethical concerns. Each individual member must understand organizational expectations and his/her role in forwarding the goals and upholding the values of the organization.

Lee's study identified the impact that language within an organization can have on communication of values. He noted that the resurgence in the language of healing and caring (as opposed to scientific or technical vocabularies) communicated values of Catholic Pacific Healthsystem. He points out that language choice represents how values are set and makes the mission explicit. This observation can also be applied to educational organizations such as schools of nursing. Nancy said that she had observed some of her colleagues referring to students as "kids," telling them that they did not "think critically." She learned that some students had been reprimanded in front of other nurses in the clinical area. One faculty member even yelled at the students. Obviously, such situations may cause students to doubt whether they are valued or respected. One student told Nancy, "I am trying so hard, and nothing I do satisfies her. I can't stand being yelled at anymore." What does the language of faculty communicate to students about the values and the mission of the organization? When students talk about the fact that faculty want to get rid of them, does this reflect the mission of the organization?

Lee notes also that language can be a tool to reconfigure social position and that his ability to "toss about the language of managed care contracting and the economics of physician reimbursement and banter about 'DRG creep' and the significance of Medicare waivers" mattered to the field informants in operations and administration with which he interacted for his study (p. 109). This insider knowledge of the language can also work to the detriment of employees in an organization. In the case presented here, one secretary told Nancy about a faculty member who asked her to type a handout for a pathophysiology course and then after a few minutes of frustrated explanation said, "Oh, never mind. You obviously don't understand the language. I'll just type it myself." The language that faculty members use in their interaction with both staff and students reflects their own values and, by extension, the values of the organization. As observed in Lee's study, language both in policy and in procedure constructs the representation by which the public identity of the organization is presented (p. 107).

How does one identify problems that an ethical organization should address? Bruhn (2004) notes that organizations tend to act like individuals with bad habits. It is often only after a diagnosis of lung cancer that a smoker quits smoking. It is similar with organizations. There are warnings about the behavior of organizations and their members, just as there are about the consequences of smoking, but too often people ignore them. Some warning signs that an ethical culture may be lacking in an educational organization may be expressions by employees of feeling unappreciated and assertions of scapegoating, abdication of responsibility, guarding turf, abuse of power and privilege, and disengagement as well as frequent turnover and poor satisfaction ratings on surveys.

An ethical working environment is the result of ethical leadership supported by ethical systems. Petrick and Quinn (1997) paraphrase Socrates's famous line, suggesting that, "Just as the unexamined personal life is not worth living, the unexamined work life is not worth working" (p. xi). As educational healthcare organizations struggle to grow, it is imperative that they examine the work environment and identify measures to build and maintain ethical organizations to meet the increased demand for practitioners, shorten their preparation time, and establish increasingly complex community partnerships.

Building and Maintaining an Ethical Organization

Potter (1996) defines organizational ethics as "the intentional use of values to guide the decisions of a system" (p. 4). Silva (1998) notes that in any attempt to change the values of an organization, the existing organizational culture must be dealt with directly. Although the organization's leadership is important, it is not enough. The most prevalent sources of ethical action are the everyday actions of members, which although seemingly of minimal consequence, build to create the ethical culture (Taft, 2000).

One approach to enhance efforts to build an ethical culture is for the organization to develop its own code of conduct. One study found that 92% of 169 major companies surveyed (two-thirds of which were Forbes 500 companies) had a formal code of ethics (Murphy, 2003). It is not enough, however, for organizations to adopt codes; they also must outline specific processes for addressing ethical issues. Members of organizations want and need clear definitions of what is expected of them. In Lee's study, the tactics of mission integration sought to tie values to hospital operations in order to diffuse ethical practice across the system and make ethical reflection part of organizational identity beyond a formal code. As Lee argues, the "Process for Ethical Decision-making" at Catholic Pacific Healthsystem offers one model for institutionalizing ethical reflection and practice in a social process.

What can be done about unethical organizational cultures? First, it is important to conduct a formal assessment to clarify and articulate the organization's values and link them to the mission and vision. Once the analysis is complete, the institution must focus on building a solid ethics infrastructure that permeates all aspects of the institution, including an effective communication system, appropriate education, and creation of structures to encourage and monitor ethical practices (Silva, 1998).

A survey of 2,000 members of the American Organization of Nurse Executives identified questions that nurse executives might ask to address key ethical problems in their organization (Cooper, Frank, Hansen, & Gouty, 2004). These questions emphasized that employees may incur personal risk in addressing ethical issues within an organization. Instances of "whistleblowing" have occurred when employees have found no satisfactory procedures in place within the organization to address serious concerns and have therefore taken their story to the media. Whistleblowing, however, suggests an ethical failure at the organizational level and should not occur if there are effective internal procedures in place (Fletcher, Sorrell, & Silva, 1998). In an educational organization such as a school of nursing, faculty without tenure may be at risk for raising ethical concerns. Organizations must create a culture in which all members are valued and have a sustained voice in shaping institutional policies. To accomplish this, there must be mechanisms in place for members to be heard by decision makers at all levels in the organization (Cooper, Frank, Hansen, & Gouty, 2004).

An Ethics of Articulation in Healthcare Organizations

Sister Carol Taylor, Director of the Center for Clinical Bioethics at Georgetown University, asserts that to establish an integrity-based organizational ethics program, the organization must be able to articulate its intentional use of values that are linked to its conception of the good (Taylor, 2000). She notes that as a leader, one needs to find a critical distance to step back and see what needs to be done. The integrity-based strategy is characterized by a conception of ethics as a driving force of an enterprise. Ethical values shape the search for opportunities, the design of organizational systems, and the decision-making processes used by individuals and groups. They provide a common frame of reference and serve as a unifying force within the organization.

Too often persons in healthcare leadership positions tend to micromanage or ignore ethical issues or allow legal concerns to override ethical decisions. When executives micromanage, they may be unable to see their organization as a whole. It is the responsibility of all members of the organization, however, to maintain an ethical climate in the workplace. The decline of collective responsibility and civic engagement has resulted in an unwillingness of people to make moral claims on one another and, thus, reluctance to express their convictions when someone does something that is wrong (Bruhn, 2004).

As noted in Lee's study, it was the practice at Catholic Pacific Healthsystem for an individual to read a "reflection" before a meeting that called committee members to the task at hand in the context of an organization founded on religious values that were directly related to the organizational mission (p. 110). If schools of nursing adopted this practice at faculty meetings, how might it affect the articulation of values within the organization? If Nancy had read a reflection at the faculty meeting about the secretaries' feelings of disempowerment, would faculty have been more receptive to her concern? Organizations need to explore creative ways to open dialogue among employees to address ethical concerns.

Lee's study is about "corporate citizenship, not in the sense of a hospital as a business entity, but corporate in the sense of a collective subject acting in the social world" (p. 75). His analysis asks, are Catholic healthcare practices distinctive? What can non-Catholic healthcare organizations learn from this study? In the case of Catholic Pacific Healthsystem, the organization's Catholic legacy offered a model for ethical praxis in both the Catholic and secular facilities, building on common ground as not-for-profit providers. As Lee documents in the interplay between system and local facilities, one important consideration is the need to listen to voices at all levels within the workplace. Members of an organization may unwittingly dominate through privileged position, class, ethnicity, age, or gender. Subtle oppression may operate at the edge of awareness, where it is easy to ignore. In an effort to keep up with the many demands in the workplace, we may find ourselves in a condition that Fiumara (1990) calls "benumbment" (p. 84), feeling too busy to listen. Creating ethical spaces within an organization provides for listening to voices too often silent and provides an essential articulation of the organization's values.

References

Bruhn, J. (2004). The ethic of "The Organizational Good": Is doing the right thing enough? *The Health Care Manager, 23*(1), 4–10.

Cooper, W., Frank, G. L., Hansen, M. M., & Gouty, C. A. (2004). Key ethical issues encountered in healthcare organizations: The perceptions of staff nurses and nurse leaders. *Journal of Nursing Administration, 34*(3), 149–156.

Fiumara, G. C. (1990). *The other side of language: A philosophy of listening.* New York: Routledge.

Fletcher, J. J., Sorrell, J. M., Silva, M. C. (1998). Whistleblowing as a failure of organizational ethics. *Online Journal of Issues in Nursing.* Retrieved November 5, 2005, from http://www.nursingworld.org/ojin/topic8/topic8_3.htm

McCurdy, D. B. (2001). Creating an ethical organization. In M. B. Holstein, M. Mitzen, & P. B. Mitzen (Eds.). *Ethics in community-based elder care.* New York: Springer.

Murphy, P. E. (2003). *Trend in ethics codes: Addressing both compliance and values.* Presented at the Southern Institute for Business and Professional Ethics 2003 seminar, "Building a better code of ethics." Retrieved January 2005, from http://www.southern institute.org/Resources-GoodBusiness-Content(26).htm

Petrick, J. A., & Quinn, J. F. (1997). Management ethics: Integrity at work. Newbury Park, CA: Sage.

Potter, R. L. (1996). From clinical ethics to organizational ethics: The second stage of the evolution of bioethics. *Bioethics Forum, 12*(2), 3–12.

Silva, M. C. (1998). Organizational and administrative ethics in health care: An ethics gap. *Online Journal of Issues in Nursing.* Retrieved November 5, 2005.http://www.nursingworld.org/ojin/topic8/topic8_1.htm.

Taft, S. H. (2000): An inclusive look at the domain of ethics and its application to administrative behavior. *Online Journal of Issues in Nursing.* Retrieved November 5, 2005, from http://www.nursingworld.org/ojin/topic8/topic8_6.htm.

Taylor, C. (1999). National Conference on Managing Health Care Costs Challenges to Ethics and Quality. Arlington, VA. Retrieved January 2005, from http:www.marymount.edu/ethics/proceedings/12.html.

Taylor, C. (2000, April 4). *Organizational ethics and advanced practice nursing.* Presentation to Advanced Clinical Nursing class, College of Nursing and Health Science, George Mason University.

4

Teleology, the Modern Moral Dichotomy, and Postmodern Bioethics in the 21st Century

JOHN PAUL SLOSAR

It could be suggested that the turn of the 21st century, the beginning of the new millennium, would have been a fitting occasion by which to mark the beginning of the postmodern era of bioethics. In its current form, bioethics began as a critique of traditional medical ethics conceived as the customary practices of physicians rooted in the Hippocratic tradition. Medical ethics in this previous form survived for more than two millennia until only a few decades ago, when intellectuals and academics outside of medicine began to critique some of its central moral tenets. The majority of these thinkers were philosophers and theologians who critically examined the moral character of the medical profession as manifested in the creeds recited at medical school graduations and adhered to by physicians dogmatically, if not unconsciously, in their noble efforts (Jonsen, 1998, pp. 23–24). These critiques reflected diverse moral perspectives that previously had been considered as having little relevance to the practice of medicine. These moral perspectives, which have begun to reshape the moral character of medicine, are largely influenced by modern moral theory.

The way in which modern moral theory has begun to reshape the moral character of medicine can be illustrated by considering a case and the commentaries of two bioethicists:

At age seventy, Mrs. R. had become severely disabled by cardiac failure due to a damaged mitral valve. In an attempt to restore her quality of life to what it was prior to the cardiac failure, she underwent valve replacement surgery. Twelve hours after the surgery, however, her cardiac output began to drop and became insufficient. Despite attempts employing a variety of means, treatment in the ICU did not restore her cardiac output to a sustainable level. With appropriate informed consent, Mrs. R. had an experimental cardiac assist device implanted in her chest. A few hours after this surgery, her cardiac output began to fall again. Though she was on a respirator and receiving fluids, everyone involved in her treatment agreed that Mrs. R. would not survive through the night. Since Mrs. R. was conscious and vaguely alert, her physician treated her for pain with morphine (with consent again). After turning off the respirator and cardiac assist device, her physician gave her another dose of morphine. When Mrs. R. continued to show signs of pain and discomfort, jerking at intervals and furrowing her brow, her physician had the nurse draw up 10 cc of potassium chloride and, with the consent of the family, injected it into her intravenous line. Within minutes, Mrs. R. lay still and the cardiac monitor showed no heartbeat. (Adapted from Levine, 1989, pp. 144–145)

In providing moral analysis of this case, two bioethicists arrive at conflicting conclusions. One morally vindicates the physician's actions, while the other condemns them. According to the former, "My opinion is that [the doctor] did nothing morally wrong. . . . Upon determining . . . that further interventions were turning futile and useless, [the doctor] did the humane thing. He provided a quick, painless death, a good death." (Levine, 1989, p. 145). According to the other commentator, the physician's actions cannot be justified because the physician acted to end the patient's life despite the medical profession's code of ethics, civil law, and the duty to "cherish" life (p. 145).

The commentator who vindicates the physician saw nothing morally wrong with the physician's actions because, in this case, that commentator places the emphasis of moral evaluation on pragmatic results. From this perspective, the moral value of an action is determined by its resulting state of affairs, and the physician's action was perceived to have a good outcome, namely, a quick and painless death, "a good death." On the other hand, the commentator who condemns the action of the physician places the primary emphasis of moral evaluation on principles of moral obligation as rooted in the customs of the profession, the laws of society, and any intrinsic value of human life. From this perspective, adherence to these constraints on human action takes priority over the outcome or result of the act as the basis for moral evaluation. These moral views constitute a common polarity found in the acculturated moral reasoning of contemporary society. On one hand, people seem to act based on the choices they think will result in the most good. On the other hand, people also seem to do that which they think is the right thing to do, no matter what the outcome might be. Some people may recognize the moral significance of both results and principles, but place more emphasis on one rather than the other (Kavanaugh, 2001, pp. 73–77). While these observations provide some insight into everyday moral reasoning, they also reflect the nature and character of modern moral theory.

The Modern Moral Dichotomy and Bioethics

Modern moral theory has been dominated by a conception of ethics as the intellectual search for a single, monistic, rule-governed procedure of decision making that is applicable to all moral problems. The predominant theories have generally been either consequence based or duty based in nature. Accompanying this dominance has been the idea that all cognitivist ethical theories that employ rules derived from more fundamental principles can be classified as either consequentialist or deontological. Consequentialist theories, such as utilitarianism, posit the nature of an action's moral value to be its consequences, that is, its resulting state of affairs. As Samuel Scheffler describes it in *Consequentialism and Its Critics,* "Consequentialism in its purest and simplest form is a moral doctrine which says that the right act in any given situation is the one that will produce the best overall outcome, as judged from an impersonal standpoint which gives equal weight to the interests of everyone" (1988, p. 2). Accordingly, an action is judged as right or wrong in proportion to the degree its consequence(s) promote some version of the principle of the good. In its most general form, the principle of the good states that those actions that are morally valuable and therefore ought to be pursued are those that maximize good consequences.

In contrast, deontological theories such as Kantian ethics posit the nature of moral value to be the conformity of an agent's will or motive and its resulting action with some duty or rule of right action. In this framework, any considerations regarding consequences are irrelevant insofar as moral value is seen as inherently tied to some set of duties or rules of right action (Broad, 1930, p. 207). The source of these duties or rules of right action will differ according to different types of deontological theories, but the determinant of moral value is always the adherence to some form of moral law, duty, or rule. Deontological theories place the emphasis of moral evaluation on some principle of right action rather than on a principle of the good. In their most general form, principles of right action state that actions are morally valuable insofar as they and their motives are in accordance with some moral law, obligation, or duty that is defined independently of any considerations regarding an action's consequences.

It should be noted that, as conceived in this way, the principle of the good and the principle of the right are formal principles. The principle of the good obliges one to maximize good consequences, but the principle itself does not specify what constitutes good consequences. In fact, there are many different competing conceptions of what constitutes those good consequences that ought to be maximized, for example, the happiness principle, preference satisfaction, and utility maximization, to name only a few. So, too, while the principle of the right obliges one to act in accordance with some duty, rule, or law, the principle itself does not say of what this duty consists nor exactly what type of action it entails. As such, these principles are intended as generalizable and universal maxims that provide a foundation from which action-guiding moral rules can be derived once the substantive content of the principles has been specified.

The underlying assumption of this modern conception of ethics is that there is a single source of moral value that can be fully specified by one supreme principle. Indeed, the central task of modern moral theory has been the justification of a single theory that makes either some version of the principle of the good or some version of the principle of the right always and everywhere, in every circumstance, normatively fundamental. Traditionally, this supreme principle has been conceived either as some variant of the principle of the good, understood in consequentialist terms, or as some deontological principle of right action. While some modern moral theorists refer to all ends-centered theories as "teleological," they are most often talking about ends-centered theories that posit the state of affairs resulting from an action as the determinant of that action's moral status. This equivocation has led to the widespread misconception that all teleological theories are fundamentally consequentialist (Broad, 1930, pp. 206–207; Frankena, 1973, p. 14). The view that all cognitivist, principle-based ethical theories can be classified as either deontological or consequentialist and the propensity to give either the principle of the right or the principle of the good fundamental normative status is what I refer to as "the modern moral dichotomy." This modern moral dichotomy has for the most part persisted in contemporary moral theory and has had significant influence on the development of bioethics.

A significant problem with the modern moral dichotomy and its underlying conception of moral theory as monistic is that the sources of moral value are actually heterogeneous (Nagel, 1979, p. 134). This heterogeneity of moral value implies that which principle really is most fundamental in the concrete circumstances of a particular decision to act is dependent, at least partially, on the situational particulars of those circumstances. The subsequent implication is that monistic theories, unless restricted to one particular type of decision making narrowly construed, are inadequate for mediating conflicts between the principles of the good and the right and their derivative rules. Such conflicts often arise when considerations of consequences and of duties compete for the attention of our moral sensibilities, as in the case described above. This conflict between the principles and their derivative rules often gives rise to a plurality of good reasons that justify incompatible actions. In such cases, an agent may also be faced with a decision that will necessarily violate either the principle of the good or the principle of the right. Such conflict cannot be adjudicated by appealing to a higher order principle, since the good and the right are principles of the highest order within this conception of ethics.

Within bioethics, the modern moral dichotomy manifests itself in two ways. The first way is that the principles of the good and the right often conflict with one another in the different circumstances in which morally perplexing healthcare decisions must be made. Such conflict occurs at both the individual and societal levels of decision making in bioethics. At the individual level, tension between the two principles arises in the clinical context of the physician–patient relationship. The very goal of the clinical encounter is to bring about the best possible outcome for each particular patient. Yet physicians and other care providers engage the patient within a labyrinth of diverse value perspectives, professional codes of ethics, institutional-specific policies, state and federal regulations, and a tort system of liability. These elements of the practice of medicine combine to constitute a variety of deontological constraints that must be taken into consideration as physicians strive to bring about the best possible outcomes for their patients (Veatch, 2000, pp. 709–718). At the societal level, conflict between the principles arises because of prior and unresolved tension within the more general moral theories applied to particular problems. For example, such conflict manifests itself in the divergent views regarding social policies addressing such issues as the legality of abortion and public funding for human embryonic stem cell research.

The second way the modern moral dichotomy manifests itself in bioethics is in the influence it has had on the development of some of the more predominant theories of bioethics. Some of these theories have been developed, in part, as a response to some inadequacies of the monistic and deductive dimensions of modern moral theory. For example, Tom Beauchamp and James Childress have argued that deductive moral theories rely on an oversimplified conception of moral reasoning that cannot sufficiently capture the complexity required by difficult cases, that they fail to acknowledge the heterogeneity of moral value and the way in which competing principles must be balanced in individual cases, and that such theories cannot account for the fact of moral pluralism and incommensurable conceptions of the good life (1994, p. 13). In response to these inadequacies, the more predominant theories of bioethics have purposely avoided the search for moral truth. In place of any objective moral reality, these theories rely on either an inductive or a coherentist method of justification independent of any comprehensive theory of moral value. In either case, the result is an approach to bioethics that is thoroughly relativistic. A third, also predominant, alternative has been to abandon altogether the idea that reason can justify any moral propositions and assert the principle of permission as the only possible foundation for bioethics. Ultimately, we are left with a thoroughly subjective view of morality in which bioethics is simply a tool for analyzing competing but irreducible moral claims—a kind of map for illustrating how certain starting points lead to corresponding conclusions that hold no moral relevance for those who disagree on the starting points (Engelhardt, 2004, p. 10).

If the search for moral truth is not an essential part of bioethics, then any guidance bioethics has to offer will be only a matter of social custom at best or arbitrary at worst. But where should those who want substantive normative guidance from bioethics turn in the postmodern world? If one turns to modern moral theory, then one gains the objectivity of a deductive method of justification but is left with the seemingly irresolvable conflict between the fundamental principles of the right and the good. If one turns to the postmodern approach, then one simply finds a method of peaceful conflict resolution with very few, if any, substantive normative constraints. What seems to be needed is some method that shares the strengths of modern moral theory and those methods of bioethics that were developed in response to its weaknesses. Such an alternative would have to rest upon a stable foundation and have sufficient normative strength to avoid the tendency to relativism, but it would also have to transcend the pitfalls of the modern moral dichotomy. The central thesis herein is that a contemporary appreciation of Aristotle's teleological approach to ethics, conceived as distinct from modern moral theory per se, offers such an alternative and could be useful for addressing current and emerging issues of bioethics in the 21st century.

The Nature of Modern Moral Theory

Consequentialism and deontology are two distinctly modern frameworks of moral philosophy. As such, they share a common methodological nature. In this common nature, ethics is approached as a systematic study that will bring about the philosophical illumination of universal practical principles that, once discerned, provide the basis for the norms of human action. The underlying assumption is that there is a single source of moral value that can be fully specified by one supreme principle and that moral judgment consists in the intellectual application of rules derived from such a principle. Once this supreme principle has been articulated, all other moral principles are assigned normative significance only insofar as they are derivative of the supreme principle. The formulation and justification of such principles rely primarily on abstract, philosophical reasoning. Their nature, their form, and their authority rest on corresponding arguments that justify them.

Within this framework, the *praxis* of ethics has become a primarily intellectual endeavor in which moral judgment consists in the application of normative rules within the concrete particulars of a given situation. The goal of modern moral theory in general has been to derive an explicit procedure of rule-governed decision making (Larmore, 1987, p. 4). Ethical theories that rely on general principles and their derivative rules, together with an appropriate appreciation of the relevant facts of a given situation to justify particular moral judgments, are known as deductivist or top-down theories. Utilitarianism and Kantianism are paradigms of this modern conception of normative moral theory.

The paradigmatic status of Kant's ethics and utilitarianism is not an accident of modernity. Rather, it rests on explicit and critical philosophical inquiry regarding the nature of moral value and human reason. In the *Groundwork of the Metaphysics of Morals,* for example, Kant argues that the only thing that can be good without qualification, independently of any empirical contingencies, is a good will. As he argues, the goodness of the will is not dependent upon the results it is successful in attaining, but only in what it wills to be attained (Kant, 1785/1996, p. 62). As Kant further argues, a good will is one that wills that which is in accordance with the moral law, a law that pure practical reason determines and dictates for itself. According to Kant, if moral law is to be binding, then it must apply universally and unconditionally. Thus, moral value can be found only in the a priori fitness of one's maxims. One's maxims, then, are to be tested against the categorical imperative for universality. In its simplest form, the categorical imperative dictates: act only on that maxim which you can at the same time will that it become universal law (1785/1996, p. 73). In other words, according to the categorical imperative, one ought to do only those actions that follow from a principle or rule of right action that one could will all people to use as the basis of their actions in similar circumstances. According to Kant, pure practical reason has the function of testing one's maxims and is itself the source of the moral law.

This procedure of testing one's maxims is the Kantian way of judging whether or not an action is morally right. That one's maxims accord with the categorical imperative is also a necessary though not sufficient condition of a good will. If one's will is to be morally good, it must additionally meet the condition of acting out of reverence for the moral law. This criterion is articulated in the principle Kant calls "the universal ethical principle": act in conformity with duty from duty (1785/1996, p. 522). A good will, then, is one that acts both in accordance with the moral law and for the sake of the moral law, and moral value can only be attributed to those actions that are consistent with Kant's formulation of the principle of the right: namely, the categorical imperative. In this way, moral goodness is in Kant's view derivative of the principle of right.

The guiding notion of Kant's procedure is that moral value is singularly located in the exercise of pure practical reason. The principles of pure practical reason are intended to be sufficient to determine, through a rule-governed process, how and what ought to be done within the particular circumstances of an action. While this rule-governed process involves several formulations of the categorical imperative, these are only various formulations of a single moral principle. As Kant writes with regard to the three formulations of the categorical imperative, "the [above] three ways of representing the principle of morality are at bottom only so many formulae of the very same law, and any one of them of itself unites the other two in it" (1785/1996, p. 85). These principles do not reflect multiple sources of value but only one fundamental source, namely, pure practical reason. This monistic conception of value is at the heart of the Kantian project and illustrates the modern view of moral judgment as consisting in the intellectual application of rules derived from a fundamental normative principle intended to specify the sole source of moral value.

The theory of act utilitarianism, particularly as conceived by John Stuart Mill (1859/1987), also exemplifies this modern emphasis on the theoretical formulation of general principles and the intellectual application of rules derived from such principles. For utilitarianism, however, the principle that specifies moral value is not concerned with the agent's a priori will but with the distribution of the effect of the consequence(s). Within this perspective, the maximization of the net balance of aggregate happiness is the fundamental source of moral value. The guiding norm is "the happiness principle": it is always right to do that action which maximizes the greatest overall happiness as judged from an impersonal standpoint. Accordingly, moral judgment consists in making calculations based on the commensurability of values as required by the happiness principle.

Within this perspective, the claim that the happiness principle is the fundamental moral norm is determined and justified through philosophical inquiry independently of the situational particulars of action. While the situational particulars will influence one's decision of what should be done in order to satisfy the happiness principle, *that* one should satisfy the happiness principle is determined prior to considerations of the circumstances in which the action is to be performed. In other words, the utilitarian regards moral judgment as the assessment of the capacity of specific actions to promote the happiness principle, which is the only rationally acceptable value according to the utilitarian view (Clarke and Simpson, 1989, p. 4). The implication is that the happiness principle is the only possible source of moral value whatever the circumstances of action might be. The main task of utilitarian ethics has been the search for, and development of, a universal calculus of satisfactions (Nussbaum, 1993, p. 242).

Whereas for Kantian ethics proper moral judgment depends on the cognitive recognition of universal maxims that constrain one's a priori will, such judgment for the utilitarian depends on calculating and weighing the value of particular consequences within a given situation. While dichotomously opposed in this manner, both procedures are intended to ensure proper moral response to situational particulars through the intellectual application of decision making rules. Within this framework, the less general of these rules are derived from more general ones, which in turn rest on a single, fundamental principle intended to specify the nature of moral value. Thus, the shared tendency of Kantianism and utilitarianism is to posit one principle, formally the principle of the right or the principle of the good (respectively), as ultimately fundamental.

This shared tendency has given rise to a widely accepted contemporary classification of top-down moral theories as either deontological or teleological (in the consequentialist sense). This twofold classification is what John Finnis has referred to as "the grand modern bifurcation of ethics into 'teleological' and 'deontological': the ethics of ends and the ethics of duty" (1983, p. 84). Most recently, the perpetuation of this division within contemporary moral theory can be largely attributed to John Rawls and his view concerning the status of the principles of the good and the right in ethics:

The two main concepts of ethics are those of the right and the good; the concept of a morally worthy person is, I believe, derived from them. The structure of an ethical theory is, then, largely determined by how it defines and connects these two basic notions. Now it seems that the simplest way of relating them is taken by teleological theories: the good is defined independently from the right, and then the right is defined as that which maximizes the good. (1971, p. 24)

According to this classification, all teleological theories are consequentialist, since right action is defined as that which maximizes an independently defined good. Thus, the division is between theories that make consequences and those that make duties the most basic moral concepts. Essentially, then, moral value from the modern perspective can be realized only in actions that either result in a good state of affairs or those that accord with rule-based obligations. All other moral concepts must be conceived of in terms of the relationship assigned to the principles of the good and the right. Thus comes what I refer to as "the modern moral dichotomy."

This twofold division has been the subject of some criticism, which holds that some reasonable moral theories, including Platonic, Thomistic, and Aristotelian ethics, make neither consequences nor duties their most basic moral concepts (Finnis, 1983, p. 84). The modern conception of deductive ethics has come under attack by contemporary thinkers for another reason as well. This line of criticism focuses on the modern conception of ethics as a monistic, principle-based process of rule-governed decision making. As Charles Larmore has argued, the modern conception of moral judgment as the mere application of rules is too simplistic, with regard to some duties, to account for its true function. According to Larmore's account, the way in which some obligations are to be fulfilled cannot always be specified by means of a given rule. In Larmore's words, "moral duties like courage, generosity, and benevolence are duties whose rules appear too schematic to settle by themselves when those duties are incumbent upon us and how they are (in a moral sense) correctly to be carried out" (1987, p. 6). The underlying idea is that, even when a practical principle specifies the relevant moral value, the way in which some obligations are to be met and to what extent those obligations are binding are *further* dependent on the situational particulars and one's understanding of the relationship between those particulars and the principle itself.

In some cases, then, the derivative rules of a practical principle will be insufficient to determine the appropriate manner in which an action is to be performed and the extent to which specific obligations are binding. At some point, moral judgment must consist in the ability to go beyond what principles alone can tell us about duties (Larmore, 1987, p. 9). To put it another way, a principle may specify a relevant source of value, but deciding how to fulfill the conditions of that principle in action is not always a rule-governed process. The circumstances of a given situation sometimes require the exercise of a more complex form of moral judgment. Still, it could be objected that even a utilitarian or Kantian would admit that a more complex form of judgment is necessary for the application of the principle they posit as normatively fundamental. However, the point is not that the utilitarian or Kantian would deny this claim but that these views by their very nature do not accord a sufficient normative role to an adequately complex conception of moral judgment.

Another concern with monistic, rule-governed theories is that they fail to acknowledge the possibility that two principles could justify contrary choices of actions with no rule-governed basis for resolving the conflict (Hampshire, 1983, p. 155). So long as any rule-governed decision procedure is posited, so is an ideal solution to any moral problem (Urmson, 1975, p. 118). From the monistic perspective, all conflicts can be resolved by simply giving normative considerations of some values and principles a derivative status to some other, more fundamental principle. Thus, monistic theories assume that all moral values are reducible to a single unified source. In contrast, Thomas Nagel argues that irreducible moral conflicts are an undeniable reality of human life because moral values are fundamentally heterogeneous and not all values represent the pursuit of a single good. The possibility of different but equally valid reasons for valuing an action is what Nagel refers to as the "fragmentation of value." This fragmentation arises out of the complex nature of human beings and corresponds to different types of moral reasoning, such as reasoning from an outcome or agent-centered perspective (Nagel, 1979, pp. 132–134). More simply, reasons for valuing certain actions can be formally different but equally valid from different moral perspectives.

The implication of this fragmentation of moral value is twofold. First, it gives rise to a plurality of incommensurable moral values and incommensurable conceptions of the good life. In other words, the fragmentation of moral values is one reason moral pluralism exists in the first place. The fact of moral pluralism presents challenges to the modern conception of moral theory insofar as it posits both a variety of different but equally valid conceptions of moral value and different conceptions of moral rationality (MacIntyre, 1988). That moral pluralism entails different conceptions of rationality is precisely what gives rise to different but equally valid visions of the nature of moral value itself. These competing visions are each valid when considered within particular frameworks of rationality that posit unique standards that act as the ultimate moral criterion by which to evaluate competing moral visions, for example, feminist, critical theory, and deconstructionist conceptions of rationality. Accordingly, this fact of pluralism leaves us with no readily apparent way to choose between competing accounts of morality.

The second implication of the fragmentation of moral value is that moral value itself cannot be reduced to one fundamental basis nor specified by a single principle. This heterogeneous nature of moral value creates a significant problem within the dichotomous framework of modern moral theory. If two conflicting principles are those intended to specify a fundamental source of value, the conflict cannot be adjudicated by appealing to a higher order principle (insofar as the right and the good are principles of the highest order within this conception of ethics). For example, if Kantian universality and the maximization of the greatest good both represent valid reasons for favoring different actions in the same circumstances, further appeals to the theories themselves will do little to aid our decision of what to do. If such fundamental disagreements are to be settled, then it will have to be from a perspective that is neither primarily Kantian nor primarily utilitarian, neither primarily deontological nor primarily consequentialist.

The Contemporary Response and Bioethics at the Close of the 20th Century

For some moral theorists, the unavoidable recognition of these implications of the fragmented nature of moral value, among other historical and philosophical considerations, are indicative of a definitive failure of the "Enlightenment project." Contemporary moral theories, postmodern or otherwise, can to a large degree be characterized as a response to the heterogeneous nature of moral value and the fact of moral pluralism. John Rawls, for example, recognizes the problem of conflict between fundamental principles, which he refers to as "the priority problem," and tries to develop his theory of political justice in light of it. His response is to lexically order the first principles of practical reasoning and develop even more elaborate procedures for practical decision making. Rather than making one principle fundamental and assigning a derivative status to the other, this Rawlsian method of lexically ordering principles requires that one principle be considered only after the conditions of the other principle have been met (Rawls, 1971, pp. 40–45). This method of lexically ordering the principles of the good and the right allows for considerations regarding the full significance of both principles. Thus, Rawls need not justify one of the principles as being normatively more fundamental than the other, but only provide reasons why the conditions of one principle ought to be satisfied before the other.

Rawls's method of justifying his lexical ordering of the principles relies on a process of "reflective equilibrium" aimed at achieving coherence between considered moral judgments and principles in conjunction with "the original position," which is an ahistorical hypothetical-choice situation entered into by stepping behind the "veil of ignorance" (Rawls, 1971, pp. 17–21). The basic idea is that individuals enter into the original position by imagining themselves devoid of any knowledge of particular contingent characteristics of the self that often set people at odds with one another and impede rational choice. Once cloaked in this veil of ignorance, individuals will be able to bring their choice of a specific lexically ordered set of principles (of justice) into coherence with their considered moral judgments, or intuitions, through a process of revising and refining both the principles at hand and their intuitions in light of each other.

For Rawls's purposes, this method of justification is more appropriate than that of the deductive method of modern moral theories for two reasons. First, Rawls's theory is not intended to be foundational in the sense of consequentialism or pure Kantianism. Rather than making one principle the exclusive foundation of morality, Rawls posits a lexical ordering of the principles of the good and the right. The justification of the order of the principles only requires that it is coherent with our settled moral convictions. This method of justification has the advantage of allowing for appeals simultaneously to our moral intuitions in the weighing of the principles of the good and the right and to a structured process of rational deliberation.

A second reason that reflective equilibrium is more appropriate according to Rawls is that he only intends his theory of justice to be political, not metaphysical. In other words, Rawls intends his theory to be grounded in a justification that can be accepted by people who hold diverse comprehensive worldviews and incommensurable conceptions of the good (1985, pp. 221–226). Three aspects of Rawls's theory distinguish it as political rather than metaphysical. To begin with, it is intended as a moral theory that only applies to political considerations regarding justice. In other words, Rawls's theory is concerned only with the subject matter of the proper structure of social and economic institutions as they form a coherent system. Second, the theory is intended specifically to apply to a certain type of political consideration, that of a democratic constitutional society. Third, Rawls intends his theory to be "freestanding." According to Rawls, a freestanding theory is one that is neither derived from nor presented within the context of a specific comprehensive moral doctrine, though it is supported by one or more comprehensive theories

(1993, p. 13). The goals of Rawls's theory are thus prudently constrained and present a more refined view of what a moral theory can and should do in light of the failure of the Enlightenment project, the heterogeneous nature of moral value, and the fact of moral pluralism.

An alternative response to modern moral theory is illustrated in H. Tristram Engelhardt, Jr.'s theory of bioethics. According to Engelhardt, the failure of the Enlightenment has bequeathed to postmodern secular ethics a relativism and nihilism that cannot be overcome by reason alone in the world of secular morality. This world of secular morality is comprised of the interaction of moral strangers. Moral strangers are simply any members of a pluralistic society who do not share common commitments to a single vision of the good life and to the same metaphysical views (Engelhardt, 1996b, p. 9). The limits of secular morality, then, need to be established in light of the concepts of moral intimacy: namely, moral stranger-hood, moral friendship, and their correlative levels of moral content. In Engelhardt's view, these limits turn out to be the lowest common denominator of morality by which moral strangers could agree to subject themselves to inherently coercive moral authority. Accordingly, the foundation of secular morality is the negative right to be left alone, and the first principle of secular bioethics is the principle of permission (1996b, pp. 102–122).

Engelhardt's response to the failure of reason to establish a canonical conception of the good is partly an attempt to save bioethics from relativism and partly an attempt to save it from nihilism. Engelhardt attempts to do this via two different and logically independent lines of reasoning. First, Engelhardt invokes a distinction between metaphysics and epistemology (Wreen, 1998, p. 74). According to Engelhardt, there may in fact be only one true moral code (disclosed first and most clearly to Orthodox Christians, more obscurely to other Christians, even more obscurely to non-Christians, and so on), but it is not discernable or accessible through reason alone. But if this is the case, then the world of moral intimacy is primarily characterized by relativism that stems from our inability to discover the one true moral code through reason. Engelhardt's second line of defense, then, is to argue for a proceduralism founded on universally binding moral authority consisting of mutual agreement, consent, and peaceful conflict resolution. As Engelhardt writes, "if one wishes to resolve moral controversies without a mere appeal to force, and if all do not listen to God so as to be united in one religion, and since reason cannot disclose a canonical moral vision, the only source of common moral authority among strangers will be consent" (1996a, p. 339).

To understand the role that the principle of permission plays in justifying particular actions within Engelhardt's theory of secular bioethics, all one need do is consider what he would say in response to the case of nonvoluntary euthanasia considered at the beginning of this chapter. Regarding euthanasia for the once-competent patient, Engelhardt writes:

Indeed, the principle of permission does not bar terminating the life of an individual who was once competent and (1) who is not competent and (2) will not again be competent (3) where it appears by clear and convincing evidence that the person would have wished not only to be allowed to die but to have death expedited in the circumstances in question. (1996b, p. 354)

Insofar as one can infer that the family believed the patient would have wanted death expedited in the circumstances in which she found herself, the physician can be said, according to this line of reasoning, to have been justified in the direct killing of his patient insofar as he did not violate the principle of permission in any way.

Engelhardt's theory is representative of how the postmodern response to modern moral theory and to the modern moral dichotomy has influenced the methodological debates that are shaping the field of bioethics. This debate concerning justification has led some to describe the current state of bioethics as an intellectual war zone in a state of methodological upheaval, in which defending a moral principle puts one at risk of "taking a sniper's bullet" (Daniels, 1996, p. 96). In addition to Engelhardt and others who share his view, there are three principle combatants on this battleground. First, there are those who are often dubbed "theorists" and defend some version of the deductive model of justification within the modern conception of ethics. Then there are casuists, who insist that moral justification properly proceeds from an adequate appreciation of the situational particulars of cases, independent of a more general and comprehensive theory regarding the nature of moral value. Third, there are the proponents of "principlism," who maintain that the practical conclusions of bioethics are best justified by appealing to mid-level principles that are rooted in the "common morality" and accepted at face value without any appeal to more abstract ethical theories.

The revolution in which bioethics began its advance away from medical ethics traditionally conceived was formally initiated in the late 1970s with the publication of the first edition of *Principles of Biomedical Ethics* by Tom L. Beauchamp and James F. Childress. Working from the perspective of modern moral philosophy, Beauchamp and Childress recognized that there were significant limitations in the traditional method of deductive justification, particularly as applied to the complex clinical environment of medicine. According to Beauchamp and Childress, the deductive model of justification does not adequately capture how moral reasoning and justification proceed in complicated cases, and its linear conception of moral judgment is oversimplified. In particular, Beauchamp and Childress note that the deductivist model fails to fully account for the fact that principles must be specified and balanced in their application to individual cases, that it potentially leads to an infinite regress of justification, and that it cannot accommodate a plurality of equally valid but competing conceptions of moral value (1994, pp. 16–17).

As an alternative, Beauchamp and Childress put forth and argue for a set of mid-level prima facie principles intended to function as surrogates for more comprehensive moral theories. This set of mid-level principles is comprised of four principles: respect for autonomy, beneficence, nonmaleficence, and justice. According to Beauchamp and Childress, these principles are firmly grounded in a universal common morality and can be brought to bear on individual cases through a process of specification and balancing. In the absence of any general theory of the nature of moral value, Beauchamp and Childress recruited the coherentist method of justification that is at the heart of Rawls's method of reflective equilibrium for use within their approach to bioethics. They claim that the coherentist method of justification goes hand in hand with the specification of moral principles, which is the process of developing and shaping norms both conceptually and normatively to connect them with concrete action guides and practical judgments. As they write, "Specification as a method must be indissolubly connected with a larger model of coherence that appeals to considered judgments and to the overall coherence introduced by a proposed specification" (1994, p. 31). That this process of specification is intended to bring the principles into coherence with "considered judgments" also illustrates the intimate connection between this method and the common morality. According to Beauchamp and Childress, the considered judgments found among the socially approved norms of human conduct constitute the common morality from which this method derives its normative force. Within this framework, the common morality acts as a substitute for any more comprehensive theory of the nature of moral value that would in the deductive model of moral reasoning function as the justification for normative claims. While this method has certain advantages over the modern deductive approach, it is also problematic for three interrelated reasons.

The first problem with principlism as laid out by Beauchamp and Childress arises from their reliance on a set of prima facie principles superficially related to one another and divorced from any underlying unified theory of moral value. As some authors have argued, this method amounts to little more than a checklist or collection of "chapter headings" that represent suggestions and observations that should be kept in mind when attempting to resolve difficult cases (Gert, Culver, & Clouser, 1997, p. 86). The problem with this checklist approach is that the principles often conflict with one another with no identified means of resolving such conflicts. This problem arises out of the fact that Beauchamp and Childress have removed the principles from their original context as part of more comprehensive normative theories. In their original context, these principles functioned as "effective summaries" of the more comprehensive theories that generated them (Gert, Culver, & Clouser, p. 75). Once removed from this context, however, there is no systematic relationship between the principles nor inherent priority ranking among them. Rather than resolving or avoiding any conflict between fundamental principles that might arise out of the inherent tension created by what I have referred to as the modern moral dichotomy, the method of principlism seems only to amplify this inevitable potential for conflict by adding more principles into the mix with no underlying theory of moral value to guide us in their application.

A second problem with the approach of Beauchamp and Childress is that there is no clear indication of how the principles should be specified and applied in particular situations. Again, this problem seems to arise from the fact that the principles have been abstracted from the more comprehensive theories that provided the original context in which to understand and apply them. The principle of respect for autonomy, for example, will have a very different meaning and varying practical implications depending on whether one conceives of autonomy in Kantian terms of a categorical law that the will (pure practical reason) imposes on itself or as the capacity for self-determination, as Mill conceived it (Wildes, 2000, pp. 67–68). Likewise, one will reach very different conclusions depending on how one specifies the principles of beneficence, nonmaleficence, and justice. This problem is exacerbated by the fact that the common morality will not always clearly indicate how a particular principle ought to be specified.

The third problem with principlism arises out of its reliance solely on coherentism as a method of justification. Reliance solely on a coherentist method of justification requires one to assume that the considered judgments or moral intuitions that constitute the starting points of justification are themselves justified. If these starting points are not in themselves justified, then there is nothing about the process of coherence justification that would justify them or provide normative support for the conclusions based upon them. In other words, even though there may be coherence among moral beliefs, the process of bringing those beliefs into coherence with one another does not itself offer any way of judging whether or not those beliefs are correct. The genocide imposed upon the Jewish people of Nazi Germany was perfectly coherent with the Nazi's considered judgment that Jewish people are less than fully human. However, this coherence is clearly not itself a justification for the atrocities of Nazi Germany. While coherence may be a necessary element of moral reasoning in general, and of specification in particular, it is not itself a sufficient means of justification. As Edmund Pellegrino describes it, coherence "is a logical requirement of defensible moral reasoning, but not a quality of the moral rectitude of the conclusion of that reasoning procedure" (2000, p. 667). Thus, if one relies solely on a coherence method of justification with no other means of normatively examining one's starting points, then the best one can hope to achieve is a sophisticated process of consensus building that will never move beyond relativism.

Rawls, on the other hand, is able to minimize the concern of relativism in his use of reflective equilibrium by the way in which he constrains the nature and purpose of his theory. As previously noted, Rawls's theory is explicitly only intended to be a political theory of justice applied to the basic institutions of a democratic society. By confining his theory to this narrowly constrained purpose, Rawls has taken steps to ensure that the considered judgments that function as the starting points of his justification are already well established and accepted as legitimate considerations for the type of theory in which he employs his coherence method of justification. For example, if there is significant agreement or it is self-evident that opportunities to hold offices of power within a democratic society should not be limited to certain individuals arbitrarily, then bringing the principles that govern the structure of democratic society into coherence with that moral intuition will indeed justify structuring them accordingly. And so it does, since such considered judgments are integral to what it means for a society to be democratic in the first place. Of course, whether or not a democratic society is the type of society that will be most just could be considered a matter of debate, but one with which Rawls himself is relatively unconcerned. Rather, Rawls assumes that such a society is just and intends his theory only to be applicable within such a society and reasonable to those members of society that accept his starting points. Insofar as Rawls's theory is "freestanding," and not intrinsically connected to any particular theory of the good life or thick conception of the good, his theory and its justification need not rest on any particular comprehensive moral theory and worldview that may not be shared by all members of a democratic society.

While the coherence method of justification is well suited to Rawls's narrowly constrained task, questions of bioethical matters most often extend beyond the freestanding considerations of how best to ensure fair treatment of the members of a democratic society. Many bioethical questions, particularly those in the clinical environment, are intimately connected to individual life plans, one's own religious beliefs, incommensurable conceptions of the good, and diverse world perspectives that provide meaning for those who are most affected by a decision to act. Furthermore, these questions often entail no clearly self-evident or widely agreed upon considered judgments, nor self-evident moral intuitions integral to the subject matter. It is not clear, for example, whether the 5- to 7-day-old human embryo is a human person deserving of moral protection and respect or whether it is merely some form of preembryonic genetic material to be used for the betterment of postnatal sentient human beings. Nor is it self-evident that killing a person who is immanently dying, as in the case we have been considering, is a nonmaleficent and appropriate response to pain and suffering. The coherence method of justification, however, provides no method for resolving such questions on a fundamental level. Thus, it seems that while there is much to be gleaned from the Rawlsian perspective, and coherence is a logical requirement of moral reasoning, the method of coherence justification will not provide

much normative guidance in cases in which there is fundamental disagreement concerning our considered judgments, value priorities, and
specification of the principles of biomedical ethics.

   These problems can be illustrated by considering again the case of
the physician who ended his patient's life to relieve her suffering. Beauchamp and Childress themselves have argued that the act of voluntary
euthanasia can be justified in particular cases (though the practice cannot
be justified as a matter of social policy) if the individual desires death
more than other goods. In their words, "If a person desires death rather
than life's more typical goods and projects, then causing that person's
death at his or her autonomous request does not either harm or wrong
the person" (Beauchamp & Childress, 1994, p. 236). Accordingly, if the
family's surrogate consent accurately reflected her desire, then the physician's actions in the case of Mrs. R. were justified. However, this conception of harm and the corresponding conception of nonmaleficence
are implicitly based on a particular theory of rationality found in the consequentialist framework that posits preference satisfaction as the good
that should always be maximized. According to some competing theories,
it may be possible to harm an individual by satisfying a desire that person
may experience more strongly than others. For example, the physician
who writes a prescription for the drug seeker who comes to the Emergency Department complaining of phantom pain or for the patient with a
viral infection who desires antibiotics may still cause harm to that person,
even though the physician satisfies the patient's desire.

   These considerations raise two concerns. First, it appears that the approach of Beauchamp and Childress is not as free of comprehensive theories of moral value as they would like to believe. Rather, this approach
simply does not require any one particular theory of moral value as the
basis for specifying and balancing the principles of biomedical ethics. In
specifying and balancing the principles, decision makers are free to pick
and choose among existing theories of moral value as they please. Second, it is not at all clear that the conception of nonmaleficence Beauchamp and Childress use to justify individual instances of voluntary euthanasia is consistent with the "common morality." Almost all established
religions, whether Roman Catholicism, Protestantism, Judaism, Islam, or
Orthodox Christianity, hold as one of their major tenets that life is in itself
a good that should never be directly acted against (though this belief may
not always entail a moral requirement to use every available means to

prolong life as long as possible). Large segments of society made up of individuals belonging to one of these major faith traditions will likely have a very different understanding of nonmaleficence. According to this understanding of nonmaleficence, the physician in the case in question did in fact cause morally unacceptable harm to the patient, even though her family consented to it on her behalf. Beauchamp and Childress seem to acknowledge the potential for conflict of this nature when they write, "Those who believe it is sometimes morally acceptable to let people die but not to take active steps to help them die must therefore give a different account of the wrongfulness of killing persons than the one we have suggested" (1994, p. 236). However, their approach does not provide any method for resolving fundamental conflicts regarding the nature of harm and, therefore, does not appear to get us much beyond many of the problems of the modern conception of ethics as a monistic deductive process of decision making.

Another of the combatants on the battlefield of bioethics is casuistry. Stemming back to the Roman Catholic Manualist tradition of the 16th century, casuistry as a moral method is rooted in the deontological framework of morality that accompanied the rise of nominalism. However, as a moral method, casuistry does not explicitly depend on any particular theory of the nature of moral value as do more modern deontological theories, for example, Kantianism. Rather, casuists are by definition skeptical of principles and theories that are divorced from history, precedent, and the circumstances of actual cases. The primary advantage of casuistry, according to its proponents, is that it reduces the need for lofty abstract principles and comes closer to the way in which actual decisions are made in concrete cases.

In the place of general theories regarding the nature of moral value and their derivative principles, the method of casuistry posits considerations of paradigm and analogous cases as the proper starting points of moral analysis and practical reason (Jonsen & Toulmin, 1988, pp. 24–28). This case comparison is done to discern whether it is more or less probable that an action, such as euthanasia, would be morally licit or illicit according to whatever standard of law is being used to make that determination. In the case of Mrs. R., for example, this comparison would be done to discern whether or not the act of ending her life to relieve her pain and suffering would fall under the concept of murder from a legal perspective or, from a theological perspective, of killing as specified by the fifth commandment. Next, the circumstances and other facts of the case would be considered. With regard to the case at hand, these considerations would minimally include: the degree of pain Mrs. R. was experiencing; her present and future quality of life; her proximity to death; whether the family had the rightful authority to consent to euthanasia on her behalf; whether there is a morally relevant distinction between direct killing and allowing to die; and whether the physician was acting out of mercy or with maleficent intent. Finally, the probability of the moral status of the act based on cumulative arguments would be considered before arriving at a final resolution.

One difficulty with casuistry, as with principlism, is that the way all of these relevant considerations are taken into account will vary due to the different perspectives from which one addresses the relevant questions (Wildes, 2000, p. 89). The possibility of conflicting conclusions then arises, in part from the fact that there is no underlying theory of moral value to guide decision making within the deontological framework in which casuistry situates itself. Within the deontological framework of morality, the only reason one has to be dutiful and follow the rules is because those duties and rules have been put forth by some lawmaking authority. Within the context of casuistry, the criteria of morality are merely traced back to the will of some lawmaker, whether that lawmaker is God, the government, pure practical reason, or the autonomous individual (Ashley & O'Rourke, 1997, p. 147). Such criteria, however, cannot provide the reason why the rules of that authority rather than some other authority should be followed in the first place. Conflicting resolutions to a particular case may arise, then, depending on what authority and to what set of rules one adheres. The implication for casuistry is that it begins to lose its credibility among competing notions of right and wrong, particularly once divorced from its original theological context (Pellegrino, 2000, p. 662).

Regarding its method of justification, casuistry employs neither a coherence nor a deductive model of justification. Rather, casuistry relies on an inductive method of justification. This method of justification proceeds on the assumption that principles and rules are not justified by an ahistorical examination of the nature of moral value, but on a sufficiently rich appreciation of the contexts of particular cases and judgments. Rather than appealing to universal principles as the basis for generalizable rules, particular judgments in themselves are generalizable through analogy.

The underlying idea is that paradigm cases provide more foundational, normative guidance than do principles (Keenan & Shannon, 1995, p. 223).

Though distinct, the inductive method of justification shares some of the same weaknesses as the coherence method of justification. As in coherence justification, there is nothing inherent in inductive reasoning or the method of casuistry itself that assures one conclusion is morally more sound than another. As with coherence methods of justification, casuistry and its inductive method of justification stands in need of some fundamental basis by which to judge the moral rectitude of its conclusions. While there might be some general agreement concerning the resolution of certain paradigm cases, this general agreement could be about a decision that is itself wrong. With no intrinsic normative standards, casuistry itself is in need of some more comprehensive theory about the nature of moral value that would provide some context and foundation upon which to rest its normative conclusions. As James F. Keenan and Thomas Shannon describe it: "Casuistry has no purposes intrinsic to its logic or method. The context in which it is employed provides the purpose. Thus casuistry never stands free of its context or its practitioners" (1995, p. 229). Without a firm foundation, casuistry runs the risk of being merely another process of consensus building between individuals who already share the same moral starting points.

In surveying the battleground of bioethics, a trend emerges. This trend is a pronounced retreat from the search for moral truth. This trend is largely due to the fact that contemporary moral theories have relieved ethics of the theoretical weight bearing down from lofty questions concerning the nature of moral value. The influence of this contemporary conception of moral theory has set bioethics on a trajectory in which it is increasingly becoming merely a sophisticated process of consensus building. This trajectory fits well with the postmodern view of ethics as a process-oriented means of peaceful conflict resolution within a world of moral strangers. While conflict resolution and consensus may at times be admirable goals for bioethics, if bioethics as a normative endeavor is outmoded, then one need not look to the field for any substantive guidance. Indeed, if this trend continues, then we will likely find ourselves in a world of morality in which our norms are dictated by technical proficiency and the only limits are "gross manifestations of moral violence" (Pellegrino, 2000, p. 669).

An Aristotelian Alternative

Aristotle's ethical theory is teleological in a sense quite different from that of consequentialist theories of ethics. For Aristotle, the fact that ethics is teleological means that both the first principles from which action proceeds and the end at which it aims are the final cause of all human action; the final cause being the end, purpose, and good for which something exists or is done (trans. 1984a, II, 3, 194b33–195a). In an ontological sense, the final cause is that form of perfection toward which all individual beings as members of a particular natural kind, or species, naturally tend in their development. The name given to this ultimate end is often translated as "happiness." This translation, however, can be misleading. A better translation may be that of "human flourishing." This translation seems closer to Aristotle's conception of the ultimate end, which included both the notion of behaving well and the notion of fairing well over an extended period of time (MacIntyre, 1998, p. 59). The concept of "happiness" in common English usage, however, usually connotes a transient state of elation or joy.

As Aristotle made clear, the ultimate end is not some state of affairs that results from actions of a certain nature (as the state of elation does), but this end—insofar as it is self-sufficient and final—consists in activity itself, namely, activity of the soul in accordance with virtue (1984b, I, 2, 1098a17–19). The fact that the attainment of the ultimate end is constituted by activity and is not merely some transient state of affairs distinguishes the Aristotelian conception of human flourishing from any modern conception of "happiness." More importantly, this conception of the ultimate end clearly distinguishes Aristotle's theories from any modern conception of teleology (conceived in terms of consequentialism) insofar as the ultimate end can only be attained through an ongoing pursuit that unfolds over the whole of a unitary life. In contrast to the modern moral framework, which has been primarily concerned with the relationship between moral obligations and individual actions isolated in time, Aristotle's teleological perspective is more concerned with the way in which individual actions constitute necessarily interrelated and continuous elements of a unitary story that reflect a person's moral character, disposition, and lived conception of the good. As Alisdaire McIntyre describes it, this teleological approach is best understood in the sense of the medieval conception of a quest, that is, a continuous narrative journey, a unitary story, within which its hero is confronted with various harms, dangers, temptations, and distractions that provide the context in which its goal is to be properly understood and appreciated (1984, p. 219).

For Aristotle, progress on this quest cannot be measured simply by the external consequences of one's actions. Rather, Aristotle holds that virtue is a disposition to choose the mean between two extremes and that some actions never admit of a mean, for example, theft, adultery, and murder (1984b, II, 6, 1107a9–14). In this way, Aristotle's theory shares more in common with deontological theories of ethics than with consequentialist theories. However, there are some important differences between Aristotle's conception of ethics and the modern conception that make it altogether distinct.

One way in which Aristotle's ethics can be distinguished from more modern conceptions of moral theory is that the theoretical precision sought in the latter is absent in the former. According to Aristotle, the fact that contingent human actions are the subject of ethical inquiry gives moral reasoning a unique character that distinguishes it from other types of reasoning. Accordingly, *praxis,* the type of activity employed in ethical decision-making, is not subject to the same truth requirements as is *theoria,* which must always accord with the principles of a theoretical science, such as geometry. The principles of ethics do not depend on universal, eternal, and necessary connections for their truth as do those of *theoria.* Within the Aristotelian framework, then, ethics does not entail understanding and explaining phenomena through a schema of precise principles and laws as the sciences do. Nor will ethical prescriptions specify a certain course of action with theoretical precision. If ethical prescriptions are to guide action appropriately, then they must not be stated as absolutely or unalterably true. The implication is that any general counsel arrived at through ethical inquiry is contingent upon the situational particulars and, therefore, open to revision and later qualification (Broadie, 1991, p. 20).

This obscurity, which for Aristotle is inherent in ethics, reflects the limited role that principles and their derivative rules can have in determining how one ought to live. In light of this limited role, Aristotle extols a type of moral judgment that is not itself a rule-governed process. On this account, moral judgment consists of a kind of "situational appreciation" that is more akin to perception and a complex responsiveness to the particulars of a concrete situation than to principle-based reasoning

(Wiggins, 1976, pp. 40–43; Nussbaum, 1985, p. 153). Because this conception of moral judgment is not itself principle based or rule governed, it provides a framework in which one is able to adjudicate conflicts between would-be fundamental moral principles. Within the Aristotelian framework, the emphasis on right reasoning is switched from the intellectual application of derivative rules to the ability to internalize, from a scattered range of particular cases, a general evaluative attitude that is not reducible to rules or precepts (Burnyeat, 1980, p. 73). This ability is achieved through the development of the virtues, which are character traits that a human being needs in order to live well and flourish (Sherman, 1991, pp. 244–251). In this way, the intellectual powers of moral reasoning presuppose and grow out of the habits of a well-formed character. While this internalization retains a cognitive element, the theoretical justification of universal principles and the intellectual application of derivative rules are not as central as they have become in modern moral theory (Lesher, 2001, pp. 45–55).

This account of moral reasoning does not imply that ethics, as envisaged by Aristotle, is nonrational. It is rational, though primarily in a sense different from the modern notion of theoretical justifications and rule-based computations. Rather than relying solely on philosophically justified principles and the intellectual application of derivative rules, this account of ethics requires moral agents to possess a virtuous disposition along with an interest in living a good life. A virtuous disposition and the interest in living a good life are necessary because human flourishing, whatever it may consist in, is a good that can be attained only if one is prepared to subordinate some desires to others. The determination of which desires should be subordinated to others is in part based on one's conception of the good life. As Nancy Sherman describes it, "Aristotle's theory is the more abstract and programmatic end of the same process by which we, as practical agents, deliberate and arrive at some conception of good living" (1991, p. 10). While philosophical inquiry and rule-based reasoning may have normatively beneficial results, the foundation of Aristotelian ethics is not some philosophically justified principle and its derivative rules but rather the rational nature of human life itself. In other words, the foundation of Aristotelian teleology is human life itself conceived of as rational activity informed by virtue.

A second way in which Aristotle's moral teleology can be distinguished from modern moral theory is that virtue is given priority over ethical principles in general. Though ethical principles often specify valid sources of value, they are not the most basic moral concepts of Aristotelian teleology. In other words, the good and the right do not function as the only basic decision-making perspectives, and the structure of Aristotelian ethics is not determined by how it connects these "basic" concepts. Rather, the structure of Aristotle's moral teleology is founded on a conception of moral value as grounded in the shared rational nature of human life and realized most fully in the perfection of one's own life as constituted by virtuous activity.

One reason virtue is of such importance within the Aristotelian framework is that it signifies the integration of well-formed states of character that enable one to live in accordance with a conception of the good life. Virtue is necessary in this way because it enables its possessor to respond to concrete situational particulars that influence action on a level of perception at which ethical principles and their derivative rules can be of little help. At first glance, it might seem that this Aristotelian conception of moral judgment is merely a kind of moral intuition, since moral responsiveness occurs on a quasi-perceptual rather than a theoretical level (Rawls, 1971, pp. 38–40). However, within the Aristotelian framework, practical reasoning developed through habituation is on a par with, though different from, intuition and induction within scientific reasoning (Burnyeat, 1980, p. 73).

It may still be objected, however, that Aristotle's theory is not that different from consequentialist theories because the virtues are only instrumental in achieving an independent normative principle of the good conceived in terms of human excellence (Rawls, 1971, p. 325). On this account, the good is defined independently of the virtues, and the virtues are defined as that which maximizes the good. Accordingly, human excellence is deemed intrinsically valuable, and the virtues are only extrinsically valuable. This interpretation makes Aristotle's theory distinguished from utilitarianism only in what it posits as the end to be maximized, namely, human excellence. However, this interpretation places too much emphasis on the evaluation of action as determined by an abstract, fundamental principle. That type of ratiocination concerning action fails to capture the relevant moral fact that virtuous activity is itself partly constitutive of the good within the Aristotelian framework of teleology (Watson, 1990, p. 452).

Within Aristotle's teleological framework, the moral significance of virtue is most appropriately understood in terms of how it is best for a human being to be. This claim about how virtue should be understood is what Gary Watson refers to as the *claim of explanatory primacy* (1990, p. 460). This claim distinguishes Aristotelian ethics from modern moral theory in that there is no further commitment to an intrinsic value independent of the virtues upon which their moral significance depends. However, this is not to say that the virtues are foundational to all other moral concepts. That interpretation does not take sufficient account of the teleological aspect of perfecting one's rational nature, which is of primary concern within the Aristotelian framework of teleology.

It is only within the context of a conception of the good life, conceived as activity that perfects one's rational, that is, characteristically human, nature that one can gain an appropriate understanding of the value of virtue. Without such a context there would be no reason to believe that the virtues are morally valuable in the first place. While virtuous activity itself is a necessary element of human flourishing, one must first be capable of living a characteristic human life before one can be said to live a flourishing human life (Nussbaum, 1995, pp. 80–81). Thus, the concept of a characteristically human life together with a conception of a perfected version of that life constitutes a continuum of value. At the beginning of this continuum, the minimum threshold of moral value is constituted by human life itself, insofar as it is the most fundamental basic good required for all other basic goods. Those basic goods that enable further characteristic human functioning, then, are of increasing moral value, while living a perfected version of that life, for which the virtues are required, is of ever more increasing value.

The implication of a "perfected version of a characteristically human life" is that moral value is not singularly derived from the virtues themselves nor from human excellence itself. Instead, the notion of human excellence arises from an interdependent relationship between the virtues and what it is to live a characteristically human life in accord with one's rational nature. In other words, the concepts of virtue and a characteristically human life are reciprocally dependent upon each other for their meaning and normativity. If either is to have moral significance, the concepts must inform each other. What makes an action morally valuable will depend in part on what kind of life is characteristic of humanity, and what is a good human life will be determined partially by one's own personal characteristics and virtue.

That a conception of human excellence is derived from the reciprocal relationship between characteristic human functioning and virtue implies that moral value is intimately connected with that which enables us to live the kind of life that is appropriate to the kind of beings we are. As biological creatures, for example, we value food because it satisfies our physiological needs and cultivates our ability to realize our physical capabilities (whatever those may be). Nutrition satisfies a need that must be fulfilled if one is to be capable of characteristically human functioning and a minimal level of well-being (Sen, 1992, p. 39). Under this broader category of well-being, many needs in addition to physiological ones must be satisfied. Psychological and social needs will also have to be met if one is to be capable of sustained characteristic human activity.

This basic level at which moral value consists in meeting the needs required for characteristically human functioning is what John Kekes refers to as the level of primary goods. As Kekes describes them, "primary goods are the satisfactions of needs by exercising the capacities included in the description of the facts of human nature" (1995, p. 21). These goods are not primary, however, in the Rawlsian sense of being prior within a lexical ordering. The point is not that they should be given priority, but that they are primary due to the innate structure of human life. In this sense, the primary goods and their value are not choice-inclusive facts (Lachs, 1995, pp. 228–233) and do not depend on our desiring them, nor do they depend upon individual-specific, full conceptions of the good for their moral relevance. Though the particular capabilities required for characteristic human functioning may be exercised and their correlative needs satisfied in varying ways, they are universal and essential characteristics of the human person (Nussbaum, 1992, pp. 205–214). Some examples of universal and essential primary goods are: proper nourishment and shelter, freedom from unnecessary pain, affiliation with other human beings, and the freedom to exercise practical reason (Nussbaum, 1995, p. 83). Though different societies and cultures may have various ways of exercising these capabilities and satisfying their correlative needs, all societies and cultures must do so if they are to survive and ultimately flourish.

Whereas the satisfaction of needs required for characteristic human functioning constitutes a basic level of moral value that is universal, the unique satisfaction of these needs through practical reason constitutes a higher and more individual-specific level of moral value. Kekes refers to

the goods that are possible at this higher and less objective level of functioning as secondary goods (1995, p. 22). At this level, practical reason is
architectonic. That is, practical reason allows us to discern, prioritize, and
achieve moral value in ways that are unique to us as individuals (Finnis,
1983, pp. 72–74).

The implication of this architectonic status of practical reason is that
secondary values are constituted by the more complex and elaborate
satisfaction of the primary goods in ways that are appropriate to us as
unique individuals. Once one is capable of characteristically human activity, then the unique cultivation of that characteristically human activity
has increasing value. This increasing value consists not of characteristically human activities, but of those activities that have themselves been
realized in a way beyond being merely characteristic. In this way, the realization of secondary values constitutes advancement toward one's own
conception of human flourishing. This relationship between secondary
and primary goods reflects the reciprocity between characteristic human
functioning and virtue and is itself reciprocal. As Kekes describes it:

The choice of secondary values depends on such evaluations of their suitability to
our character and circumstances as are already in place. In this way, by a process
of reciprocal adjustments, increasingly finer assessments of our character, interdependent interpretations and reinterpretations of the nature and suitability of
our possibilities, we make what we believe is a good life for ourselves. The making and the living of it, however, are not two processes, but one. We make a good
life by living well, and we live a good life only if we make it good. (1995, p. 24)

Within the Aristotelian framework of teleology, this conception of the
good as perfected characteristic human activity does not function as the
foundation for a systematic, rule-governed decision-making process per
se. Rather, this account of the good functions as a regulative ideal for analyzing practical problems to say which evaluative principles apply, and
how (Nagel, 1979, p. 139). Its normative value is that it allows us to be
able to understand how fundamentally different types of moral value are
relevant to particular considerations. Understood in this way, this conception of the good acts as a general guide that is operative within a conception of moral judgment as a kind of quasi-intuitive yet fully cognitive
"discernment of perception" that grows out of the developmental process
through which the virtues are acquired. From this perspective, the primary focus of moral evaluation is not whether the action in question is

consistent with either the principle of the good (conceived in consequentialist terms) or with the principle of the right, though both will remain relevant. Instead, the primary focus of moral evaluation is whether a person's choice of action considered in all its dimensions reflects an appropriate moral disposition toward the good and fosters human flourishing in oneself and in others.

The practical implication of this teleological understanding as contrasted with that of the modern conception of ethics can be illustrated by considering for a final time the case of the physician who acted to end his dying patient's life in order to relieve her suffering. In this case, neither the consequentialist approach nor the deontological approach offers much normative guidance insofar as each merely identifies competing values that arise out of different perspectives of moral evaluation, for example, outcome centered versus act centered. Still, both perspectives can be considered valid and morally relevant, which is why both arguments carry some moral weight in the first place. Moreover, it can reasonably be presumed (given the circumstances of the case) that the physician's primary motivation was compassion for his dying patient. However, from the Aristotelian teleological perspective with its emphasis on virtue, the moral evaluation of the physician's action does not rest only, or even primarily, on these considerations. Rather, from this teleological perspective, the moral evaluation of the physician's action depends primarily on whether that act, and a corresponding predisposition toward acts of a similar nature, would be consistent with virtue and conducive to the human flourishing of physicians and their patients.

From this perspective, we can say that the act of killing the patient to end her suffering was contrary to virtue. As considered herein, a virtuous act is one that either promotes basic goods necessary for characteristic human functioning or eliminates some barrier that inhibits characteristic human functioning, for example, unnecessary pain. Though the physician's action did end the patient's pain, it did so not by eliminating the pain itself, or the experience of pain, but by destroying the basic good of the patient's continued existence. This is not to say that one may never intentionally act contrary to a basic good but that one can be justified in doing so only if it is to preserve or restore another basic good of equal or increasing moral value. While which basic goods are of increasing or secondary value is largely dependent on individual specific and content-full conceptions of the good, continued human existence is a universal and necessary condition for the pursuit and attainment of all other basic goods. Insofar as continued human existence is a necessary condition of all other basic goods, actions that destroy human existence neither preserve nor restore other basic goods. The point is not that the physician robbed the patient of further opportunity to pursue other higher goods, but that his action arose directly out of a failure to recognize the very basis of moral value in action. A resulting moral problem for the physician himself is that a disposition to perform such acts will not be conducive to the physician's own ability to recognize moral value, to choose the good, and to live a flourishing human life. While a single choice of action contrary to the basic good of continued human existence would not preclude the physician from leading an overall good life, the recurring choice of such acts would, given enough time, limit the physician's ability to discern and choose virtuous actions, which are themselves in part constitutive of the good.

Postmodern Bioethics and Teleology

One essential and distinguishing element of Aristotle's teleological conception of ethics is that it is rooted in a particular conception of what it means to be a human person with an embodied rational nature. By definition, then, Aristotle's conception of teleology is a form of ethical naturalism, the view that moral claims can be rationally supported by appeals to human nature. Reading today's secular bioethics literature, one might get the impression that ethical naturalism is dead. Regarding the hope that human nature might again serve as a moral guide, for example, Daniel Callahan writes, "unfortunately, it is hard to think of a once-robust tradition—that of natural law or naturalism—that is much more down at the heel. Even pragmatism and stoicism, also long ago pronounced dead, have staged a recent comeback" (1996, p. 21). However, the second coming of ethical naturalism is not likely within the current culture of bioethics.

There are elements of ethical naturalism that could be seen as problematic given the pluralistic context in which the questions of contemporary biomedical ethics must be addressed. Such objections can be found in both the political theory of John Rawls and the bioethics of H. Tristram Engelhardt, as previously considered. The underlying commonality of these critiques is the inability of reason to establish a single dominant conception of the good and a universally acceptable content-full morality. The implication is that the basis of biomedical ethics within a pluralistic society cannot depend on any controversial metaphysical or theological claims, if it is to be morally acceptable. Engelhardt has been the most fervent proponent of this position within the bioethics literature.

As previously discussed, according to Engelhardt, the fact of pluralism implies that moral content is available on only two levels. These levels are those of the content-full morality of moral friends and the purely procedural morality that binds moral strangers. That these levels of morality are the only ones available further implies that moral content (and the lack thereof) and the corresponding concepts of moral intimacy are related as opposing sides of a dichotomy, between which there is no middle ground. In such a framework, however, the limits of secular morality will be excessively restrictive for two reasons. First, within his framework, the rules of respecting freedom act as the starting points, or first principles, of secular moral reasoning. Yet, as has been pointed out, "to have rules about respecting freedom or anything else is to have content" (Wreen, 1998, p. 81). As Joseph Boyle has argued, Engelhardt himself assumes either that peaceable conflict resolution is of primary importance, thereby begging the question like all the theories he rejects as justifiable according to reason, or he assumes that peaceable conflict resolution is somehow identical with the concept of morality itself (1994, p. 187).

The implication is that Engelhardt has failed to provide the ethical nihilist, or even the relativist, with any reason why peaceable conflict resolution by means of consent is morally preferable to violence. It seems that a purely content-less ethics may be just as false an ideal as that of reason's ability to establish a content-full, canonical conception of the good, and there may be little or no reason to consider either a desirable characteristic of an ethical framework for bioethics. According to the contemporary appreciation of Aristotle's teleology being offered herein, there appears to be no rational basis for the claim that the end or goal of reason in ethics is to establish a canonical vision of the good life in the first place. Indeed, one need not accept this conception of the end of reason within ethics if one does not accept the starting points of the Enlightenment project. Thus, it is only if one shares a certain amount of moral intimacy with Engelhardt, inasmuch as one accepts the underlying foundations of Enlightenment thought, that one has any reason to believe that the failure of reason to establish a canonical vision of the good life is a failure at all.

A related reason Engelhardt's framework is excessively restrictive
is that the concepts of moral strangers and moral friends do not in fact
constitute an empty moral dichotomy that has no substantive breadth
but a rich continuum in which some universal moral truths may be discerned. Engelhardt's radical distinction between moral friends and moral
strangers gives us reason to suspect that he is assuming a particular sectarian view of community within his transcendental deduction of consent
as the foundation of morality. Such a view precludes the possibility of
there being some shared moral content within a community and amongst
individuals with some different moral and metaphysical commitments.
According to Engelhardt's conception of community as based on the concepts of moral friends and moral strangers, even Franciscan and Dominican priests cannot be considered as belonging to the same moral community since they do not share precisely the same metaphysical views. Their
own views of community, however, require that both groups view themselves as members of a larger overlapping community, namely, as Roman
Catholics. If Engelhardt's view precludes them from being part of this
larger community that is defined by overlapping values, then he is im-
porting his own view of community into his theory, which he may not do
according to the theoretical criteria of his own postmodern transcen-
dentalism (Wildes, 1997, p. 88). Like the Enlightenment project, the
postmodern libertarian project necessarily fails insofar as there is no
such creature as a purely content-less morality—procedural, formal, or
otherwise.

Contra Engelhardt, there may be some shared moral content, some
common conception of value, that does not imply nor entail a single conception of human flourishing. There may also be a third way—in addition
to that of divine revelation and reason alone—of discerning this shared
moral content that binds even moral strangers. For example, a philosophical anthropology of experience and history could be used to achieve reasonable agreement about the universal and essential traits of the human
form of life and their corresponding value. According to Martha Nussbaum, the universal and essential traits of the human form of life can be
discerned through the examination of the myths and stories of different
cultures despite the turn away from a metaphysical realism. As she argues:

Indeed, if, as the critics of realism allege, we are always dealing with our own
interpretations anyhow, they must acknowledge that universal conceptions of the
human are prominent and pervasive among such interpretations, hardly to be

relegated to the dustbin of metaphysical history along with rare and recondite philosophical entities such as the Platonic forms. (1995, p. 69)

Such an anthropology would not be merely an empirical study but a philosophical enterprise that is grounded in the common experiences of all human beings. This anthropology would not yield a full "canonical" conception of the good (nor must it be intended to) but only a "thick, vague" conception that identifies moral value at the level of essential traits that are characteristic of human life. This conception of the good is "vague" because it does not specify which capabilities must be engaged for a life to be the best possible of human lives. Rather, it specifies the functional capabilities that one must possess if one is to be *able* to live the life one judges to be the best kind of life. In this way, it leaves room for a plurality of competing visions of the good in which value is determined, in part, by one's full conception of the good and other subjective considerations, such as one's psychological and character traits, cultural-specific socialization, religious beliefs, etc. Though this anthropology necessarily involves empirical observations regarding the structure of human nature, it is also open to interpretation of these observations in light of social constructs. The latter do not present an insurmountable challenge to the universality of this anthropology, for its propositions are derived from common human experience as it unfolds in the history of all humanity across spatio-temporal and cultural boundaries (Nussbaum, 1995, pp. 70–71).

Within this framework, the moral relevance or significance of the values that correspond to such essential and universal traits of human life do not depend on any particular conception of rationality. Rather, their moral relevance only depends on the claim that some material conditions are necessary and some needs must first be satisfied before one can live a characteristically human life and attain other secondary goods, whether one is working with an Enlightenment, a feminist, a critical theory, or a deconstructionist conception of rationality. Indeed, even a libertarian must agree that some needs and conditions must be fulfilled in order for individuals to exercise those capacities that give negative rights their moral significance. However, it may still be the case that, even though these values are universal, not everyone will recognize them as such.

While a thick, vague conception of the good necessarily consists of claims regarding the essential capabilities and dispositional traits of human nature, to which there may not be complete agreement, a system of morality between moral strangers could rely only on those claims to which some reasonable amount of agreement can be achieved. More simply, the philosophical anthropology described above could be open to some rules of inference, such as rules of procedural neutrality. Building on the thought of Jurgen Habermas, Charles Larmore has suggested that such liberal political neutrality can be achieved through the use of "a universal norm of rational dialogue" (1987, p. 53). This conception of neutrality depends upon a kind of dialectical conversation that proceeds from and, as necessary, returns to neutral ground for the purpose of continuing moral dialogue. Controversial beliefs concerning basic goods could be set aside for the purpose of resolving dispute or, if there is no resolution to be found, bypassing the matter on which that dispute is founded. Yet, only those beliefs that prove to be most controversial would have to be put aside and only temporarily so. As Larmore writes with regard to such controversial beliefs, "one can remain as convinced of [their] truth as before, but for the purposes of the conversation one sets [them] aside" (1987, p. 53). In this way, an element of rational advantage and consensus, that is, of liberal procedural neutrality, can be built into an Aristotelian account of moral teleology for the postmodern world.

This appreciation of Aristotle's teleological framework is in agreement with Engelhardt's view that consent is a necessary element of ethics in the postmodern world, but does not reduce ethics to consent alone. Within this framework, consent is a normatively rich concept to the extent that it is through peaceful conflict resolution, rather than conflict resolution via violence, that we as morally free and rational creatures will not be deprived of the material conditions necessary for characteristically human functioning. In other words, the very foundation of consent in any morally robust sense is the fact that there are some common human needs that must first be satisfied if we are to function in ways (when luck is on our side) that constitute some approximation of human flourishing, according to our own full-content vision of the good. In this sense, this framework provides a reasonable basis, where Engelhardt's cannot, for responding to the ethical nihilist as to why consent is preferable over violence as a means of conflict resolution.

Teleology and Human Nature in the 21st Century

Perhaps an even more ominous objection to ethical naturalism is the claim that, because we will soon have the ability to refashion our genetic constitution as we see fit, there is no objective human nature that could act as the guiding normative force. As Engelhardt argues, "the likelihood that we will be able to refashion our human nature reveals how few general secular moral constraints there are to guide us. Paradoxically, the more we are able to reengineer our human nature, the less guidance is available" (1996c, p. 47). The explicit assumption upon which Engelhardt's argument rests is that within the 21st century we will have the ability to reengineer human nature so radically that there will be numerous species identifiable with the genus *Homo.* In his words, these species "could be identified as distinct not merely through the absence of cross-fertile mating, but through reference to substantial differences that would be the result of refashioning human nature in pursuit of human well-being" (1996c, p. 48). One implication of this line of reasoning is that if we can indeed change human nature as we see fit, then there is no one objective human nature that can provide any normative guidance.

The ability to reengineer human nature to the extent that Engelhardt speculates will likely come about (if at all) through germ-line gene therapy, in which a gene residing in cells within the reproductive system is either replaced or altered so as to create a change in the genome of both an individual and that individual's offspring. In principle, genes could be transferred into the gametes of adult human beings, into human zygotes, or preimplantation embryos created through in vitro fertilization (Walters & Palmer, 1997, pp. 61–66). While germ-line gene therapy presents the possibility of preventing damage during fetal development due to inherited diseases, because it would be performed at the earliest stages of development, it also has the potential to be used for the purpose of genetic enhancement. Genetic enhancements aimed at physical size, need for sleep, aging, memory, aggression, and general cognitive ability could impact human capabilities in three different spheres of functioning: physical strength and longevity; intelligence or, at least, components of intelligence; and behavior (Walters & Palmer, 1997, pp. 101–108). Though the technical capability to effect such enhancements is still somewhere in the future, it is not a very big leap to imagine a scenario like Engelhardt's in which there are some human beings who can imbibe pint after pint of stout while consuming tomes of Aristotle on very little sleep and, most likely through some unforeseen side effect of the germ-line gene transfer, would be unable to procreate successfully with other human beings.

Still, arguments regarding the malleability of human nature and its subsequent inability to provide any normative guidance are not unique to the 21st century. Indeed, such possibilities would seem to lend support to an older version of the same objection that human beings do not have an essential nature but create their own subjective essence. Take, for example, Jean-Paul Sartre's famous dictum that "existence precedes essence." According to Sartre, this statement means that:

If man, as the existentialist conceives him, is indefinable, it is because at first he is nothing. Only afterward will he be something, and he himself will have made what he will be. . . . Not only is man what he conceives himself to be, but he is also only what he wills himself to be after his thrust toward existence. Man is nothing else but what he makes himself. (1957, p. 15)

Though from different lines of thought, Engelhardt and Sartre's arguments would seem to lead to the same conclusion, namely, that human nature is essentially what we will it to be and, therefore, normatively vacuous.

However, the problem with this existentialist view of nature and essence is that it downplays, if not misses altogether, the significance that existence itself holds for the possibilities of what the human person may make of him- or herself. The existence that "precedes essence" is not some kind of blank slate with which we are free to do as we please, at least not without putting that very existence in some jeopardy. Rather, existing as a human being necessarily and simultaneously entails certain characteristics, without which we would not exist as human beings, for example, embodiment of a certain kind, human understanding, and free practical reasoning. Though we may will to manifest our existence in different ways, these characteristics are predetermined and objective and provide an organic unity to our lives (Lee, 1988, pp. 135–151). It is implausible, then, to expect that certain basic human goods could be changed or eliminated no matter what we will our essence to be or how we alter the human genome.

Moreover, the fact that through germ-line genetic engineering we may soon be able to alter human nature so radically that there would be several different species recognizable as falling under the genus *Homo* implies neither that there was no objective human nature to begin with nor that it offered no normative guidance. The fact that we may choose to disregard any normative guidance that an objective human nature has to offer, and thereby create new human natures, does not itself imply that there is no objective human nature here and now. It is perfectly consistent to hold that there is an objective human nature and that the same will to power through which we may choose to ignore its normative guidance is part of that human nature. In other words, the fact that we can and might actually choose to ignore any normative guidance offered by human nature does not in itself imply that there is no objective human nature nor that it is normatively vacuous.

But if human nature can be changed, then why should it have any normative force in the first place? From a teleological perspective in the Aristotelian sense, we might reply that the basic goods, whose content depends on the structure of human nature, are nothing less than the very opportunities for human flourishing. As Henry B. Veatch describes it:

Given a definition of goodness . . . in terms of a thing's actuality or perfection, it becomes possible to give an explanation of just how or why the properties of a thing can be the source of its goodness or value: they are just insofar as they are properties that evidence the perfection or complete actuality of the thing in question. (1962, p. 109)

The implication is twofold. First, the teleological conception of human nature provides a hermeneutic lens through which we can evaluate the moral status of prospective ways of altering the human genome. That is, the human nature that we all share here and now, and the basic goods correlated with what it means to function in characteristically human ways, can provide some basis for determining whether particular altera-tions to the human genome are consistent with a reasonable conception of human well-being and, therefore, ought to be pursued or not. Second, were our nature to change, so would the basic goods associated with that nature. While the basic goods and our duties might be different if our human nature was, or becomes, different, this change itself would not imply the absence of the teleological nature of these goods.

So what, then, are we to make of Engelhardt's concern that in the fu-ture there may be multiple species that belong to the genus *Homo* but are incapable of interspecies propagation? While such species would still belong to the genus *Homo,* they simply would not be human in the sense that we have recognized the human person throughout history and across our various cultures. Due to the absence of the potential to propagate the species *Homo sapiens,* they would not be of the same natural kind and would not have the same recognizable human nature. Rather than con-cluding that there is no human nature, we might conclude that human nature can be the basis for moral norms, but that these norms simply would not apply to those individuals whose nature has been so radically altered that they are incapable of propagating our species. Since the nature of any new species would be different from that which we recognize as our own human nature, so, too, would be the content of their specific duties and norms. Still, if there were to be some commonality between the human natures of the different species, then there would be some common basic goods shared as well.

While many of the changes that we might expect to occur through genetic germ-line reengineering, such as changes in normal levels of health, IQ and the need for sleep, would not be morally relevant at the fundamental level of basic goods, it is not reasonable to expect that basic goods such as knowledge, practical reason, and friendship would lose their value because of these changes. Neither do the potential differences between the species preclude the possibility of ethical naturalism or a teleological ethics, for, while there may not be any interspecies propagation in Engelhardt's scenario, intraspecies sexual procreation would retain its teleological value and remain a basic good of every variety of human life. If the human genome were to be altered so radically that at least some of the basic goods of human life would not still be recognizable as basic goods, then it is dubious that we would be able to even recognize those new species as belonging to the same genus.

If, then, there is an objective human nature, and we choose to heed the normative guidance it has to offer, what does it tell us about how we ought to employ the medical technologies that may emerge over the course of the 21st century, such as germ-line gene therapy? First, the basic goods of human life and the concept of characteristic human functioning can provide the basis for a normatively robust conception of health and disease. A robust understanding of human nature understood in its teleological context can provide a conceptual foundation for Norman Daniels's definition of health as "species-typical functioning" (Daniels, 1985, pp. 26–32). While reason alone will not disclose to us what specific types of functions should be counted as species-typical in the absence of universally settled moral convictions regarding this point, a teleological understanding of human nature as described herein could provide the framework and context in which some consensus regarding this point can be achieved. Once achieved, this definition of health can provide the basis for distinguishing between gene therapy aimed at curing or preventing disease and genetic enhancement aimed at improving the capacities of healthy individuals (Anderson, 1989).

In turn, this distinction could also be useful in making policy decisions, such as those regarding resource allocation. For example, we as reasonable members of society and of a moral community that shares some moral intimacy might agree that those who have existing therapeutic options available to them to restore some element of characteristic human functioning should have a certain amount of priority on our healthcare resources. Certain limits would then arise regarding how much, if any, of our public resources would be dedicated to those emerging genetic interventions that are determined to be enhancements rather than therapies. Moreover, we might also agree that government-funded research should be limited to gene therapies and not enhancement interventions, which would be of benefit only to those already capable of a reasonable level of characteristic human functioning.

Genetic interventions on the human germ-line, whether therapeutic in nature or as a form of enhancement, also give rise to questions regarding the adequacy of consent as the sole normative constraint on collaborative moral ventures such as would be required to make germ-line gene therapy a reality. For what we do to the germ line, we also do to future generations—generations that have no way of consenting to how we may alter the human nature they otherwise would have had. Given that we cannot have an adequate understanding of the potential harms that may result until it is too late and real harm has been done (Walters & Palmer, 1997, pp. 82–83), adequate consent for genetic germ-line human subject research seems nearly impossible. While it may be objected that reason alone is incapable of establishing an obligation to obtain the consent of future persons, germ-line genetic interventions will most likely be performed on actual human life in its earliest stages of development.

Though postmodernists, among others, may be hesitant to allow the human zygote, preimplantation embryo, or early fetus the moral standing of postnatal, sentient, and fully autonomous persons, even some moral strangers of diverse value perspectives but with similar metaphysical presuppositions would agree that the destruction or other harm to preimplantation embryos in research is incompatible with the kind of respect that should be given to early human life. I would argue that such views would be consistent with the contemporary appreciation of Aristotelian teleology offered herein. Within this Aristotelian framework, if preimplantation embryos are human life, only at a very early stage, then this early human life has the same "telos" as the more developed or actualized members of the same natural kind. In other words, interfering with one's ability, present or future, to actualize the capabilities that are characteristic of that form of life without consent would be no less a moral harm, simply because the actualization of those capabilities has not been achieved. In this way, the same rational grounds that provide the normative force of consent as a constraint on action between fully autonomous individuals also provides the same rational basis for constraints on actions impacting human life in its earliest stages, at least within the teleological perspective offered herein.

Conclusion

Clearly, a thick but vague conception of the good rooted in a concept of characteristic human functioning will not provide answers to all, or even many, bioethical questions and conflicts, particularly in the absence of an actual dialogue regarding the corresponding primary values. Likewise, there will always be a role for consent within a postmodern world inhabited by moral strangers. While the absence of a canonical conception of the good appears to be an indisputable fact of the moral geography in the postmodern world, a thick but vague conception of the good understood in its teleological context can provide the basis for some universal negative obligations of a deontological nature. In other words, while we may not be able to specify any single objective account of human flourishing for all individuals, we may be able to say what would not objectively count as or contribute to human flourishing. Moreover, there is no basis for believing this to be a failure of reason rather than a necessary and perhaps even desirable result of human complexity.

Reference List

Anderson, W. F. (1989). Human gene therapy: Why draw a line? *Journal of Medicine and Philosophy, 14,* 681–693.

Aristotle. (1984a). *Nichomachean Ethics* (W. D. Ross, Trans.). In J. Barnes (Ed.), *Aristotle: The complete works.* Princeton, NJ: Princeton University Press.

Aristotle. (1984b). *Physics* (W. D. Ross, Trans.). In J. Barnes (Ed.), *Aristotle: The complete works.* Princeton, NJ: Princeton University Press.

Ashley, B., & O'Rourke, K. (1997). *Health care ethics: A theological analysis* (4th ed.). Washington, DC: Georgetown University Press.

Beauchamp, T., & Childress, J. (1994). *Principles of biomedical ethics* (4th ed.). New York: Oxford University Press.

Boyle, J. M. (1994). Radical moral disagreement in contemporary health care: A Roman Catholic perspective. *Journal of Medicine and Philosophy, 16,* 183–200.

Broad, C. D. (1930). *Five types of ethical theory.* London: K. Paul, Trench, Trubner.

Broadie, S. (1991). *Ethics with Aristotle.* New York: Oxford University Press.

Burnyeat, M. F. (1980). Aristotle on learning to be good. In A. Rorty (Ed.), *Essays on Aristotle's ethics* (pp. 69–92). Berkeley: University of California Press.

Callahan, D. (1996). Can nature serve as a moral guide? *Hastings Center Report, 26*(6), 21–22.

Clarke, S., & Simpson, E. (1989). The primacy of moral practice. In S. Clarke & E. Simpson (Eds.), *Anti-theory in ethics and moral conservatism* (pp. 1–16). Albany: State University of New York Press.

Daniels, N. (1985). *Just health care.* Cambridge, England: Cambridge University Press.

Daniels, N. (1996). Wide reflective equilibrium in bioethics. In L. W. Sumner and J. M. Boyle (Eds.), *Philosophical perspectives on bioethics* (pp. 96–114). Toronto: University of Toronto Press.

Engelhardt, H. T. (1996a). Bioethics reconsidered. *Kennedy Institute of Ethics Journal, 6,* 336–341.

Engelhardt, H. T. (1996b). *The foundations of bioethics* (2nd ed.). New York: Oxford University Press.

Engelhardt, H. T. (1996c). Germ-line genetic engineering and moral diversity: Moral controversies in a post-Christian world. *Social Philosophy and Policy, 13*(2), 47–62.

Engelhardt, H. T. (2004, September). *The birth of bioethics critically reassessed.* Paper presented at the Distinguished Speakers Series at Saint Louis University, Saint Louis, MO.

Finnis, J. (1983). *Fundamentals of ethics.* Washington, DC: Georgetown University Press.

Frankena, W. (1973). *Ethics* (2nd ed.). Englewood Cliffs, NJ: Prentice-Hall Publishing.

Gert, B., Culver, C., & Clouser, K. D. (1997). *Bioethics: A return to fundamentals.* New York: Oxford University Press.

Hampshire, S. (1983). *Morality and conflict.* Cambridge, MA: Harvard University Press.

Jonsen, A. (1998). *The birth of bioethics.* New York: Oxford University Press.

Jonsen, A., & Toulmin, S. (1988). *The abuse of casuistry.* Berkeley: University of California Press.

Kant, I. (1996). *Groundwork of the metaphysics of morals* (M. J. McGregor, Trans.). Cambridge, England: Cambridge University Press. (Original work published 1785)

Kavanaugh, J. F. (2001). *Who count as persons? Human identity and the ethics of killing.* Washington, DC: Georgetown University Press.

Keenan, J., & Shannon, T. (1995). *The context of casuistry.* Washington, DC: Georgetown University Press.

Kekes, J. (1995). *Moral wisdom and good lives.* Ithaca, NY: Cornell University Press.

Lachs, J. (1995). *The relevance of philosophy to life.* Nashville, TN: Vanderbilt University Press.

Larmore, C. (1987). *Patterns of moral complexity.* Cambridge: Cambridge University Press.

Lee, P. (1988). Human beings are animals. In R. George (Ed.), *Natural law and moral inquiry* (pp. 135–151). Washington, DC: Georgetown University Press.

Lesher, J. H. (2001). On Aristotelian episteme as understanding. *Ancient Philosophy, 21,* 45–55.

Levine, C. (Ed.). (1989). *Cases in bioethics: Selections from the Hastings Center Report.* New York: St. Martin's Press.

MacIntyre, A. (1984). *After virtue: A study in moral theory* (2nd ed.). Notre Dame, IN: University of Notre Dame Press.

MacIntyre, A. (1988). *Whose justice? Which rationality?* Notre Dame, IN: University of Notre Dame Press.

MacIntyre, A. (1998). *A short history of ethics: A history of moral philosophy from the Homeric age to the twentieth century* (2nd ed.). Notre Dame, IN: University of Notre Dame Press.

Mill, J. S. (1987). *Utilitarianism.* New York: Prometheus Books. (Original work published 1859)

Nagel, T. (1979). *Mortal questions.* Cambridge, England: Cambridge University Press.

Nussbaum, M. (1985). The discernment of perception: An Aristotelian conception of private and public rationality. *Proceedings of the Boston Colloquium on Ancient Philosophy, 1,* 151–201.

Nussbaum, M. (1992). Human functioning and social justice: In defense of Aristotelian essentialism. *Political Theory* 20, 2 (1992): 202–246.

Nussbaum, M. (1993). Non-relative virtues: An Aristotelian approach. In M. Nussbaum & A. Sen (Eds.), *The quality of life* (pp. 242–269). New York: Oxford University Press.

Nussbaum, M. (1995). Human capabilities, female humans. In J. Glover & M. Nussbaum (Eds.), *Women, culture and development* (pp. 61–104). New York: Oxford University Press.

Pellegrino, E. (2000). Bioethics at century's turn: Can normative ethics be retrieved? *Journal of Medicine and Philosophy, 25,* 655–675.

Rawls, J. (1971). *A theory of justice.* Cambridge, MA: Harvard University Press.

Rawls, J. (1985). Justice as fairness: Political not metaphysical. *Philosophy & Public Affairs, 14,* 223–251.

Rawls, J. (1993). *Political liberalism: The John Dewey essays in philosophy.* New York: Columbia University Press.

Sartre, J. P. (1957). *Existentialism and human emotion.* New York: Philosophical Library.

Sen, A. (1992). *Inequality reexamined.* Cambridge, MA: Harvard University Press.

Scheffler, S. (1988). *Consequentialism and its critics.* Oxford: Oxford University Press.

Sherman, N. (1991). *The fabric of character: Aristotle's theory of virtue.* Oxford, England: Clarendon Press.

Urmson, J. O. (1975). A defense of intuitionism. *The Proceedings of the Aristotelian Society, 75,* 111–119.

Veatch, H. B. (1962). *Rational man: A modern interpretation of Aristotelian ethics.* Bloomington: Indiana University Press.

Veatch, R. M. (2000). Doctor does not know best: Why in the new century physicians must stop trying to benefit patients. *Journal of Medicine and Philosophy, 25,* 701–721.

Walters, L., & Palmer, J. G. (1997). *The ethics of human gene therapy.* New York: Oxford University Press.

Watson, G. (1990). On the primacy of character. In O. Flannagan & A. O. Rorty (Eds.), *Identity, character and morality* (pp. 449–470). Cambridge, MA: MIT Press.

Wiggins, D. (1976). Deliberation and practical reason. *Proceedings of the Aristotelian Society, 76,* 29–51.

Wildes, K. (1997). Engelhardt's communitarian ethics. In B. Minogue, G. Palmer Fernandez, & J. E. Reagan (Eds.), *Reading Engelhardt: Essays on the thought of H. Tristram Engelhardt, Jr.* (pp. 77–94). Boston: Kluwer Academic.

Wildes, K. (2000). *Moral acquaintances: Methodology in bioethics.* Notre Dame, IN: University of Notre Dame Press.

Wreen, M. (1998). Nihilism, relativism and Engelhardt. *Theoretical Medicine, 19,* 73–88.

An Ancient Ethics for 21st-Century Healthcare

Slosar argues that today's ethics, both in healthcare and elsewhere, gives individuals a choice between two unsatisfying alternatives: a deontological ethics like that of Kant, or a consequentialist ethics like that of Mill and other utilitarians. These two models for ethics have been dominant for so long that they tower over all ethical discussions. Even attempts at new ways of thinking in ethics inevitably situate themselves as responses to one or both of these models, and often thus become trapped in the same limited options these two models offer. Slosar searches for a way out of this bind, a way out of the dominance of deontology and utilitarianism over our ethical thinking; and he finds the answer not by looking forward but backward to the father of systematic ethics in the West: Aristotle. Through Aristotle, Slosar hopes to recover a teleological ethics that offers us a glimpse at the in-between that helps us make decisions when deontological and utilitarian ethics cannot.

It may be helpful to look in more detail at Aristotle's thinking on how one can become a moral person and perform moral acts. For Aristotle, these two goals are inescapably intertwined; one cannot perform moral acts without being a moral person, and one cannot become a moral person without making a habit of practicing moral acts (2000, II, 1–2). A person who wishes to become moral must also put her desires in order, training herself to desire to do moral acts. In this way, Aristotle completes a happy circle for the moral person: If her desires are in order, she will desire to do moral acts; this desire will motivate her to perform those acts; when she does perform them, she will be satisfying her own desires, and will therefore be not only moral but fulfilled as well.

When a person finds herself in a situation where a moral decision must be made, she can draw on these desires and habits to help guide her. In addition, while forming these moral habits, she will have acquired practical experience; this practical experience can help her determine the right thing to do if she is faced with a complicated situation. Using her practical experience, she then looks to Aristotle's concept of the mean; the right action, Aristotle says, is that which accords with the mean between the extremes of excess and deficiency, relative to the person and the situation.

This model of ethical decision making can provide guidance in situations where deontological and utilitarian ethics may lead to conflicting or inconclusive results. For example, Janet is an emergency room nurse faced with a dilemma. A family has been in a car accident, and Janet is overseeing the treatment of the father, Mr. L. She knows that the rest of the family did not survive the accident. Mr. L.'s condition is critically unstable. He asks Janet, "Is the rest of my family okay?" Janet faces a dilemma: Lie to her patient, thus violating a trust, or tell him the truth and risk harming his health and his chance at pulling through.

In this situation, Kantian ethics gives no leeway. It is always wrong to lie; one has a duty to tell the truth always. Kantian ethics, as Slosar points out, gives no consideration to relationships or circumstances. While this answer for Janet may be refreshingly clear and certain, it is alarming in its lack of attention to the particulars of the situation. Furthermore, one could argue that Janet is also bound by her duty as a nurse to preserve the health of her patient, in which case she has two binding duties that conflict with each other. On the other hand, utilitarianism teaches Janet to look to the consequences and maximize the net good. This seems easy at first: Surely she should spare Mr. L. any danger by lying to him. However, what if Janet looks at the bigger picture? How much is she hurting her relationship with Mr. L. or with future patients by being willing to lie to them? How much is she affecting the future status of nurse–patient trust in general? Also, what if Mr. L. can handle the truth? If telling him the truth would not in fact harm his health, then that is clearly the best thing to do. And herein lies the problem with utilitarianism: To calculate the net good, Janet needs to be able to see the bigger picture, short term and long term, and she needs to be able to predict consequences (e.g., the result of telling Mr. L. the truth), which, in this case, she cannot accurately predict.

Enter Aristotle. His ethics allows Janet to take into consideration the particulars of the situation, including her own desires and capabilities.

Since the virtue in question here is honesty, Janet thinks of what the extreme excess of honesty would be in this situation: To tell Mr. L. flat-out, "Your family did not survive." On the other hand, the extreme deficiency of honesty would be to lie: "They're fine." By considering these two extremes, both undesirable, and employing her practical experience and wisdom (acquired both in her personal and professional life), Janet can seek an action that falls in the mean, in the right spot between the extremes. This type of deliberation calls for creativity rather than Kantian rule following or utilitarian calculation of the good. This creative approach may lead Janet to some compromise, such as an attempt to avoid the question: "You just worry about getting better," or "I'll ask the other nurses when we're done taking care of you."

However, Aristotelian ethics need not lead to a compromise just because it seeks the mean. As Aristotle says, sometimes the mean (i.e., the right thing to do) is close to the extreme (2000, II, 6). Employing her practical experience and drawing on her moral habits and moral character, Janet can adjust her behavior as the situation unfolds. If avoiding the question results in further questions and agitation from Mr. L., her practical wisdom may lead her to gently tell him the truth, or it may lead her to lie to him, with a promise to herself to apologize and explain her actions to him once he is stable. In this way, Aristotelian ethics allows Janet to constantly reevaluate the situation and to draw on that valuable tool of professional experience and judgment that neither Kantian nor utilitarian ethics gives heed to.

Kantian or utilitarian ethicists may object to the above example, insisting that a creative solution such as artfully avoiding the question is well within the parameters of both Kant's deontological principles and the utilitarians' happiness principle. Saying "You just worry about getting better" does not cause Janet to lie, and it may be the best way to achieve the greatest net happiness. However, neither Kantian nor utilitarian ethics provides a way to search for that in-between solution. Kant tells Janet, "Do not lie," not what to do in a complicated situation where lying might seem best. Utilitarians tell Janet to maximize the net happiness, but without a way to calculate consequences on a large scale; this advice is not overly helpful, nor does it offer a method of *finding* the action that will maximize the net good.

If Aristotle's ethics, as Slosar suggests, can offer us methods and answers that the two modern paradigmatic schools cannot, then why has contemporary ethics consistently overlooked that option? Slosar argues that "the paradigmatic status of Kant's ethics and utilitarianism is not an accident of modernity. Rather, it rests on explicit and critical philosophical inquiry regarding the nature of moral value and human reason" (p. 145). In other words, contemporary ethics looks to these two models because they best fit our idea of what ethics should be. One thing these two models offer us that Aristotle does not is a clear-cut, systematic decision-making process. We know the principle we're following—the categorical imperative or the happiness principle—and we act in accordance with that principle. We can perform Kant's test of universalizing the maxim behind our actions or we can calculate the consequences of our actions and determine net happiness. In Slosar's words, "While dichotomously opposed, . . . both procedures are intended to ensure proper moral response to situational particulars through the intellectual application of decision-making rules" (p. 147). Aristotle's ethics, in contrast, is much messier. Aristotle explicitly does not want to tell his readers *what to do.* He wants to tell them *how to be.* In an era when technology, managed care, longer life expectancy, and many other factors make healthcare ethics more complex than ever, we are understandably drawn to the ethics that will tell us what to do no matter what. As Slosar states, "the central task of modern moral theory has been the justification of a single theory that makes either some version of the principle of the good or some version of the principle of the right always and everywhere, in every circumstance, normatively fundamental" (p. 141).

Slosar argues, however, that Aristotle's ethics can provide more guidance than we might at first think. Aristotelian ethics does not condemn us to each individual making her own decisions based on her own standards, Slosar would say, because we are all human beings and therefore share a common concept of the good based on our needs and desires as human beings. Even among people of diverse backgrounds or cultures, Slosar claims, we can at least find a "thick, vague" conception of the good in common. Anthony Weston makes a similar point, insisting that even when views of the good seem absolutely opposed, the disagreement is likely to be more one of facts than of values (2002, p. 8). For instance, two nurses in Janet's situation might make different decisions about the right thing to do, but that disagreement might be because of their different assessments of the *fact* of Mr. L.'s health. Such may also be the case in bioethics issues such as stem-cell research. A man who utterly opposes any stem-cell research may in fact share the same core values as a man who supports the research, but they disagree on the facts. The opponent believes that life begins at conception (a judgment about facts), whereas the proponent believes life begins some time later; it is likely that they both agree that human life is to be respected and preserved when possible. If Weston's claim of disagreement over facts rather than values is accurate, then Slosar's claim that we as a society can look to a shared "thick, vague" conception of the good as guidance for Aristotelian deliberation seems quite feasible. As Slosar states, we should be careful in giving heed to Engelhardt's concept of "moral strangers"; we should not exclude the "possibility of there being some shared moral content within a community and amongst individuals," even if they do have "some different moral and metaphysical commitments" (p. 172).

Slosar suggests that "controversial beliefs concerning basic goods could be set aside for the purpose of resolving dispute or, if there is no resolution to be found, bypassing the matter on which that dispute is founded" (p. 174). Turning again to Weston, such a strategy could lead vehemently opposed parties to a practical, feasible, and positive solution. If activists on both sides of the abortion debate were to put aside slogans such as "God Hates Abortion," "Abortion Stops a Beating Heart," and "If You're Against Abortion, Don't Have One," they could find the common ground in their shared belief that we should work together toward a better society where "every child [is] a wanted child" (2002, p. 64). Moreover, Slosar argues that even when disagreements do arise about basic goods, we can turn to rational dialogue that "proceeds from and, as necessary, returns to neutral ground for the purpose of continuing moral dialogue" (p. 174). Similarly, Weston argues that dialogue should start with the assumption that "each side is right about *something*" (2002, p. 52). Difficult matters are difficult, Weston says, precisely *because* each side has a valid point. For instance, the issue of assisted suicide is difficult because "freedom from pain matters, and autonomy matters, and also respect for life matters. *Both sides are right*" (2002, p. 54).

If both sides are right, then the only way to a solution is dialogue, and Slosar argues that this dialogue will fare best in the context of an Aristotelian, teleological concept of the good. Though Slosar does not explicitly invoke Aristotle's teacher, Plato, his emphasis on dialogue is certainly in accordance with that other ancient thinker, as well as *his* teacher, Socrates. As captured in Plato's immortal works (written, significantly, in dialogue form), Socrates is a model ethicist who believes all searches for the good must take place through dialogue, in a respectful exchange of ideas. Socrates believes that "human beings are simply more resourceful this way in action, speech and thought" (Plato, 1992, 348d).

Let us turn one more time to Janet. Following Slosar's model of ethics—dialogue within an Aristotelian framework—Janet will make her decision in the case of Mr. L., and her decision will be based on her professional experience along with her own moral character and habits. Ideally, Janet will also find an opportunity soon to discuss her decision with colleagues, and maybe even with Mr. L. himself. By engaging in such a dialogue, Janet can explore her own concepts of the good and learn more about how others see the good, and perhaps how others would have acted in her situation. The next time Janet faces a moral dilemma in her work, she will have this additional experience—including the decision, the outcome, and the dialogue—to draw on; and this experience, combined with her moral character, will help her determine the right thing to do. The ethics of Plato and Aristotle are ancient, true, but they offer possibilities for 21st-century healthcare that allow us to find and explore the in-between left by those two looming modern models, Kantian and utilitarian ethics.

References

Aristotle. (2000). *Nicomachean ethics* (T. Irwin, Trans.). Indianapolis, IN: Hackett.
Plato. (1992). *Protagoras* (S. Lombardo & K. Bell, Trans.). Indianapolis, IN: Hackett.
Weston, A. (2002). *A practical companion to ethics.* New York: Oxford University Press.

5

Reflections of Moral Dilemmas and Patterns of Ethical Decision Making in Five Clinical Physical Therapists

BRUCE H. GREENFIELD

Introduction

Physical therapists, like all healthcare workers, make value judgments about the clinical care of their patients. Often, however, values between patients, physical therapists, and other healthcare workers conflict, challenging the moral obligations (duties) of the physical therapists to do the right thing. Although a code of ethics provides a moral framework for physical therapy (American Physical Therapy Association [APTA], 2002c), some physical therapists may find the principles contained in codes of ethics too abstract or impersonal to address their day-to-day moral concerns and issues. Referring to codes of ethics, Liaschenko and Peter (2004) write, "Codes of ethics are the primary means for expressing the values and regulating the conduct of professionals in relation to their clients. . . . Yet we find professional ethics and codes of ethics to be of limited use in the everyday morality of practitioners and their work environments" (p. 489).

Purtilo distinguishes between morality and ethics. Morality, writes Purtilo, "is concerned with relations between people and how, ultimately, they can best live in peace and harmony" (1999, p. 7). Ethics, conversely, "is a systematic reflection on morality" (Purtilo, 1999, p.12). Ethical considerations about one's moral position occur in the presence of a moral dilemma. A moral dilemma occurs in the presence of conflict when one must decide a course of action by balancing two or more values that are both held dear (Purtilo, 1999). I will argue in this paper that the moral dilemmas physical therapists face as well as physical therapists' ethical decision making are embedded in their daily practice experience, reflective of what Liaschenko and Peter (2004) describe as the "housekeeping issues that make up most of health care work that are largely ignored or invisible" (p. 491).

A particular purpose of this research was to examine how physical therapists process moral dilemmas in practice, as compared to the theoretical framework of normative ethical decision making. Physical therapy is a health profession that specializes in the evaluation and treatment of patients with physical impairments to restore function and prevent disability (APTA, 1997). In order to meet its professional responsibilities, physical therapy has moved toward greater autonomy within the field of healthcare. The board of directors of the APTA wrote in its 2002 statement, "autonomous physical therapist practice is characterized by independent, self-determined professional judgment and action" (APTA, 2002d, p. 14). In addition, the APTA vision statement supports advanced education with a clinical doctorate degree: "Physical therapy by 2020 will be provided by physical therapists that are doctors of physical therapy. . . . Physical therapists will be practitioners of and will hold all privileges of autonomous practice" (APTA, 2002b, p. 1).

As an indication of physical therapists' growing autonomy, data show that more than half of the states now allow physical therapists direct patient access in order to evaluate and treat patients without a physician's referral (APTA, 2002a). As of 2004, there were 111 physical therapy programs that offered a Doctor of Physical Therapy (DPT) degree versus 98 that offered a Master of Physical Therapy (MPT) degree, indicating that 53% of physical therapy programs now offer the DPT (APTA, 2004). As physical therapists gain more autonomy in healthcare, they are forced to take greater responsibility without the oversight of physicians to determine the type, nature, and course of patient treatment. Professional autonomy requires that physical therapists identify ethical issues that arise in practice and implement ethical decision making (Clawson, 1994; Magistro, 1989). Guccione's survey of the clinical practices of New England physical therapists identified moral dilemmas related to patient autonomy, interprofessional relations, and resource distribution (Guccione,

1980). Because moral dilemmas frequently occur in the course of patient care, the practice of physical therapy is a moral as well as a clinical
endeavor.

The concern with the inability to fully understand how physical therapists act as moral agents in clinical practice is the basis for this study. I
argue that physical therapists lack a depth of understanding about the
complexities of morality and ethics in their own lives and in the lives of
their colleagues. Researchers have done surveys of physical therapists
asking questions about moral dilemmas. To date, no research fully ex-
plores the professional life stories of physical therapists in order to
understand their own morality and ethics. Some elements of moral practice have been posited in the literature (Barnitt, 1998; Blackner, 2000;
Clawson, 1994; Guccione, 1980; Magistro, 1989; Purtilo, 1999; Triezenberg, 1996; Wise, 2000) but the research is sometimes conflicting. Raz,
Jensen, Walter, and Drake (1991) carried out in-depth interviews to examine the values, perceptions, and experiences of 10 female physical
therapists as they related to their professional development. They argued
that female professionalism differed from the traditional male professional model and proposed a theory of gender-based professionalism related to caring that reflected the data from female participants' interviews. On the other hand, Wise (2000) sampled 10 physical therapists,
including three men, and found that both male and female participants
focused on caring as central to their weighing factors in making decisions.
Jensen, Gwyer, Shepherd, and Hack (2000) examined the dimensions of
clinical expertise across genders with 12 physical therapists categorized
as experts and found that caring and commitment to their patients was
paramount, with each focusing on the role of personal advocacy for their
patients. These studies found the values of caring and responsiveness to
be central to the practice of physical therapy, but the Jensen et al. study
suggested that these values may be related to expertise, rather than to
gender. Research studies reviewed suggest that ethical decision making is
more complex than can be explained by a normative approach and that
the process is centered upon individual circumstances for patients and
particularities of a case. However, very little research presents physical
therapists' own stories to describe what constitutes a moral practice and
individual constructs of morality and ethics in the profession.

For this study, I used an interpretative narrative approach to describe
the moral dilemmas that physical therapists face in daily practice and

ways in which they make ethical decisions in the presence of these dilemmas. This interpretive approach was selected in order to understand better the experience of moral dilemmas and ethical decision making from the physical therapists' perspectives. I used in-depth interviews to answer the following questions:

1. What are the moral dilemmas faced by physical therapists?
2. How do physical therapists make ethical decisions?

Overview of the Problem

Medicine is a profession characterized by specialized knowledge and skills and by a value system that presumably guides its practitioners in making ethical decisions (Baker, Caplan, Emanuel, & Latham, 1999; Etzioni, 1969; Freidson, 1990; Purtilo, 1979; Reiser, Dyck, & Curran, 1977; Siegler, 1979). Purtilo (1999) indicates that the values of healthcare workers are based upon the fiduciary responsibility of the healthcare worker to the public, noting that when a person is placed in a position of special trust, that person should consider the best interests of the other party (p. 190).

Wylie (1998) argues that ever since there have been patients and healthcare providers, there has been ethical discourse in professional training, in the clinic, and in various medical journals. This discourse has influenced practitioners who direct the practice of healthcare. As Engelhardt (1996) explains, "Medicine is the medicine of the people. . . . Medicine is the agent of the people. It is engaged in their behalf. It is restrained by obligation to respect the wishes of persons and directed by the goal of doing good" (p. 276).

If healthcare is a moral profession, what provides the moral orientation of health care professionals? What does it mean to practice a normative morality and ethics? How does such morality and ethics compare to a nonnormative approach? How do these orientations direct moral judgments? What do these orientations fail to tell us about the moral practice of physical therapy? For most healthcare professions, these concerns led to a code of ethics, which defines the values and the moral principles of the profession. The philosophical underpinnings of morality in healthcare are contained within codes of ethics. Codes of ethics are rooted in Western culture, from the secular polytheism of Hippocrates and Plato, through the monotheistic Judeo-Christian tradition, to the 18th century

British and Scottish moralists (Reiser, Dyck, & Curran, 1977; Reiss, 2000). They
are normative documents that define the probity of activities and etiquette of
health caregivers toward their patients. A normative morality assumes a belief in
universal and ideal moral principles and values (Beauchamp & Childress, 2001).
Codes of ethics are also legal, political, and moral documents that define a
profession's scope of practice to the public.

The APTA Code of Ethics is the source of principles that prescribe
the moral obligations that physical therapists ought to follow in practice
toward each other and toward the public. In practical terms, the code of
ethics is the moral construct for the profession of physical therapy that
codifies good and bad behavior and right and wrong action. Therefore,
the code of ethics in the healthcare context of physical therapy, based as it
is in principilism, follows a model of morality that is normative. There are
important questions, however, about the role of a code of ethics in present
day clinical practice. First, how do the principles codified in the code of
ethics account for moral concerns and issues that physical therapists face
on a daily basis? Second, how do physical therapists use the code of ethics
to make ethical decisions in the presence of moral dilemmas?

Beauchamp and Childress (2001) explain that the purpose of a normative document is to establish obligatory moral standards for everyone
in the profession. These moral standards are framed as professional duties (Purtilo, 1999). Failing to abide by these standards is to engage in im-
proper conduct. With respect to the APTA's Code of Ethics, Guccione
(1980) states that the code may be seen as a guide for ethical judgments
of physical therapists by describing professional ideals and defining some
of the limits of morally acceptable behavior in the profession (p. 1264).
Limentani (1999) argues that the advantage to be gained from codes of
ethics is having a common vocabulary about the ethical nature of practice. This observation is not insignificant in light of Engelhardt's (1996)
observation about the meaning of ethics and morality: "There are numerous ambiguities at the very root of ethics. There is not even one sense of
ethics, but a family of senses. To answer moral questions, one must first
be clear about the meaning of morality and about the kind of morality at
stake" (p. 33). Therefore, a worthy goal of codes of ethics is to clarify a
moral language for its professional members.

The bases of normative morality in physical therapy include, but are
not limited to, beneficence, nonmaleficence, justice, and autonomy.
Autonomy is the moral principle holding that the right of a patient to

make decisions for him- or herself is paramount (Beauchamp & Childress, 2001). The philosophical underpinnings of these principles trace back to the moral idealism of the ancient Greeks. This moral idealism presupposes a universal truth about what is the right and good way to live. For example, Heraclitus (trans. 1979), writing before Socrates and Plato, held that:

Thought is common to all. Men must speak with understanding and hold fast to that which is common to all, as a city holds fast to its law, and much more strongly still. For all human laws are nourished by the one divine law. For it prevails as far as it wills, suffices for all, and there is something to spare. (p. 499)

This universal truth was later embodied in Judeo-Christian ethics. Eighteenth-century philosophers such as Kant secularized universal moral laws as categorical imperatives (Kant, 1785/1994). Seventeenth- and 18th-century Scottish and English physicians, such as Gregory and Percival, transformed moral laws into etiquette of gentlemanly practice (McCullough, 1998; Percival, 1794). Their writings formed the basis of the 1847 American Medical Association (AMA) Code of Ethics. In 1935, the APTA, then the American Physiotherapy Association, adopted its first Code of Ethics and Discipline, based on the medical code of ethics (Purtilo, 1997). Given these philosophical underpinnings, the principles in the current APTA Code of Ethics reflect a Western tradition of universal morality.

Limitations of Codes of Ethics

Despite the presence of codes of ethics, several authorities raise concerns about their use as a moral framework for clinicians, citing that codes give no specific guidance and give confusing guidance about ethical decision making (Davis, 1998; Engelhardt, 1996; Guccione, 1980; Limentani, 1999). These concerns warrant a discussion because they raise the deeper issue about the relevance of normative morality and ethics in a society that is ethnically and religiously diverse.

Codes' Lack of Guidance

Limentani (1999) argues that the use of principles as prima facie duties contrasts with actual duties. Prima facie duties are duties that all humans must fulfill in a general sense, all things being equal (Purtilo, 1999). But prima facie duties are not absolute, since particular principles applied to a moral dilemma may be equally compelling to an individual. That is, individuals are left with the problem of providing justification of their moral decisions as either good or right in a particular situation. The code of ethics does not describe how physical therapists apply moral principles in the presence of a moral dilemma. Rather, physical therapists must call upon their personal beliefs to establish moral justification for making decisions. At some point in time they must decide which principles or courses of action (to solve a moral dilemma) are appropriate in a particular situation. This may be problematic if physical therapists' values contrast with those in the APTA Code of Ethics (Appendix A). As Guccione (1980) states:

Conflict between personal values and professional values, or between the profession's values and society's attitudes, may easily arise. The professional organization's declaration of its values sometimes is helpful in these instances. However, beyond this declaration, each physical therapist must decide what he values as a health professional. (p. 1268)

It is important to be mindful, in other words, that professional organizations are aggregates of individuals whose perspectives and beliefs may be as diverse as the communities they serve. Professional organizations tend to pass down moral principles to guide their current practitioners. But until practitioners understand what their own values are, and how their values integrate into clinical practice and ethical decision making, the possibility of unresolved value conflict between the profession and its members exists.

Codes' Conflicting Guidance

Limentani (1999) argues that codes reduce morality to a list of principles that may raise unrealistic expectations about their scope in solving new and complex moral dilemmas. Limentani explains that principles sometimes may conflict with each other and will require further judgment to arrive at a moral conclusion (p. 395). For example, Clawson (1994) describes how moral dilemmas might evolve when principles contained in the APTA Code of Ethics are in conflict. This may occur when a patient does not follow his/her recommended course of treatment, despite the positive benefits of receiving the treatment and the negative ramifications of not receiving the treatment. The situation involves a conflict between patient autonomy and clinician responsibility of beneficence or nonmaleficence. Although the APTA Code of Ethics contains principles of autonomy and nonmaleficence, it offers no guidelines about how to apply these principles in specific situations. The physical therapist may be faced with the need to make an ethical decision with no apparent clear-cut resolution of the dilemma.

Barnitt (1998) surveyed the moral dilemmas of practicing occupational and physical therapists using a structured questionnaire and found that occupational therapists faced most moral dilemmas in mental health facilities, whereas physical therapists faced the majority of their moral dilemmas in acute care settings. Moral dilemmas arose over issues of treatment appropriateness and effectiveness, difficult patients, unfair allocation of resources, and unprofessional and incompetent staffs. Barnitt warned against relying on moral principles alone to identify and solve moral dilemmas.

It seems advisable that research into ethical practice in healthcare should integrate data about principles held by moral agents with data about the practice setting in which ethical principles emerge. If the data about moral principles only are collected, Barnitt (1998) warns, "the possibility of assuming that normative ethical theory is supported is high, that all moral standards of every time and place can be rationally ordered and explained by reference to some set of fundamental principles" (p. 198). In other words, to apply principles to moral dilemmas still entails the need for a person to make his or her own assessment (judgment) in order to decide how the foundational moral, professional, religious, or political theories held by individual clinicians are compatible with a particular principle (Limentani, 1999, p. 396). The next section describes the normative approach to ethical decision making and its limitations.

Normative Ethical Decision Making

Normative ethical decision making identifies and justifies moral principles that resolve moral dilemmas. Most of us are required to make daily moral decisions. A need for ethical decision making occurs when a moral dilemma arises. The theory of ethical decision making associated with normative ethics is deontology (Beauchamp & Childress, 2001). A deontological ethics is a deductive decision-making approach based upon solving specific moral dilemmas from general moral principles. Deontologists such as Kant (1785/1994) describe a universal, common morality whose process of justification includes an appeal to rationality. The criticism of deontology is that it fails to reconcile conflicting duties, overemphasizes laws or rules, and underemphasizes relationships (Engelhardt, 1996). For example, deontologists fail to tell us how to resolve two conflicting possible actions, each of which conforms to a principle of a deontological code of ethics.

Suppose a physical therapist realizes the patient he is treating would benefit greatly from at least four more sessions, and she might be harmed if the therapy were stopped immediately. However, the therapist also realizes that the patient can now pass the HMO's set of criteria that would classify her as no longer in need of therapy. The therapist could fill out the assessment form properly and end the patient's treatments, or he could "fudge" results on the form and make it seem that his patient is not doing as well on the tests yet as she actually is. In this example, a deontological approach leaves the therapist with at least two problems. The deontological ethics ignores the therapist's relationship with his patient and the importance of that relationship to both of them; and it leaves the therapist with two conflicting duties: 1) Care for his patient to the best of his ability, and 2) Never lie. Furthermore, since the APTA Code of Ethics does not rank or indicate a hierarchy of principles based upon their perceived relative importance to each other and the profession, physical therapists often are forced to interpret the relative values of those principles within the context of a particular dilemma.

Nonnormative Morality and Ethics

Davis (1998) argues that ethical codes are broadly written and provide general principles that serve only as boundaries of moral behavior. They do not provide professionals with specific answers to all moral dilemmas, making the use of normative morality and ethics problematic (Engelhardt, 1996). Nonnormative morality assumes that there is moral pluralism, which precludes a universal notion of what is good and right. Pluralism refers to multiple moral communities that share their own customs, values, notions of right and good, and patterns of ethical decision making (Beauchamp & Childress, 2001). Nonnormative ethics includes an analysis of the language, concepts, and methods of reasoning in the investigation of a moral dilemma (Beauchamp & Childress, 2001). Nonnormative ethics does not claim that there are preestablished methods to solve a moral dilemma.

The interpretive element of making ethical decisions in the presence of new and changing moral dilemmas was the thesis of Johnson's *Moral Imagination: Implications of Cognitive Science for Ethics* (1997). Johnson argued that traditional Western morality misses the imaginative activity that is crucial to human moral deliberation. He stated that a priori rules or normative principles convey meaning only from our interpretation of them, and all interpretation is irreducibly imaginative. Johnson argued further that morality can never be merely a matter of obeying restrictive rules because those rules discount imaginative exploration in the presence of changing environments and situations that are new and compelling.

Much earlier than Johnson, Dewey (1960) described the contingent nature of moral principles. Moral principles are, according to Dewey, imaginative ideals for reflecting on our own activities. They are not as Western moral tradition often portrays them—crystallized and universal ideals. Dewey argued that moral principles guide the individual in the analysis of good and evil elements in a specific context (Dewey, 1960, p. 141). In other words, moral principles are coincidental to experience, which Dewey defined as a process of reflective inquiry. Thus, principles are always changing and evolving. Morality becomes educative. In this sense, morality is learning the meaning of what we do and what our actions mean, and explaining that meaning in our actions.

Consequently, unlike normative morality and ethics, nonnormative morality and ethics seek to understand what people value and do, rather than what they ought to value and do. Consequently, normative and nonnormative morality and ethics may potentially produce a tension between the ideals of a profession's morality contained in a code of ethics and the morality and ethics of its individual members. The basis of this tension is the distinction between a moral society and moral communities (Engelhardt, 1996). Engelhardt contrasts a moral society with moral communities, explaining that:

Community is used to identify a body of men and women bound together by common moral traditions and/or practices around a shared vision of the good life, which allows them to collaborate as moral friends. Society is used to identify an association that compasses individuals who find themselves in diverse moral communities. (p. 7)

Thus, a profession provides a moral and ethical framework for its members. However, this framework does not necessarily inform us about the moral and ethical perspectives and behaviors of its members. The premise of this study is that individual perspectives about morality and ethics, whether they are normative or nonnormative, are embedded and consequently uncovered within a particular lived experience. I explore this premise through in-depth interviews of 5 physical therapists.

Methodology

This qualitative study explored the life and clinical experiences of 5 physical therapists in order to understand what characterizes morality and ethical decision making in the clinical practice of physical therapy.

Interpretative Narrative Approach

This study used an interpretive narrative approach to address the research questions. In this approach, the participant uses a narrative structure to describe an experience and the researcher and the participant mutually interpret the experience (Gilbert, 2002). An interpretive narrative approach has its philosophical roots in phenomenology (Koch, 1995). The phenomenological movement known today originated at the end of the 19th century and early 20th century in the work of Husserl and Heidegger (Spiegelberg, 1994). Both of these philosophers rejected positivism, the epistemological belief that phenomena are observable facts or events that can be predicted according to reproducible scientific laws (Shepard, Jensen, Schmoll, Hack, & Gwyer, 1993). From the perspective of positivism, evidence is rooted in an objective reality that can be manipulated and reproduced by the researcher. Phenomenology arose as an attempt to understand the phenomena of human activity from the viewpoint of the person being studied. A scholarly and in-depth discussion of Husserlian and Heideggerian phenomenology is beyond the scope of this chapter. An interested reader may refer to Herbert Spiegelberg's

The Phenomenological Movement (1994) and George Steiner's *Martin Heidegger* (1987). However, certain phenomenological concepts that are traceable to both Husserl and Heidegger have evolved to currently influence present-day interpretive narrative approaches to inquiry and are briefly reviewed here.

Phenomenologists posit that human beings are meaning-making individuals. According to Husserl, all consciousness is intentional and the world gives itself to consciousness, which confers on it meaning (Noddings, 1995). Therefore, Husserl argues, we as human beings are conscious of experiences as we live them and are constantly making meaning of the world as we experience it. Through understanding the structure of consciousness of the world and individual meaning making, we can understand human experiences and, ultimately, human meaning about those experiences. Heidegger asserts that we cannot escape interpretation, that we as humans are part of a hermeneutic circle that involves continual interpretation and reinterpretation of experiences. In this paradigm, reality is represented as a particular point of view, in contrast to positivistic notions of reality as truth. Because knowing is embedded in experience, experience provides the context for understanding elusive phenomena such as morality and ethics.

The concern with knowing in context based on phenomenological assumptions about the nature of reality and the nature of knowing has led researchers in recent years to search for appropriate methods in which a description of one's experience can be reproduced, explored, illuminated, and gently probed. One form of meaning construction frequently identified in qualitative interview data is the story, or narrative (Mishler, 1986). Narrative inquiry embodies the phenomenological belief that individuals make sense of their world through stories.

The interpretative narrative approach offered several advantages for this study. First, by telling a story, the participants could make sense of their world by describing what matters most to them. Second, the story gave the researcher access to the contextual elements of the experience, thus avoiding abstraction. Third, the participant used narrative to bring diverse elements of experience, thought, and feeling together in a unified whole, a process that is particularly relevant in capturing the phenomena of morality and ethics in all its dimensions. A story requires participants to remember what occurred in the situation in terms of their concerns, in their own language and understanding of the situation. The storyteller is, in effect, telling the researcher what is perceived, worth noticing, and what concerned him/her about the situation.

Therefore, these stories of participants are told in their own words and with minimal probing by the researcher. Benner, Tanner, and Chesla (1996) write that narrative accounts of actual situations provide a more direct access to practical knowledge than do general questions about beliefs, ideology, theory, or typical behaviors in practice (p. 355). Seidman (1998) suggests that by presenting the participants' stories, the researcher opens up the possibility of readers connecting their own stories to those presented in the study.

Participants

The participants in my study were 5 clinical physical therapists who were licensed and had at least 7 years of experience. I wanted experienced physical therapists because I wanted to examine how clinical experience affects morality and ethical decision making. I limited the number of participants in order to do multiple interviews of each participant, to explore multiple experiences of each participant's practice.

I used a process of purposive sampling to recruit participants for this study. Patton (1980) describes purposive sampling as a strategy that facilitates understanding of select cases without needing to generalize to all cases (p. 100). In other words, for purposive sampling, the researcher may choose the cases from which he or she may best learn. I selected the participants in consultation with three faculty members in a university physical therapy program. Two of the faculty members were actively practicing physical therapists, as well as academicians, and one was the educational program's clinical coordinator.

Candidates were identified as potential participants who would be open to sharing their personal and clinical stories during the in-depth interviews. Specific criteria for selection for this study were: (1) 7 or more years of clinical practice; (2) actively involved in direct patient care at least 75% of the time; (3) geographically located in a region close to the investigator; and (4) willing to commit to an ongoing process of personal interviews and data interpretation. Five participants were chosen for this study, which included two males and three females (Table 5.1). Barbara was the only participant who was classified as a minority (African-American).

Table 5.1 Participants' Demographics

PSEUDONYMS	TOM	BARBARA	LAURA	SAM	JULIE
Gender	male	female	female	male	female
Age	41	48	49	51	56
Years of Practice	11	27	27	27	34
Practice Setting	Hospital-based, outpatient clinic—orthopedics	Corporate-owned private practice—orthopedics	Rehabilitation/Physical therapist–owned private practice	Corporate-owned private practice—orthopedics and sports	Acute care (hospital)—neonatal unit
Formal Course Work in Morality and Ethics	Four-hour continuing education course	Four-hour continuing education course	Four-hour continuing education course	Four-hour continuing education course	None
Entry-Level Degree	MA in physical therapy	BS in physical therapy	BS in physical therapy	BS in physical therapy	BS in physical therapy

Data Gathering

As researcher, I obtained approval for the research study from my university Institutional Review Board. I made initial contact with all the potential participants by telephone. After I explained the study and the procedure and determined that the potential participant was interested in participating, I arranged a time for the first interview. I presented a consent form to be signed prior to conducting the first interview.

I used a modification of Seidman's (1998) three-stage, in-depth interview process. Multiple interviews for each participant were used to enhance credibility. I tape-recorded the interviews, each of which lasted approximately 90 minutes. The first interview was a focused history. My task was to build rapport and to ask the participants to describe important aspects of their practice. For example, I asked them to tell me about experiences in their lives that shaped their values.

The second interview took place within 1 week of the first interview and detailed the participants' current experiences. Participants were asked to reconstruct their daily clinical experiences, including, but not limited to, their interactions with patients. I asked participants to provide detailed examples of several care scenarios. Questions for the first two interviews were purposely not scripted; rather, the participants were given a broad, open-ended question asking them to describe experiences that were important to them (for whatever reason) in their own words. By not specifically guiding the participant, I was able to keep in check my bias about what I considered significant.

The third and final interview took place approximately 2 months after the second interview and consisted of probe questions to gain insights and to provide additional layers of depth and understanding of each participant's experiences. Examples of probe questions included:

1. How did you reach a decision? Would you respond the same way again?
2. What were your priorities during the experiences?
3. Did your priorities change during the experience? If so, how?
4. What principles, if any, guided your behavior in this situation?

Issues of Trustworthiness

According to Lincoln and Guba (1985), the issue of trustworthiness in qualitative research relates to whether the presentation of the data is consistent with the participants' experiences. That is, are the data worth paying attention to? Has the researcher faithfully reinterpreted the experiences of each participant to reflect his or her own interpretations? Lincoln and Guba describe four characteristics of trustworthiness: transferability, credibility, dependability, and confirmability.

In contrast to external validity, in which the researcher's goal is to generalize findings to a larger population, transferability is a process performed by the readers of the research. Readers read and reflect on the data and compare them to the specifics of an environment/experience with which they are familiar. If there are enough similarities between the readers' experiences and the participants' stories, readers may be able to infer that the results of the research would be similar to their own situation. The narrative approach to data collection gives background and context to allow the reader to get a clear sense of what the participant is communicating, thus enhancing the possibility of transferability.

Credibility relates to the truthfulness of the research findings. In this study, I attempted to enhance credibility through a process of member checks, a process of reciprocal interpretation of the data with each participant. The use of multiple interviews and memos added a thick description, or additional layers of interpretation to the data.

Finally, dependability and confirmability relate to the repeatability and objectivity of the findings. That is, were the data collected systematically to ensure that the interpretation, themes, and subthemes were consistent with the data? In the same way that records stemming from an inquiry are used to conduct an inquiry audit, this study used records of transcribed interviews (validated by both the researcher and the participants) and systematized and cross-referenced significant statements, themes, and subthemes to the original documents. In addition, in order to keep my bias in check, I kept a diary, recording my choices about methodological decision making and my thoughts and reactions to the participants' stories.

Data Analysis

After transcribing the interviews, I made copies of each transcription and filed the original in a secure place. I sent a copy to the participants to read for accuracy and to suggest corrections or clarifications (first member check). This collaboration between researcher and participant continued throughout the analysis and interpretation of the data.

Data analysis was carried out in a series of steps. Each transcript was read several times. First, I marked in pencil on the copy what I perceived were significant statements about the participants' morality, including their core values. Second, next to each marked statement, I wrote a memorandum indicating why I thought the statement was significant. Third, I compiled a written list of these significant statements and labeled each significant statement with a notation system that designated its original place in the transcript. This labeling allowed me to retrace the context of a statement for accuracy and additional interpretation.

Fourth, I sent a clean copy back to participants and asked them to mark significant statements related to their values and beliefs with written explanatory memorandums next to each (second member check). This process lent a check on my bias and added a level of interpretation and depth to the study. Fifth, after the participants returned their transcripts, I checked their significant statements and their comments against my notes and made a final determination of significant statements. The process of choosing the significant statements from both the participants and my own coding affirms the role of judgment in the process of analysis. Marshall (1981) calls this part of the analysis the dark side of the process, or the time when one may lose confidence sorting out what was important. Seidman (1998) indicates that it is important that researchers acknowledge that in this stage of analysis they are exercising considerable judgment about what is significant.

Sixth, I clustered the formulated statements together to create themes and subthemes. A theme was a unifying category that reoccurs across all interviews. A category is a specially defined division in a classification system (Rosch & Lloyd, 1978). Although classical theory of category structure is based on the idea that categories are defined by lists of features that an entity must possess if it is to count as a member of that category, Rosch and Lloyd (1978) caution that there typically is a great deal of internal structure to a category. In other words, not every member of a category may be central to our understanding of a given category—some members of a category may more prototypically possess the qualities of that category than others. Subthemes consisting of life histories of the participants that appeared to have influenced their moral development were also identified. Finally, I rechecked the themes and subthemes against the original data and with each participant to control for any interpretative errors. The subthemes are not described here but are reported in a larger study (Greenfield, 2003). Discussion in the following section is organized around two major themes: ethical issues and moral conflicts, and ethical decision making.

Ethical Issues and Moral Conflicts

The participants recounted ethical issues and moral conflicts related to patient care and to the organization of their clinical practices. Probing and questioning led the participants to uncover value conflicts embedded in these experiences. I have focused the discussion of this data around the categories of providing interventions without scientific support, determining professional responsibilities when physical therapy goals conflict with a patient's and/or a family's goals, and determining appropriate treatment, even in the face of conflicting goals of the healthcare system.

Providing Interventions Without Scientific Support

Nascent professions, such as physical therapy, have historically fashioned their professionalism on the medical model (e.g., the AMA) and have sought to gain acceptance partly by emulating those values. The struggle of physical therapy to achieve the status of professionalism, as defined by the traditional, Western model, has resulted in value conflicts among its practitioners (Raz et al., 1991). This struggle is evident in the participants' stories. The profession calls for evidence-based practice paradigms while practitioners struggle to identify effective interventions and moral identities that prioritize caring, context, and relationships over autonomy, money, status, and efficiency.

Sam talked about his concern over providing interventions without scientific support:

Has physical therapy ever been shown to be therapeutic? Well, there is a hot issue with that. I don't think there has been a proven way, or anything that we do in medicine, that has been shown to change the path of back pain. So here we are, in this dilemma. We're treating somebody without any substance. While I'm treating him and I am taking from the insurance company, I have to earn a living. So, to me, that is the biggest moral issue of my profession. I am working in a profession that really has not shown me [*sic*] to make a difference.

Sam went on to explain how he addressed this concern in practice:

If I really thought this patient would be hurt more, or have more pain and suffering, then I would see them twice a week or three times a week, which I've done
that. Um, I had a doctor call me the other day to see if I would treat this indigent
patient free. I said, "OK, send him over," I didn't hesitate.

Sam justifies performing an unproven treatment in order to earn a
living but his personal advocacy for the patient is clear. Production of evidence for interventions often lags behind practice itself. Barnitt (1998)
reports a similar moral dilemma in her survey of occupational and physical therapists. The value conflict is whether the desire to help the patient
(beneficence) outweighs the risk of potentially causing harm (malefi-
cence) by using an untested treatment. Moreover, there is a dilemma of
justice or fairness about using a treatment on a patient that may not be efficacious yet asking the patient or his or her insurance company to pay for
the treatment. This raises the issue of the importance of informed consent in medicine. Interestingly, Sam did not mention that he informs his
patients about the lack of scientific validity of certain treatments.

This moral dilemma raises larger issues about the nature of professional practice. Healthcare providers in Western societies have always
been ambivalent about how much evidence is enough to justify practice.
The traditional model of Western professionalism has been drawn from
the practice and ideology of professions such as medicine (Etzioni, 1969).
Values associated with this model are professional autonomy, status,
respect, and commitment. Specialized knowledge is valued based on a
positivist assumption that there are external truths to be discovered
through a process of objective, scientific methods of inquiry.

Determining Responsibilities When Professional Goals Conflict with Patient or Family Goals

Participants discussed how it was sometimes difficult to sort out their
own sense of professional responsibilities when confronted with conflicting goals from patients and/or families. Laura was frank in her reflection
on the difficulty of determining treatment for a patient whom she viewed
as noncompliant:

It's the patient that whines and doesn't want to do anything and puts full responsibility on you. Then my demeanor immediately changes to one of indifference.

[I tell the patient], "These are the goals and this is what you do. Quite frankly, if you don't do it then you're wasting my time, your time." I get that direct.

She continued:

In another case that wasn't mine but another physical therapist's, the physical therapist was continually supporting the patient's notion that her back was weak. She was seeing this patient for over 10 years because the patient and the physical therapist got implanted in their heads that the patient's back was weak, when in fact, the patient travels all over the world.

In spite of her frustration with patients who she saw as noncompliant, however, Laura was able to articulate a philosophy for dealing with noncompliant patients:

When the patient begins to give excuses—I mean, they are having a problem at home or they're stressed or something, I tend to give into it and justify it sometimes, and maybe back off today. When I should have made more of a statement to structure them. I tell the patient, "Let's find a constructive way out of this situation because you've got to continue to move forward."

Laura was able to disengage herself emotionally from the patients she viewed as noncompliant, but she tried to find a constructive way to help them move forward with treatment. She acknowledged her own frustrations but the patient's well-being remained central to her decision making.

Laura also described a situation where the patient attempted to use the goals of the psychologist to challenge goals of the physical therapist, resulting in the judgment of the treating physical therapist being called into question:

It so happens this particular patient had been treated by a psychologist for over 10 years. Obviously, she had not made any gains with the patient because she's still dependent and very into her condition. Okay, here's the scenario: The physical therapist starts to initiate a discharge of this patient; this patient reacts. The first person the patient contacts is her psychologist, who calls the physical therapist and says, "She needs to continue physical therapy." And the result is that the physical therapist has to defend her position to the psychologist. Now the physical therapist's supervisor was contacted when the psychologist thought she wasn't getting anywhere with the treating physical therapist. That was inappropriate in and of itself.

Laura described another case, when a patient tried to manipulate the physical therapist trying to discharge her:

This was an ethical situation that I was just confronted with. I thought it was rather simple, but a physical therapist who's trying to discharge a patient. The primary physician was contacted who had referred her. He had not realized the length of time of treatment, and had supported the decision for discharge. The patient was then going to manipulate and go to another orthopedist who she had seen in the past, and who had referred her in the past, but who had not referred her recently. So that the therapist questioned me, "Should I send my discharge note to this orthopedist also?" My response was "Yes." The dilemma was the therapist thought she was going behind the patient's back by sending this note to the orthopedist, versus, you know, you're doing this ultimately for the benefit of the patient. We recognized this as a moral dilemma. The therapist said it might be ethically okay for the ultimate care of the patient and for the benefit of the patient to write a letter to the orthopedist, because the patient is a dependent personality and she's playing off healthcare providers with each other.

Julie described a situation where she was faced with the need to go beyond "professional training" to find a way to advocate for a family:

I told you the stories of the initial families that I got involved with. There were three or four families with devastating disabilities, and there were three or four families that adored these children, and just wanted everything going for them. I was just sort of awestruck about how they coped. I had my book learning about what to do. But I came across the dilemma about a family wanting to take charge with their child. There was an orthopedic surgeon who wanted to have one surgery after another and the family wanted to go to the Grand Canyon, camping with their child. I developed the idea that I should become the advocate trying to help the family work the system, and going with what the family wanted to do. And nobody in professional training told me I would have to do that.

Julie's account illuminates the tension between making the healthcare system respond to patient needs and using the system in ways that are harmful by fostering patients' dependence on physical therapy or by wasting scarce resources. Participants' stories suggested that physical therapists often find themselves in the middle between patients, families, and other healthcare professionals, causing them to struggle with how to identify their professional responsibilities in the face of conflicting goals with others on the healthcare team. Within this struggle, physical therapists must confront the dilemma of determining appropriate treatment.

Determining Appropriate Treatment When Professional Goals Conflict with Healthcare System Goals

Many of the participants' stories focused on the underlying tension between defining themselves according to the values inherent within the healthcare system and defining themselves according to their own core values. Stories encompassed concerns related to working the system, fiscal responsibilities, and sustaining personal caring.

WORKING THE SYSTEM

Participants described how they needed to identify creative ways to ensure that patients' needs were met, even within the constraints of the healthcare system. Julie's example above shows how she was able to "work the system" to meet patient and family needs. Sometimes the creative decision making involved "bending the rules" to ensure that patients' needs were met. Barbara told a story about a particular patient whose insurance for a primary injury had expired, but who had developed a secondary condition:

I have a situation like this with a lady with a brachial plexus injury. She had a gunshot wound to the shoulder that resulted in a brachial plexus injury. [This] Black female, middle class, [had] a totally nonfunctional upper extremity. So we went two months. She's doing better in rehabilitation. She's starting to get some functional return. But she still is pretty nonfunctional. . . . She had to go for stellate ganglion blocks. . . . And then her insurance company denied her treatment after the 60-day period.

Well, during that time period, through telephone conversations with her, she told me, "My shoulder has frozen up." During the time period of trying to get her back into therapy . . . she'd be calling saying, "I'm just getting worse, I'm getting worse, you've got to help me, what do I need to do?" I said, "Well, go to the doctor; we might be able to see you back . . . for a frozen shoulder." That's a different diagnosis.

So that's what happened. . . . Technically, she had a new diagnosis secondary to the injury. We were able to institute another program based on that. Sometimes you can do it that way. . . . You try to find ways around the rules, sometimes, without being unethical, without lying, because she did have a frozen shoulder.

In spite of the difficulties of working within the managed care system, Barbara described how she was able to identify ways to address the moral tension she experienced between obligations to the patient's care and her obligations to the organization:

I love what I do, but it's becoming more of a hassle to do it, and more of a burden. If I could go in and treat people, make them better, [and] not have to do all the other things that are associated with it, then I would. The insurance needs constant verification, [such as] how many times [do the patients] come in. So, economically, [I] have to figure out a way to get [the patient] better with the least number of visits [in order to obtain approval of the insurance company to treat this patient]. I know that there are ways of getting around [the system], but [I prefer to work] with the system, instead of against the system.

Barbara's solution to the constraint of managed care was to always keep the patient's needs central to her ethical decision making and to tread a fine line of bending, but not breaking, the rules. This strategy of striving to be morally imaginative was also reflected in stories of other participants. Julie described her perception of how the rules relate to being a moral practitioner:

I feel like it is way beyond following the rules, I mean, the rules might set the bottom line, so that you don't lose your license, you don't get into trouble, and don't get sued. But to me the rules are really down there [she pointed toward the floor]. A moral practitioner is an individual that is accepting a patient as a client, a family, where they are, without value judgment on them, [who sees them] as worthy of your best effort, as worthy of the system's best effort.

FISCAL RESPONSIBILITIES

Corporate practices have developed in recent years to centralize physical therapy practices into conglomerates that compete for managed care contracts. The result is that many previously privately owned corporate, nonhealthcare managers now run physical therapy practices. Potential clashes may occur between corporate owners' focus on the bottom line and physical therapy practitioners' focus on patient care needs.

Tom struggled with his perceptions of the care needs of his patient and how they conflicted with financial expectations of the healthcare system:

A conundrum case . . . This is where our reimbursement for this patient was very small, and this was very frustrating to me, because this patient was obviously in dire need, and she was primary support for her family. I thought to myself that she is a high-level musician, and this is a person's life. You know, and I felt responsible for her well-being and her future. And I did get her back performing again, but never to the level that she had before, but it took literally three years. My manager was somewhat supportive, but kind of telling me that I really needed to think about this situation. And I realized as time went on that he was right. I was becoming an enabler. I had developed too much of an emotional bond with this patient. My manager finally sat down with me and calculated out the number of visits and how much money we had actually lost. And it was several thousand dollars that we had lost, in terms of her reimbursement. . . . So you know from a variety of ethical standpoints, I was trying to figure out what's the best way to go, and I struggled with this case.

In this particular case, Tom struggled with continuing to support this patient, emotionally and psychologically, even though the practice was losing money. He labeled himself as an enabler, worrying that he had developed too much of an emotional bond with the patient, despite describing the patient as "in dire need." Tom's account highlights the difficulties of seeing clinical situations through the lens of fiscal responsibilities. That is, because of the cost of prolonged care, the success Tom initially describes is recast as a liability and Tom's engagement with the patient is reduced to emotion.

The physical therapist has a fiduciary responsibility to the employing organization (be it healthcare agencies or insurance companies) to avoid unnecessary or prolonged treatments. Clearly, practicing in a responsible manner is important to ensure that services are available over time to those in need. However, the fiduciary responsibilities of physical therapists must often be balanced against their responsibilities to the patient's well-being. The participants in this study described how fiduciary responsibilities created systems that sometimes made it difficult for patients. For instance, Laura described the difficulty some patients have adjusting to the organizational schedule, which can affect their care. Laura stated:

What happens is a patient may say, well we want to see ———, or we want to see ———, or something like that. There'll be a delay getting in. They get in, and then there's a delay being able to be seen. So some people feel, Well, you know, I just can't deal with that. So they will leave.

Laura also addressed the differences in treatment goals that sometimes resulted from the type of insurance a patient had:

I mean, I'll have a couple of patients who say look, you know, I'm paying out of the pocket, and I can come, you know, four times. I may think that they need more, but it changes my focus a bit. So it is a real difference between when somebody, they're paying out of pocket, or where there's insurance, even in terms of compliance and commitment.

The issue for many of the participants was that healthcare had placed burdens on physical therapists to control costs while providing adequate care for their patients. Rates that are capitated provide health maintenance organization (HMO) patients a limited rate of remuneration per diagnostic category, despite the number of visits. Since managed care seeks to keep costs low, many providers may not want physical therapists to treat a substantial number of poor patients within their group (Weech-Maldonado, Morales, Spritzer, Elliott, & Hayes, 2001). Because of the environment in which they live, their financial situation, and other factors, the poor may be more likely to get sick and need treatment. Barbara described an example of the impact of managed care and fiscal constraints in treating patients with chronic conditions such as stroke:

Strokes. It's usually people with more chronic diagnoses [who are] neurologically involved that you know, based on your experience, they're not going to get well in two months. It's not that you need to see them three times a week for six months, but they need some type of follow-up, to make sure they're doing what they need to do. How do I handle these long-term patients with limited insurance? Well, there's someone I know that I can treat in 2 months, but we're trying to limit it to 5 to 7 visits. I do a lot of patient education, based on the individual. And I do a lot of written home instructions. So there's no excuse to say you didn't know what to do [and] I try to follow them on a weekly basis.

If there's someone that I'm suspicious that might not do well, I might have them come in twice a week. And then I get them down to once a week. So far it has worked. I mean it has worked, you know, with some limitations. So, economically, we have to figure out a way that we can get them better with the least number of visits. When it gets to the point where their 60-day period is just about ended, and I know they might need some more information and therapy, then we might go into that discussion. And we always tell them at the beginning of when they check in, when they register, that we can work with you.

Julie noted how she was affected by the financial constraints of the system in her position at a large urban hospital:

The patients have had at least a million dollars spent on them by the time they're referred to me for intervention, to get them where they can be discharged. Then the services they need to maximize what their potential is in life—those services aren't available, and yet the million dollars have already been spent to guarantee their survival. I will try my best to get them the best that is available within my constraints, but it's often not what I would ideally hope for.

Sam stated that in the presence of managed care and dealing with patients with limited insurance, the economic viability and the good of the practice takes precedence:

If you were in business, if you had your sole business, you would take the same attitude as I'm going to express now. If you're in managed care, the worst type of patient insurance is the one-dollar amount. And that one-dollar amount then, if you see them one visit you get that dollar amount, if you see them two visits you get half that dollar amount. And, we pick and choose our battles, but the patient moves along quickly into the system, then we got to minimize our utilization, their visits, and get them out of the door.

In spite of his description of healthcare as a business, however, it is clear that Sam is careful to consider his professional responsibilities toward the patient:

The only time, with the managed care constraints that it became an issue with me, [was when] one of the other therapists that works with me, is not presenting the menu [options] correctly to the patient. The patient felt that they were being pushed out the door. Patients cannot feel like they're being pushed out the door.

Sam suggests that his approach to patient care is adjusted to meet the needs of fiscal constraints imposed by managed care. He in essence uses a patient-audit metaphor that views the patient as a commodity to be manipulated in order to maximize financial rewards through a focus on organizational input, transformation of product, and output, but he is also careful to consider the patient's feelings.

SUSTAINING PERSONAL CARING

Noddings (1984) points out that caring as a moral orientation for ethical decision making involves reciprocity between the cared for and caregiver so that each acknowledges his/her role in the relationship toward each other and toward a common goal. Guilt may accompany caring when patient expectations or clinician expectations are consistently not realized. Interviews with participants in this study indicated that they struggled in the healthcare environment to continue to care for their patients and themselves.

One of the dangers of a struggle to ensure appropriate care, even in the face of conflicting goals of the healthcare system, is the potential loss of personal caring for the individual patient. Barbara described how the treatment process could threaten a personal relationship with patients:

You know, HMOs, [the patients] don't have so many visits. Okay, you know, this patient can only come 5 times. [I] give them exercises and move them along, that's what I see . . . more impersonal . . . more robotic.

Barbara recounted struggling to find a way to maintain her caring with a particularly problematic patient:

Well, I remember this one patient. He followed me everywhere . . . and it got to the point I would dream about him at night. He was a self-inflicted gunshot wound to the chest. Oh, he loved me [but] he got on my nerves. I mean, I did everything for him I was supposed to do, but you're still a human being. But some stuff you cannot leave at the door . . . because of the fact that you are human. And there's no way you can just cut it off when you step out of here.

Barbara is aware that human connection is part of her moral framework of physical therapy practice. Although her reference to the patient as "a gunshot wound," rather than as a man living with a wound, may seem to reflect a Western medical model that views the body as separated from the mind, her emotional commitment to this patient is evident.

Caring relationships involve focusing on the patient's needs, expectations, and goals as the moral basis for making ethical decisions (Branch, 2000; Fealy, 1995). Because a caring practitioner places the patient's needs as the focus of ethical decision making, caring entails risks of doing too much for the patient by minimizing the patient's role in the treatment plan, rather than developing a plan that integrates patient responsibilities into everyday activities. The case described by Tom earlier, when he came to see himself as an enabler, marked a turning point in his professional moral life, forcing him to come to terms with what it meant to be a caring practitioner in the context of his professional responsibilities:

Well, over time you need to discharge this patient because number one, she plateaued, and because I realized that I was enabling her right now, I was not necessarily helping in any kind of way, and I really started to sense the honesty in and the truth in my manager's conclusion. I was enabling, and that I was continuing that, and it got to a point where I realized that this was too emotional. I was intertwined in the emotional dysfunction. I have to realize that myself, as a person, I can no longer do this.

The participants in this study also described the need to identify boundaries between their personal and professional lives. For all the participants, taking care of oneself by spending time with their friends and family and moderating their long work hours was central to a moral practice of physical therapy. They also discussed how they used colleagues, including social workers, for professional and emotional support with difficult patients. The literature supports these feelings of stress by practitioners in caring for patients and themselves in the context of the healthcare system. Blau and colleagues (2002), in a study of 5 physical therapists, reported a similar feeling of stress and disheartenment toward their corporate controlled hospital environment, not having enough time to provide adequate patient care due to increased demands of the workplace to meet productivity and patient quotas. In fact, the burdens of "managing" managed care in a corporate environment are difficult for all healthcare workers. Leners and Beardslee (1997) found that nurses were particularly susceptible to emotional stress when they saw themselves failing to solve moral dilemmas that impacted caring for their patients. Post and Weddington (2000) reported increased stress experienced by African-American family physicians due to a shift toward managed care and the desire on their part for time for themselves away from medicine. These physicians developed coping strategies, including spirituality and kinship.

The central aspect of moral imagination is to empathize with the patient's predicament. Johnson (1997) argues that moral imagination entails the ability of one person to identify with the emotional needs of another. To do that, one must be able to reframe his or her moral perspective to fit new situations. The situations in which the participants found they must decide how to act did not come with one and only one "proper" description; the participants had to conceptualize the situation in different ways, using imaginative extensions of their own metaphorical conceptual system. That is, to be morally imaginative the participants had to figure out what the metaphors were that defined their own and others' conceptual systems, as well as be open to feelings of others.

In conclusion, all the participants identified ethical issues and moral conflicts in their daily practices. Specifically, the participants in this study described moral dilemmas with direct patient care and in relation to the organizational structure of their practices. These moral dilemmas included: (a) providing interventions without scientific support; (b) determining responsibilities when professional goals conflict with patient or family goals; and (c) determining appropriate treatment when professional goals conflict with healthcare system goals.

These findings are similar to the findings of Barnitt (1998), Guccione (1980), and Triezenberg (1996), although the participants in this study provided context and depth to the moral dilemmas. In addition, there are several moral dilemmas—most notably related to informed consent—not mentioned by the participants. The issue of informed consent is whether physical therapists should routinely inform patients about the efficacy and/or risks of a potential procedure. This issue relates to values of patient autonomy and fairness and is reported by Triezenberg (1996) to be an important future issue in physical therapy. Perhaps recent physical therapy graduates may be more sensitive to the issue of informed consent than experienced physical therapists, due to their recent exposure of this issue in their curriculum. Further research is needed to provide a clearer picture of the ethical issues and moral conflicts faced by physical therapy practitioners at different phases of their careers.

Ethical Decision Making

How then do physical therapists address the ethical issues and moral conflicts that they encounter in their clinical practice? For example, do they identify a conflict as moral at the time that they encounter the conflict? If not, how do they identify the conflict? And how do they decide to act? Do they consciously weigh factors and undergo a formal process of ethical decision making? Do they use a moral language to recognize that they are dealing with an ethical dilemma? What constitutes a moral practitioner?

None of the participants in this study had any formal training in ethics before beginning clinical practice. Unlike the clinical problem-solving models that they learned in professional school, none of the participants learned ethical decision-making models. Laura, perhaps, exemplifies the thinking of most of the participants. In response to my question about morality and ethics being part of professional practice, in a similar way as clinical decision making, she told me, "You know what? I honestly can tell you I never even thought about [ethics] until we were required to take those courses, you know, the 4-hour course [on ethics] that's required for our license." And when I asked her if she had ever read the code of ethics of the APTA, she said:

I read them years ago, but I couldn't tell you [what they are] right now. It doesn't guide me. Well, I read them, years—I mean, you know, at one point. But I can't honestly tell you when I go in the room that this is what's on my mind.

Similarly, when I asked Barbara whether she thinks about morality much in clinical practice, she said, "No. There are subtle problems you face in clinic, where you sort of act, and I am not thinking about something as moral or ethical."

Sam also indicated that he had not looked at the professional code of ethics, nor was he aware that he was making ethical decisions. He told me:

Well, when I'm making decisions about fairness, I'm not thinking, say, what would my Mom and Dad do in this situation. But I imagine, somewhere, twirling around in my brain . . . I guess if I had to be confronted with a moral decision or judgment right now I'd say, "Am I hurting somebody from this?"

When I asked Tom how he learned to make ethical decisions, he said, "I wish I can say it's an ethics course in school, but it was not." Referring to his moral judgment, he said:

I think some of that came from my Catholic upbringing, in terms of examination and formation of conscience as an important aspect in determining what is morally correct. And that also [I have] understanding or accepting of the standards . . . the APTA and the hospital standards of practice. The acceptance of those standards is the important part, because if you do not accept it then the reinforcement of those standards is somewhat weak.

The participants apparently were not aware of making ethical decisions based on a prescribed set of steps. This is consistent with the findings reported by Guccione (1980), who found that his sample of physical therapists were not aware that they were dealing with moral dilemmas. It is also consistent with Benner's work, which suggested that practitioners are likely to turn their attention to theoretical aspects of practice during a "breakdown" of an element of practice that they encounter (Benner, 1984). Benner noted that encounters with many actual situations in practice help practitioners to refine preconceived notions and to add nuances to theoretical understandings (p. 36). Since the years of practice for participants in this study ranged from 11 to 34 years, one would anticipate that all had encountered frequent situations of breakdown in practice, but it appears that they had not systematically reflected on these encounters.

Tom was the only participant who stated that he had recently read the APTA Code of Ethics or any professional document related to professional morality and ethics. Tom remembered being able to identify a particular conflict as a moral dilemma:

> I think, at the time, I recognized them as moral conflicts because I felt some turmoil in making decisions, especially when the pressure of management would say something otherwise. So I was pressured to say what are my reasons for continuing or justifying treatment. And in my heart I knew that it was something that had to be done, based on my ethics and my moral determination that made the conflict a turmoil, [and] based on my values, my morals, and my perception of what was right.

If the participants did not have formal training in morality and ethics and do not make ethical decisions based on formal principles or codes, how do they identify and address moral dilemmas? Part of the answer may be related to Johnson's (1997) idea that imaginative activity is crucial to moral deliberation and that individuals use metaphors developed from prototypical experiences to understand nonprototypical experiences. As previously noted, Johnson argued that a reliance on following rules discounts imaginative exploration of new situations.

Cognitive scientists empirically study the nature of prototype structures to gain insight into their importance for moral understanding and ethical decision making (Johnson, 1997; Lakoff & Johnson, 1999). For example, Churchland (1989, 1996) argues that certain moral and social schemas actually represent complex prototypes that exist within human neural structures. Johnson (1997) argues that prototypes are important to our moral deliberations because they represent experientially basic types of situations:

> That is, given the kinds of bodies we have, the nature of our cognition, and the kinds of physical, interpersonal, and cultural interactions we engage in, certain

types of situations will take on a special importance for us in our attempt to function successfully in our physical and social environments. (p. 190)

In other words, human prototypes are patterns of categorizing and conceptualizing things with which we commonly interact. Prototypes are both culturally and biologically determined. The chief imaginative dimension of prototypical understanding is metaphor, which structures human conceptual understanding. Humans understand more abstract and less well-structured domains, such as morality, via mappings from more concrete domains of experience, such as bodily experience or movement. Nonprototypical experiences offer new and unique experiences to a person for which he or she has no obvious metaphorical understanding.

Tom identified a moral dilemma as turmoil and "knew in his heart" what must be done. In my interview with Tom, he noted that his moral understandings evolved from oaths and rituals he learned in relatively organized and strict organizations, such as the Catholic church and the Boy Scouts, and that these beliefs were reinforced by his traditional Western upbringing. Thus, he learned that doctrine and rituals are morally good. The goals are spirituality and inner peace. An event that results in a perturbation in what he perceives as prototypically morally good is thus felt as morally bad, with internal turmoil.

Although formal reflection on the ethical decision-making process was not readily apparent, all of the participants reported conflicts and experiences in practice that resulted in a struggle to make ethical decisions. The nature of the participants' ethical decision making appeared to contain some elements of the grand theories of ethics and ethical decision-making models. For example, Tom's description of making ethical decisions implies combining consequentialism with deontology. He said:

I generally look at the different possibilities and the options, and in terms of what it is, what you are looking at. If there is something that is presented to you and you wonder whether a course of action is morally correct, you start to look at all possible options to see which is morally correct. And [you balance] what are the consequences and implications of those options.

Moreover, when I asked him how he determines if something is morally correct, he answered:

I think it just gets back to looking at standards of ethics—looking at the standards of ethics of our profession, and looking at the standards of ethics of my particular employer. And also, from just a humanitarian standpoint, treat people in an equal manner by not discriminating against people for whatever reasons. I try to look at all the particular aspects of a particular decision and the implications of different decisions that can be made.

The participants appeared to weigh moral principles through a process of imagination directed at specific situations in their practice. Tom acknowledged that his experiences with Catholic doctrine influenced his normative morality. He underwent a process of reflection—weighing his own core values, the values of the profession, and the needs and goals of the patient—to make an ethical decision that met the needs of a particular situation. He told me about a patient and the patient's family who were angry about the patient's discharge, even though all the therapeutic goals were met:

A caseworker from a particular independent living facility called me, based on some issues with a parent that was unhappy with the fact that the physical therapist had discharged their son from services at the hospital. Certain things for us had been met for discharge. And this parent was basically very angry and, you know, had called the governor's office. Part of my job is to make sure we have good ground to stand on, just making sure that we've touched base with everything, and I consult with all my resources of information: the chart, the people involved. That's what I start doing, and as I was kind of processing this, I came up with an action plan to try to appease, as best I can, an angry patient. In this case we decided to have a discharge meeting with our case managers—with them and the patient's father . . . so that we have all the parties there, and people understand what's what.

Tom used moral imagination to gauge the points of view of all relevant parties and tried to come to a compromise decision. Rules and regulations were important to Tom, but so were the concerns and needs of the disputants.

Julie described her approach to ethical decision making as, "Existentialism, where you have a set of rules, but you've got to figure out a way that you have to play fast and loose with the system." She told me, "With a new situation, I guess there is sort of a process of exploring different aspects of the gray area and all the different viewpoints and trying to sort it out in my own mind." She sees herself as an advocate of the patient. She talked about helping the patients' families to "negotiate the system," and to form a "trusted relationship with somebody there in the nursery."

Julie made it clear that she does not refer to professional documents, including the APTA Code of Ethics, to guide her ethical decisions. Instead, her construction of a moral dilemma and its solutions are based on the care and responsibility of the patient, rather than on individual rights and organizational rules. There is symmetry of findings between Julie's experiences, her approaches to ethical decision making, and the research of Gilligan (1982) and Raz et al. (1991). These authors report women's perspectives of moral judgment, based on being responsive to another individual's needs, as central to ethical decision making. Julie reported similar values in her clinical approach to patient care.

I found that all the participants in this study believed that they incorporated caring in their moral judgment, although they expressed it differently. Tom stated:

I think there is a sense of caring that goes beyond a 10-minute interview. I think there is a bond that develops between a physical therapist and patient that goes beyond the therapist interaction. There is either hand contact with someone, in terms of actually doing manual work, listening to personal problems, and also the way in which a physical therapist can actually change and affect a patient. It's a very intimate type of clinical relationship that I necessarily do not see in other healthcare fields.

Sam's approach to caring was less evident. For example, he talked a lot about his own enjoyment and about the challenge of running an organized clinic, about efficiency, about moving patients in and out of the door, about getting into the mindset of patients, and about proving the efficacy of treatment. But he talked very little about the primacy of caring. Whereaas Julie used metaphors about her professional self as "links in the chain," or a "patch in the net," Sam expressed a more impersonal view of the patient–clinician relationship. He talked about himself in the following way:

I'm not the kind of guy where, you know, I'm going to get to know you that well. . . . I wasn't a schmoozer with and I'm still not a schmoozer. . . . I'm here to do my job, and get my job done, and just go to the next one.

He said: "I enjoy having a full schedule, a difficult schedule, and have things go like clockwork, and people leave the room like they've had a good treatment." Sam, however, does show caring and moral imagination during clinical practice. He stated:

You have to be sensitive; if one was not sensitive, if one just had an ego, then I would say [to a patient], Don't go to a chiropractor . . . if I was insensitive and did not care how the patient felt about everything. . . . I put myself in that person's place. . . . I think once you put your self in that person's place, and I tend to do that when I treat patients, if I was that patient, where and how would I want to be touched?

In this case Sam uses empathy to imagine the needs of the patient. However, Sam made it clear to me that he values the rules and regulations of his organization. He talked about the impact of corporate practice on patient care:

With my own practice, I would work the same way as with corporate practice. No, I would have to say I'd probably work a little bit less harder [sic], in terms of longer hours, because I would not need to have that additional 20% that I need to make for corporate practice. I don't work longer now. I just maybe work that extra patient into my schedule whereas, obviously, in private practice I would say, I made my quota for the day . . . I don't think of fairness. That's what the rules are.

There are some conclusions that may be drawn from the ethical decision-making processes of these participants. First, the participants integrated their core values into what Johnson (1997) refers to as nonprototypical clinical situations. Nonprototypical clinical situations represent novel experiences of each participant. Each participant came to clinical practice with a core set of values that appeared to frame their initial approach to identifying and addressing a moral dilemma. But the participants' core values did not necessarily prepare them for their role in the clinical setting that involved new and different moral dilemmas. As Guccione (1980) reports, moral dilemmas are ubiquitous in physical therapy clinical practice. Each participant in this study made moral judgments about patient care in the context of clinical care. This appears to support Clawson's (1994) argument that there is no demarcation between clinical and ethical decision making.

Second, participants did not necessarily recognize that they were dealing with moral dilemmas. Guccione (1980) also reports that physical therapists may not recognize moral dilemmas, per se. Although some researchers have listed identifying a moral dilemma as a step in ethical decision making (Purtilo, 1999; Rest & Narvaez, 1994; Swisher & Krueger-Brophy, 1998), they are generally not clear how this occurs. Johnson (1997) argues that a moral framework evolves through a web of values that includes its own narrative and frame of reference. Perhaps as physical therapists become more experienced in clinical practice, their narrative changes and their frame of reference expands to make sense of individual experiences and to internalize a theoretical understanding of moral issues.

Third, the process of ethical decision making is creative, fluid, and contextual. This finding is similar to the theories of Swisher and Krueger-Brophy (1998) and Wise (2000), inasmuch as physical therapists frame ethical decisions on a contextual or situational basis. All the participants appeared to rely more and more—as their clinical experiences increased—upon communicating and understanding the patients' point of view. Thus, the participants' personal belief systems continually readjusted to accommodate new and shifting clinical expediencies.

Beauchamp and Childress (2001) describe a convergent system of ethical decision making. They describe this system as occurring neither from the top down nor from the bottom up. For example, when the process begins from the top down, then an individual enters into ethical decision making based on a set of principles integrated into the consequences of applying a particular principle in a particular situation to solve a moral dilemma. Conversely, when the process begins from the bottom up, the individual views the context and relationships first and integrates principles as they apply to that particular situation. The top-down system may be described as deductive, whereas the bottom-up system may be described as inductive. The deductive system implies a normative morality and ethics, where general principles guide decisions. Conversely, an inductive system implies a nonnormative morality and ethics, where the particular case frames the ethical decision.

Beauchamp and Childress (2001) argue that neither approach is purely practical and that an alternative approach should combine elements of both normative and nonnormative morality and ethics. They base their argument on the exigencies of individual experiences and on the unpredictable nature of one's subjective responses, as well as upon the rigidity of normative morality and ethics that fail to account for those exigencies. Instead, their approach argues for a common morality of right and wrong that must be grounded in a particular experience. Beauchamp and Childress refer to a process of considered moral judgment, where an individual judges a situation within the context of the immediate experience and within the context of basic moral understanding—and, in the case of the participants in this study, within the context of their core values.

As reported by these participants, the nature of clinical practice has changed over the years. Managed care is a prime example. Private and corporate practices present these participants with a distinct set of moral dilemmas. The participants move back and forth between normative and nonnormative morality, weighing and balancing their own core values, the values of the profession, the values of the healthcare system, and the experiences of the patient.

Limitations of This Study and Directions for Future Research

This study had limitations that could be addressed in future research. The study included a small sample, which was purposive, but not necessarily representative of APTA members. It would be interesting to examine how younger physical therapists with less clinical experience than the therapists in this sample construct their morality and ethics. For example, how do their stories differ from the older generation of physical therapists? Did they have professional ethics in their curriculum? What are their life experiences? What core values do they bring to clinical practice?

It would also be helpful to study the impact of ethnicity and culture on ethical decision making in physical therapists. In addition, as a profession we need to examine the stories of educators in physical therapy education. How do they construct their morality and ethics? How do they create a moral teaching and learning environment?

Although I attempted to ensure the trustworthiness of findings, another interviewer may not elicit the same stories and interpret them the same way. Also, this study sought the experiences and perspectives of physical therapists about their moral practice. It would be interesting in a future study to examine the experiences of patients and how they construct morality.

Implications

This study set out to tell stories of 5 clinical physical therapists who are actively practicing. These stories form the basis of their construction of professional morality:

1. None of the participants came to clinical practice with formal training in morality and ethics.
2. For the most part, participants were not aware that they were practicing a formal system of morality and ethics, although they were able to relate clinical stories that revealed that they did indeed face moral dilemmas and make ethical decisions.
3. Participants appeared to navigate through moral dilemmas with moral imagination, emotional sensitivity to value conflict, and the integration of their core values to new situations.
4. Despite each participant having a priority set of core values, each underwent a process of moral transformation that included changing patterns of caring for their patients and for themselves.
5. All the participants viewed the healthcare system as imposing moral constraints on their patient care.
6. In response to the constraints of the healthcare system and corporate practice, the participants developed strategies for coping, including caring for themselves, forming support relationships with their peers, friends, and families, and developing creative strategies to "bend the rules" for the advantage of their patients.

Implications for Clinical Practice

This study has implications for clinical practice that are relevant to physical therapy and to other healthcare professions as well. An important concern that emerges from the participants' stories is that healthcare, as it is currently constituted (managed care and corporate practice), places constraints on healthcare practitioners to offer cost-effective but equitable healthcare. Participants described the dilemma of controlling costs while providing adequate care for their patients. What are the implications of being a moral practitioner in a managed care market (versus a private pay market)?

Newman and Dunbar (2000) describe how the change from a private pay system to a managed care system that predominates in today's healthcare system has profound implications for ethical practice of healthcare. Indeed, they argue that every facet of practice of managed care is rife in moral and ethical implications as physicians and other healthcare practitioners struggle to redefine their professional autonomy in a system that calls on them to balance competitive business practices with delivery of effective healthcare. One way of understanding the moral implications associated with the current healthcare system is from the perspective of a paradigm shift that continually demands a rethinking of professional responsibilities and morality on the part of its practitioners. A paradigm shift described by Thomas Kuhn (1962) is a change from one way of thinking to another, or in healthcare, one way of doing business to another. The older paradigm (since 1970) represented a hierarchical model of healthcare with the physician at the top of a hypothetical pyramid dispensing healthcare decisions to the patient and other healthcare workers below. Physician decision making occurred in a relatively autonomous manner. Fees would be collected based on the services provided. There was little external pressure (from insurance companies) to limit the type and number of services provided by the physician. Although the potential for abuse from overcharges existed, the physician had little conflict between choosing between his or her professional well-being and the well-being of the patient. Physicians were accountable to their practice standards and to their professional organization and were less accountable to justify their clinical decision judgments and decisions to third-party payers or other healthcare practitioners.

Under this old system, there were minimal financial controls in place for physicians to be overly concerned about controlling the cost of treatment or to justify medical decisions that carried significant costs. Moral dilemmas tended to be confined to clinical decision-making processes between the physician and patient rather than to conflicts between the physician and other entities within the larger healthcare system, including insurance companies and other healthcare disciplines. Moral dilemmas involved such issues as patient autonomy in making clinical decisions, truth telling (e.g., the revelation of terminal cancer diagnosis), and end-of-life issues.

During this time period, nurses and other health professionals were striving to identify themselves as professionals, defined in part as the ability to control their own work, but it was clear that the structure of the healthcare system subordinated these professionals to ancillary roles. By the early 1990s, marketplace changes, including the increased impact of managed care, resulted in a paradigm shift in which healthcare was less hierarchically oriented and characterized by shifting relationships among providers, both individuals and organizations. Liaschenko and Peter (2004) describe a healthcare environment that frequently resulted in fragmentation of care and tension between healthcare providers, managed care companies, and patients. Moral dilemmas associated with justice increased (DuVal, Clarridge, Gensler, & Danis, 2004; Newman & Dunbar, 2000). Justice, which holds that all persons must be treated with fairness and equality, may be a concern under managed care, where limited resources may not always be allocated equitably. The business emphasis on cost control, units of work, commodity prices, economic efficiency, and profit margin resulted in a sense of identity crisis and alienation from their patients for many healthcare workers.

The complexity of the healthcare system and the competing demands that it imposes on the obligations and decision-making processes of healthcare workers can be appreciated using an organizational model. Kramer (1997) describes domains that influence a patient's and healthcare worker's experience and decision-making process. The broadest of these domains is the system of care that includes the site of care, its organizational goals, philosophy and culture, financial incentives, and continuity among services. Depending on where the healthcare worker works, the external environment of his or her organization, including its culture, its administration, and its supervisory expectations, places obligations and, at times, competing demands on the practitioner that result in value conflict. For example, an organization with a rigid bureaucratic culture that is highly structured and designed to regulate the behavior of members through a rigid and elaborate set of rules may impede independence, creativity, and flexibility of health professionals to care for their patients.

Lammers and Geist (1997) describe how institutional expectations in a managed care organization that emphasizes efficiency and values cost-effective treatment conflicts with the daily relational aspects of healthcare workers to care for their patients. Based on conflicting institutional, professional, and personal obligations, Romanello and Knight-Abowitz (2000) describe the risk to physical therapists to provide good care to their patients in the presence of incompatible demands imposed by the patient's insurance company to limit or discontinue treatment against the recommendation of the physical therapist. Risk of professional burnout can result from healthcare practitioners being overburdened with advocating for the patient in the presence of a rigid bureaucracy, engaging in political battles, and expending significant energy to fight institutional mandates that limit treatment.

In this environment, Strasser and colleagues (2005) describe how cohesive medical and rehabilitation team functioning is instrumental in fostering good patient outcomes. In particular, individual practitioners must consider moral dilemmas and make ethical decisions within the context of the hospital culture, organizational constraints, and other medical team members. In this system, Strasser and colleagues found that medical teams with rigid bureaucratic structures and limited communication were associated with less favorable patient outcomes.

One implication of the concern with the changes in the healthcare system is that physical therapists, as well as other healthcare workers, may need to be morally imaginative. Traditional methods of philosophic ethics based on applying normative principles contained in professional codes to solve moral dilemmas are, according to Pellegrino (1999), not adequate for current psychosocial, economic, social, organizational, and cultural complexities of moral dilemmas in the current healthcare system. Purtilo (2000) argues for a changing moral landscape for physical therapists that involves establishing a partnership of patients as persons (patient-centered care) as well as professional partnering of physical therapists within the larger community of citizens and institutions. Physical therapists and other healthcare workers need to be open to exploring different ways of solving moral dilemmas through a process of creativity and flexibility. Individual practitioners can be sensitive to the language of others (including the insurance provider) to discern commonalities and differences in moral frameworks in order to open up new possibilities for decision making.

This process can be taught in the classroom and nurtured in practice. For example, a course in morality and ethics can present stories of physical therapists recalling moral dilemmas associated with managed care. The students can hear how Barbara became creative in order to meet her patients' healthcare needs. They can hear how Julie relied on her peers and her patients' families for moral support in order to provide the best care for her patients. They can hear how (and why) Sam is able to navigate through the constraints of managed care, in part because his own core values of organization and efficiency most closely correlate with the values of managed care. Finally, the students can hear about the transforming process of clinical practice, and how the participants redefine what caring means toward their patients, and how it is important to care for themselves.

In addition to the concerns about the impact of the current context of healthcare on ethical decision making of physical therapists, a second important issue that evolved from this study is the conflict between the participants' values and the expectations of the profession of physical therapy. Nascent professions such as physical therapy seek to gain public and professional acceptance partly by emulating the values associated with the traditional medical model. However, the struggle of physical therapy to achieve the status of professionalism may result in value conflict among some of its practitioners. For example, the profession pushes evidence-based practice paradigms and professional autonomy, while certain members such as Barbara and Julie struggle to maintain their professional and moral identities that prioritize caring, context, and relationships over autonomy, money, status, and efficiency.

As physical therapists move toward the degree of Doctor of Physical Therapy, the question about what constitutes professional practice is an important one. In a profession dominated by women, physical therapists have an opportunity to redefine the traditional male paradigm of professionalism. Values of caring and responsiveness to patients, often delegated to the sideline, are becoming more central to an emerging, more-inclusive definition of professionalism, though this redefinition of the male professional paradigm may be made more difficult by managed care (Friedson, 1990; Pellegrino, Veatch, & Langan, 1991). Students may need to learn about the relationship between individual morality and professional morality. They may need to explore the historical nexus of the professional male model of professionalism and current and emerging models of professionalism based on care and responsiveness to patients. They may need to explore the influence of gender on professional development and identify potential areas of tension between their own values and those of the profession.

A third concern that grew out of this study is that participants in the study did not have formal education in professional ethics, rarely referred to formal documents and codes of ethics, and did not use any consistent theory or pattern of ethical decision making. Yet all reported experiences of moral dilemmas and entered into ethical decision making. How did they do this? One explanation may be the neuroethical model, which suggests that emotions and bodily experiences are part of a loop of reason (embodied reasoning). Damasio (2002) suggests that human beings develop biological neural markers in response to their prototypical (and recurring) patterns of socialization, and these neural markers enhance emotional responses during reasoning about moral dilemmas. The participants in this study appeared to use moral imagination to give rise to different ways of conceptualizing new (nonprototypical) situations. Several of the participants talked about emotions and feelings as integral to their moral sensitivity, moral motivation, and moral reasoning. This point is important for understanding moral perspectives. Common or prototypical experiences are those that are part of an individual's past experiences, embedded in the individual's current conceptual system, and are used for drawing inferences relative to some new conceptual system. Physical therapy students can be taught about the neurological basis of moral reasoning and the importance of moral imagination as extensions of one's conceptual system.

Given the lack of a conscious ethical decision-making process by participants in this study, the following question arises: What about a code of ethics? Is the APTA Code of Ethics called into question by this study, which indicates that practitioners fail to consider it? Classes in ethics can enhance awareness of the value of a code of ethics and normative ethics for physical therapy practitioners. However, findings from this study as well as literature in physical therapy and other professions suggest that although codes of ethics and normative ethics are important for healthcare professionals, practitioners also need to pay attention to the nonnormative bases for ethical decision making.

Implications for Education

What are the educational implications for professional physical therapy programs? Previous studies, as well as this one, suggest that new educational practices should be considered. Sisola (2000) reports the importance of moral judgment and reasoning skills in the development of clinical competence and emphasizes the importance and challenge of physical therapy educators to develop strategies for integrating ethics into professional training. Triezenberg and Davis (2000), responding to a lack of a specific curriculum in ethics in physical therapy programs, outline a curricular strategy to facilitate physical therapists as moral agents in

clinical practice, arguing that ethical instruction should form the philosophic underpinning of every physical therapy curriculum. The goals of
their plan are to help students develop moral sensitivity, moral reasoning,
and moral character through a combination of progressive curricular
strategies including, but not limited to, storytelling, role playing, discussion of case studies with moral issues, reviewing ethical theories, cri-
tiquing standards of professional practice, and exploring the application
of those standards to real-life situations.

One implication for educational change is the use of narrative to open
up new possibilities in professional physical therapy programs, helping to
bridge the gap between theory and practice. I believe that theory, which
provides the constructs and principles of clinical and moral management
of patients, is useful for the foundational knowledge of physical therapy
students. Theory provides a way of entering into the discourse of a profession and of exposing students to what has been and is being done with respect to patient care. However, to the extent that theory is removed from
practice, such a theory is by definition an abstraction that "falls short
of the mark in describing the particular situation" (Benner et al., 1996,
p. 308). In other words, the formalism of theory, including its language
and its assumption of constancy across patient cases, fails to account for
qualitative distinctions that are central to our understanding. Using narrative in education provides a context for understanding theory (through representing experiences) and encourages students to evaluate the effectiveness of their learning, including the integration of theory into practice.

Second, a traditional approach to professional education is rooted in
reliabilism. Reliabilism holds that a person holding a belief in a proposition is justified if and only if the belief is the product of a reliable belief-
making process. Therefore, giving a reason need never be a necessary condition for human knowledge (Boyles, 2000). Boyles argues that a reliabilist
approach to education results in a pattern of blind realism, that students
must blindly accept a belief about a proposition (without justification or
responsibility for finding the truth of a proposition). Simply put, all too
often in professional education programs, educators (and students) accept
truth based on authority figures—those historic figures in textbooks
whose knowledge has been passed through generations. In turn, many of
these authority figures too easily fall into comfortable patterns of telling
students what students think they ought to know, without engaging and
challenging the students about these beliefs. The result is a permeation of

unchallenged assumptions about the nature and scope of clinical practice, resulting in what Boyles (2000) describes as "knowing weakly" (p. 36). I am arguing for a justification of knowledge based on what Boyles refers to as a justificatory social epistemology that rejects reliabilism.

Third, a great number of physical therapy programs are based on positivism. Physical therapy students learn how to objectify and reduce knowledge and how to control for extraneous variables. This is the positivist approach to knowledge. The catchword for physical therapy education, as in some other health professions, is evidence-based practice. But what constitutes evidence remains elusive. Individuals interpret data differently. I argue that what is missing in positivism are personal experience and context that can convey a tacit knowledge that is embedded in experience (Benner et al., 1996). Sternberg and Wagner (1986) describe tacit knowledge as practical know-how that usually is not directly taught or even openly expressed. Rather, it is the kind of knowledge an individual obtains in everyday situations rather than through formal instruction. It is the knowing that is "in between and beyond," the richness and depth that is often lost through a process of strict reliabilism or empiricism.

Benner et al. (1996) argue that professional education has been rooted in the instrumental application of research-based theory as the solution to patient care problems. There are qualitative distinctions of experience that theoretical constructs and abstract principles taught in classrooms can never capture. For example, Julie described moral imagination in the clinic as "existentialism, where you have a set of rules but you got to figure out a way that you have to play fast and loose with the system." This type of experience is impossible to replicate in the classroom, and some may argue there is a good reason for that. I refer to Dewey (1925) in this context. In *Experience and Nature* he writes, "Meaning is a quality of interactions of organism and environment, it is a property of behavior. . . . When objects are isolated from the experience through which they are reached and in which they function, experience itself becomes reduced to the mere process of experiencing" (p. 15).

I believe that the emphasis is on the student to answer the question, "How do you know?" Consistent with placing justificatory responsibility for knowing on the student, the teacher also is responsible to provide the context and the experience, allowing the student to undergo a process of reflective inquiry and construction about a proposition. In this context, both the teacher and the student create experience in order to learn, and, therefore, knowing becomes a fluid and ever-evolving process. Knowing, and in the case of this study, knowing about morality, becomes contingent on an individual's experiences.

Concluding Thoughts

The stories presented in this study tell us about how physical therapists construct and understand their professional morality. If the experiences of these 5 participants are not unique it suggests that professional morality begins with a person's core values and is influenced by his or her previous life experiences. It is safe to say that, at least from a Western perspective, there are common cores of values that we share, but that those values are ordered differently, based on one's community experiences. We can also conjecture that most physical therapists undergo a process of moral transformation. This includes a process of integration and moral imagination, including a metaphorical understanding of moral dilemmas. We know that caring demands caring for oneself.

If, as the study indicates, morality and ethics are contextual, should educators even bother to teach morality and ethics? I posit that we should. First, physical therapy is a moral practice with a normative framework, and its students should learn what the formal documents are, what they say, and what their limitations are.

Second, the constraint of managed care imposes moral dilemmas for the practice of physical therapists. Students may need to learn about the managed care environment and how it impacts physical therapists. They may need to hear stories directly from physical therapists, patients, and insurance providers. They may need to listen to the language that is used to understand the different emotional responses and moral perspectives.

Third, students need to learn about the relationship between individual morality and professional morality. They need to explore the historical nexus of the professional male model of professionalism and current and emerging models of professionalism based on care and responsiveness to patients. Exploring areas of tension that may arise between physical therapists' own values and those of the profession can help them to become more reflective practitioners.

Finally, students may benefit from learning about the neuroethical model of morality and its implications for their own personal and professional morality. Understanding where prototypical understanding develops, how it is embedded in our brains and bodies, the importance of emotions and feelings in reasoning, and the semantic framing of our conceptual systems offers students a new lens through which to view the development of their ethical decision making.

I have argued that narratives reveal human meanings and concerns, moral issues, and the practical knowledge embedded in clinical experiences. Narrative reveals the language and metaphors that we use in clinical practice, avoids the sterility of theoretical abstraction and principilism, avoids reliabilism, avoids blind realism, avoids depending solely on positivism, and provides context for meaning. In addition, students who are encouraged to listen to each other's stories begin an interpretive process that may carry over toward an empathetic understanding of their patients.

Appendix

American Physical Therapy Association Code of Ethics (2002)

PREAMBLE
This Code of Ethics of the American Physical Therapy Association sets forth principles for the ethical practice of physical therapy. All physical therapists are responsible for maintaining and promoting ethical practice. To this end, the physical therapist shall act in the best interest of the patients/clients. This Code of Ethics shall be binding on all physical therapists.

PRINCIPLE 1
A physical therapist shall respect the rights and dignity of all individuals and shall provide compassionate care.

PRINCIPLE 2
A physical therapist shall act in a trustworthy manner towards patients/clients, and in all other aspects of physical therapy practice.

PRINCIPLE 3
A physical therapist shall comply with laws and regulations governing physical therapy and shall strive to effect changes that benefit patients/clients.

PRINCIPLE 4

A physical therapist shall exercise sound professional judgment.

PRINCIPLE 5

A physical therapist shall achieve and maintain professional competence.

PRINCIPLE 6

A physical therapist shall maintain and promote high standards for physical therapy practice, education, and research.

PRINCIPLE 7

A physical therapist shall seek only such remuneration as is deserved and reasonable for physical therapy services.

PRINCIPLE 8

A physical therapist shall provide and make available accurate and relevant information to patients/clients about their care and to the public about physical therapy.

PRINCIPLE 9

A physical therapist shall protect the public and the profession from unethical, incompetent, and illegal acts.

PRINCIPLE 10

A physical therapist shall endeavor to address the health needs of society.

PRINCIPLE 11

A physical therapist shall respect the rights, knowledge, and skills of colleagues and other healthcare professionals.

References

American Physical Therapy Association. (1997). *The guide to physical therapist practice (Rev. ed.).* Alexandria, VA: Author.

American Physical Therapy Association. (2002a). *Physical therapy member demographic profile.* Retrieved January 2005, from http://www.apta.org/research/survey_stat/ pt_demo.

American Physical Therapy Association. (2002b). *APTA vision sentence and statement for physical therapy 2002, 1–3.* Retrieved April 23, 2002, from http://www.apta.org/About/aptamissiongoals/vision statement.

American Physical Therapy Association. (2002c). Code of ethics. *Physical Therapy, 82*(1), 98.

American Physical Therapy Association. (2002d). Definition of "autonomous practice," amended. *PT Magazine, 10*(1), 14.

American Physical Therapy Association. (2004). *2004 fact sheet: Physical therapy education programs.* Alexandria, VA: Author.

Baker, R., Caplan, A. L., Emanuel, L. L., & Latham, S. R. (1999). *The American medical ethics revolution: How the AMA's code of ethics has transformed physicians' relationships to patients, professionals, and society.* Baltimore: Johns Hopkins University Press.

Barnitt, R. (1998). Ethical dilemmas in occupational therapy and physical therapy: A survey of practitioners in the U.K. National Health Service. *Journal of Medical Ethics, 24,* 193–199.

Beauchamp, T. L., & Childress, J. F. (2001). *Principles of biomedical ethics* (5th ed.). New York: Oxford University Press.

Benner, P. (1984). *From novice to expert: Excellence and power in clinical nursing practice.* Menlo Park, CA: Addison-Wesley.

Benner, P., Tanner, C. A., & Chesla, C. A. (1996). *Expertise in nursing practice: Caring, clinical judgment, and ethics.* New York: Springer Publishing Co.

Blackner, J. (2000). Ethical issues in rehabilitation medicine. *Scandinavian Journal of Rehabilitation Medicine, 32,* 51–55.

Blau, R., Bolus, S., Carolan, T., Kramer, D., Mahoney, E., Jette, E. W., et al. (2002). The experience of providing physical therapy in a changing healthcare environment. *Physical Therapy, 82*(7), 648–657.

Boyles, D. R. (2000). Students as knowers: An argument for justificatory social epistemology by way of blind realism. *Social Epistemology, 14*(1), 33–42.

Branch, W. T. (2000). The ethics of caring and medical education. *Academic Medicine, 75*(2), 127–132.

Churchland, P. (1989). *A neurocomputational perspective: The nature of the mind and the structure of science.* Cambridge, MA: MIT Press.

Churchland, P. M. (1996). The neural representation of the social world. In L. May, M. Friedman, & A. Clark (Eds.), *Mind and morals* (pp. 91–108). Cambridge, MA: MIT Press.

Clawson, A. L. (1994). The relationship between clinical decision making and ethical decision making. *Physiotherapy, 80*(1), 10–14.

Damasio, A. R. (2002). The neural basis of social behavior: Ethical implications. In S. M. Marcus (Ed.), *Neuroethics: Mapping the field* (pp. 15–19). San Francisco: Dana Press.

Davis, C. M. (1998). Influence of values on patient care: Foundation for decision making. In S. B. O'Sullivan & T. J. Schmidt (Eds.), *Physical rehabilitation: Assessment and treatment* (2nd ed., pp. 200–243). Philadelphia: F. A. Davis.

Dewey, J. (1925). *Experience and nature.* Chicago: Open Court Publishing.

Dewey, J. (1960). *Theory of the moral life.* New York: Holt, Rinehart & Winston.

DuVal, G., Clarridge, B., Gensler, G., & Danis, M. (2004). A national survey of U.S. Internist's experiences with ethical dilemmas and ethics consultation. *Journal of General Internal Medicine, 19*(3), 251–258.

Engelhardt, T. (1996). *The foundations of bioethics* (2nd ed.). New York: Oxford University Press.

Etzioni, A. (1969). *The semi-professions and their organizations.* New York: The Free Press.

Fealy, G. (1995). Professional caring: The moral dimension. *Journal of Advanced Nursing, 22*(6), 1135–1140.

Freidson, E. (1990). Professionalism, caring, and nursing. Paper prepared for The Park Ridge Center, Park Ridge, IL. Retrieved April 2005, from http://itsa.ucsf.edu/~eliotf/Professionalism,_Caring,_a.html.

Gilbert, K. R. (2002). Taking a narrative approach to grief research: Finding meaning in stories. *Death Studies, 26,* 223–239.

Gilligan, C. (1982). *In a different voice.* Cambridge: Harvard University Press.

Greenfield, B. H. (2003). *Practitioners' reflections of morality and ethical decision-making in physical therapy.* Unpublished doctoral dissertation, Georgia State University.

Guccione, A. A. (1980). Ethical issues in physical therapy practice: A survey of physical therapists in New England. *Physical Therapy, 60,* 1264–1272.

Heraclitus. (1979). On the universe. In W. H. S. Jones (Ed. and Trans.), *Hippocrates* (Vol. 4, pp. 460–524). Cambridge, MA: Harvard University Press.

Jensen, G. M., Gywer, J., Shephard, K. F., & Hack, L. M. (2000). Expert practice in physical therapy. *Physical Therapy, 1,* 28–52.

Johnson, M. (1997). *Moral imagination: Implications of cognitive science for ethics.* Chicago: University of Chicago Press.

Kant, I. (1994). Grounding for the metaphysics of morals. In J. W. Ellington (Ed. & Trans.), *In ethical philosophy* (2nd ed., pp. 1–69). Indianapolis, IN: Hackett Publishing Co. (Original work published 1785)

Koch, T. C. (1995). Interpretative approaches in nursing research: The influence of Husserl and Heidegger. *Journal of Advanced Nursing, 21,* 827–836.

Kramer, A. (1997). Rehabilitation care and outcomes from the patient's perspective. *Medical Care, 35*(6), JS48–JS57.

Kuhn, T. (1962). *The structure of the scientific revolution.* Chicago: University of Chicago Press.

Lakoff, G., & Johnson, M. (1999). *Philosophy in the flesh. The embodied mind and its challenge to Western thought.* New York: Basic Books.

Lammers, J. C., & Geist, P. (1997). The transformation of caring in the light and shadow of "managed care." *Health Communication, 9*(1), 45–60.

Leners, D., & Beardslee, N. Q. (1997). Suffering and ethical caring: Incompatible entities. *Nursing Ethics, 4*(5), 361–370.

Liaschenko, J., & Peter, E. (2004). Nursing ethics and conceptualizations of nursing: Profession, practice and work. *Journal of Advanced Nursing, 46,* 488–495.

Limentani, A. E. (1999). The role of ethical principles in health care and the implications for ethical codes. *Journal of Medical Ethics, 25,* 394–398.

Lincoln, Y. A., & Guba, E. G. (1985). *Naturalistic inquiry.* Newbury Park, CA: Sage Publications.

Magistro, C. M. (1989). Clinical decision making in physical therapy: A practitioner's perspective. *Physical Therapy, 69,* 532–540.

Marshall, J. (1981). Making sense as a personal process. In P. Reason & J. Rowan (Eds.), *Human inquiry* (pp. 395–399). New York: John Wiley and Sons.

McCullough, L. B. (1998). *John Gregory and the invention of professional medical ethics and the profession of medicine.* Dordrecht, Netherlands: Kluwer Academic Press.

Mishler, E. G. (1986). *Research interviewing: Content and narrative*. London: Harvard University Press.

Newman, J. F., & Dunbar, D. M. (2000). Managed care and ethical conflicts. *Managed Care Quarterly, 8*(4), 20–32.

Noddings, N. (1984). *Caring: A feminine approach to ethics and moral education*. Berkeley, CA: University of California Press.

Noddings, N. (1995). *Philosophic education*. Boulder, CO: Westview Press.

Patton, M. Q. (1980). *Qualitative evaluation methods*. Beverly Hills, CA: Sage Publications.

Pellegrino, E. D. (1999). The origins and evolution of bioethics: Some personal reflections. *Kennedy Institute Ethics Journal, 9*(1), 73–88.

Pellegrino, E. D., Veatch, R. M., & Langan, J. P. (1991). *Ethics, trust, and the professions: Philosophical and cultural aspects*. Washington, DC: Georgetown University Press.

Percival, T. (1794). *Medical ethics; or a code of institutes and precepts. Adapted to the professional conduct of physicians and surgeons*. London: J. Johnson.

Post, D. M., & Weddington, W. H. (2000). Stress and coping of African-American physicians. *Journal of the National Medical Association, 92*(2), 70–75.

Purtilo, R. (1979). Structure of ethics teaching in physical therapy: A survey. *Physical Therapy, 58*, 1109–1106.

Purtilo, R. (1997). The American Physical Therapy Association's Code of Ethics: Its Historical Foundation. *Physical Therapy, 57*, 1977.

Purtilo, R. (1999). *Ethical dimensions in the health professions* (3rd ed.). Philadelphia: W. B. Saunders.

Purtilo, R. B. (2000). Thirty-first Mary McMillan lecture: A time to harvest, a time to sow; Ethics for a shifting landscape. *Physical Therapy, 80*, 1112–1119.

Raz, P., Jensen, G. M., Walter, J., & Drake, L. M. (1991). Perspectives on gender and professional issues among female physical therapists. *Physical Therapy, 71*, 1991.

Reiser, J., Dyck, A. J., & Curran, W. (1977). *Ethics in medicine: Historical perspectives and contemporary concerns*. Cambridge, MA: MIT Press.

Reiss, O. (2000). *Medicine in colonial America*. Lanham, MD: University Press of America.

Rest, J. R., & Narvaez, D. (1994). *Moral development in the professions: Psychology and applied ethics*. Hillsdale, NJ: Lawrence Erlbaum.

Romanello, M., & Knight-Abowitz, K. (2000). The "ethic of care" in physical therapy practice and education: Challenges and opportunities. *Journal of Physical Therapy Education. 14*(3), 25.

Rosch, E., & Lloyd, B. B. (1978). *Cognition and categorization*. Hillsdale, NJ: Lawrence Erlbaum.

Seidman, I. E. (1998). *Interviewing as qualitative research. A guide for researchers in education and the social sciences* (2nd ed.). New York: Teachers College Press.

Shepard, K. F., Jensen, G. M., Schmoll, B. J., Hack, L. M., & Gwyer, J. (1993). Alternative approaches to research in physical therapy: Positivism and phenomenology. *Physical Therapy,73*, 88–101.

Siegler, M. (1979). Clinical ethics and clinical medicine. *Archives of Internal Medicine, 139*, 914–915.

Sisola, S. W. (2000). Moral reasoning as a predictor of clinical practice: The development of physical therapy students across the professional curriculum. *Journal of Physical Therapy Education, 14*(3), 26–34.

Spiegelberg, H. (1994). *The phenomenological movement* (3rd ed.). Dordrecht, The Netherlands: Kluwer Academic Publishers.

Steiner, George. (1987). *Martin Heidegger.* Chicago: University of Chicago Press.

Sternberg, R., & Wagner, R. (1986). Practical intelligence: Nature and origins of competence in the everyday world. New York: Cambridge University Press.

Strasser, D. C., Falconer, J. A., Herrin, J. S., Bowen S. E., Stevens, A. B., & Uomoto, J. (2005). Team functioning and patient outcomes in stroke rehabilitation. *Archives of Physical Medicine and Rehabilitation, 86,* 403–409.

Swisher, L. L., & Krueger-Brophy, C. (1998). *Legal and ethical issues in physical therapy.* Boston: Butterworth-Heinemann.

Triezenberg, H. L. (1996). The identification of ethical issues in physical therapy practice. *Physical Therapy, 76,* 1097–1107.

Triezenberg, H. L, & Davis, C. M. (2000). Beyond the code of ethics: Educating physical therapists for their role as moral agents. *Journal of Physical Therapy Education, 14*(3), 48–58.

Weech-Maldonado, R., Morales, L. S., Spritzer, K., Elliott, M., & Hayes, R. D. (2001). Racial and ethnic differences in parents' assessments of pediatric care in Medicare managed care. *Health Services Research, 36*(3), 575–594.

Wise, D. (2000). How practicing physical therapists identify and resolve ethical dilemmas (Doctoral dissertation, Capella University, 2000). *Bell & Howell Information and Learning Co.* (UMI No. 3002458)

Wylie, J. V. M. (1998). *In the face of suffering: The philosophical-anthropological foundations of clinical ethics.* Omaha, NE: Creighton University Press.

Bending, but Not Breaking, the Rules

The rules break like a thermometer,
quicksilver spills across the charted systems,
we're out in a country that has no language no laws,
we're chasing the raven and the wren through gorges unexplored since dawn
whatever we do together is pure invention
the maps they gave us were out of date by years . . .

Adrienne Rich, 1978

Greenfield suggests that a worthy goal of codes of ethics is to clarify a moral language for its professional members. His study raises the question: In the current context of managed care and evolving roles for healthcare practitioners, how much guidance do professional codes provide for ethical decision making? Do practitioners of physical therapy, nursing, and other health professions need to explore further the meaning of rules, traditionally charted systems, and ethical maps that guide their practice?

Pellegrino notes that professionals are confused about the obligations and moral values that ought to govern their interactions with those who seek their help (Pellegrino, Veatch, & Langan, 1991, p. vii). Greenfield points out that professions identify moral principles that are intended to guide their practitioners, but these professions are composed of individuals with diverse perspectives and beliefs. Unless practitioners understand their own values, the possibility exists for unresolved value conflicts between the profession and its members, and the codes serve as mere abstractions. The premise of Greenfield's study is that individual perspectives about morality and ethics are embedded and consequently uncovered within their particular lived experiences. Thus, if we are to understand these individual values, we must listen to the voices and experiences of practitioners.

Ethics, Caring, Science, and Technology

Most readers of this book are probably representatives of the nursing profession, which has emphasized the importance of caring in nursing. It is interesting to hear that the voices of physical therapists are very similar to those of nurses. We hear the physical therapists' concern about establishing a scientific database for their practice in much the same way that nurses struggle with establishing "the evidence" for practice. Sam articulates this seeking of science:

Has physical therapy ever been shown to be therapeutic? Well, there is a hot issue with that. I don't think there has been a proven way, or anything that we do in medicine, that has been shown to change the path of back pain. So here we are, in this dilemma. We're treating somebody without any substance. While I'm treating him and I am taking from the insurance company, I have to earn a living. So, to me, that is the biggest moral issue of my profession. I am working in a profession that really has not shown me [sic] to make a difference. (p. 207)

Benner and Wrubel (1989) propose an alternative way of viewing this situation that would seem to provide ethical guidance for nurses, physical therapists, and other healthcare professionals. They propose that the "essential relationship among caring, science, and technology" is what the professions need to figure out (p. 372). They note that nursing (and this would seem to apply also to physical therapy) could make claims for recognition, rights, and status based on its highly specialized knowledge of science and technology related to healthcare, but this would avoid the battle to gain legitimacy and status for caring. In fact, it may be caring, and its essential relationship to evidence, that guides the ethical use of technology. Sam worries about using a treatment on a patient that has not been scientifically validated as efficacious, but perhaps it is the "caring" embedded in the decision making that provides the basis for the ethical, although yet unproven, intervention.

Greenfield's participants discussed struggling to support patients, emotionally and psychologically, even after all of the physical therapy goals had been met. Tom articulated his struggles:

A conundrum case . . . where our reimbursement for this patient was very small. . . . She is a high-level musician, and this is a person's life. You know, I felt responsible. . . . I did get her back performing again, but never to the level that she had before. . . . But it took literally three years. . . . I had developed too much of an emotional bond with this patient . . . and I struggled with this case. (p. 212–213)

Greenfield notes that Tom saw himself as becoming an enabler by creating an emotional and psychological dependency that was mutually detrimental, both to the mental health of Tom and to the patient. Benner and Wrubel (1989) discuss how to find the right kind and level of involvement with patients. They point out that overinvolvement as caregiver can reflect the need to control and dominate the situation, analogous to a "leaps in" solicitude described by Heidegger (1962). Benner and Wrubel suggest that this kind of practitioner may take on the role of omnipotent rescuer, where the boundaries between self and others become blurred (p. 374). They propose that the remedy for overinvolvement is not *lack* of involvement, but rather, the right *kind* of involvement, which embodies the art of maintaining an openness and intimacy, accepting the value of one's best offering without becoming enmeshed in the need to do more and more, even if the help may not be curative (p. 376). Nodding (1984) uses the term "engrossment" to refer to this offering of caring embedded in a warm and caring relationship (p. 19).

Beyond the Rules

Barbara, a participant in Greenfield's study, stated, "You try to find ways around the rules, sometimes, without being unethical" (p. 211). If we accept that an important element of being a moral practitioner is to thoughtfully and deliberately examine the rules in order to create an understanding of the essential relationship between caring, science, and technology, it stands to reason that it may be unethical in some situations *not* to bend or even break rules. Acting from rule-governed obligations ignores the responsibility of exploring the unique context of healthcare and building a knowledge base for ethical decision making in the professions.

The classic research described by Benner, Tanner, and Chesla (1996) helps us see the importance of expert clinical practice in shaping ethical decision making for practitioners. Rubin (1996) unfolds a paradigm case of a nurse who describes her actions in giving medication to a patient to cause her death:

> She was ready to die and was dying and there wasn't a lot that could be done to prevent it anyway unless she wanted to be intubated and have a long course and probably die anyway, and opted not to be intubated and to take—what did she take?—some minor Valium or something. I've forgotten what, and stopped breathing, basically. (p. 172)

The nurse cannot recall for certain what medication she gave to cause the patient's death, the patient's condition, or her age. Rubin found that this lack of memory for details of patient situations was characteristic of the nurses who she categorized as experienced, but not expert, and reflected a peculiar form of practice that appeared to impede the development of ethical decision making. These nurses never came to experience their patients as individuals (Rubin, 1996, p. 177). They frequently made clinical and ethical judgments, but did not experience themselves as making these judgments, so that clinical knowledge and ethical judgment appeared to serve no meaningful function in their experience (Rubin, 1996, p. 173). The nurse in the paradigm case saw only a choice between the patient living in pain or helping her to die. The option of helping comfort the patient without causing her death was not considered (Rubin, 1996, p. 178). Expert nurses would certainly have explored this and other options to find an ethical and humane solution.

In fact, the nurse in the chilling paradigm case did not even consider this an ethical decision, but only a legal one, as reflected by this dialogue:

INTERVIEWER: Did you feel like you were in that gray zone?
NURSE: Well, I wondered if what I was doing was legal. And I think I must have found a way to, uh, make it okay in my mind. I mean I don't want to get sued. (Rubin, 1996, p. 181)

The nurse's response was characteristic of the lack of ethical perspectives shown by other nurses in this category identified by Rubin, in that they had no clear conception of the existence of an entity as ethical, instead reducing ethical considerations to legal ones.

In academics, ethical and clinical knowledge are often treated as separate entities, yet expert practitioners come to know that the two are inseparable (Benner et al., 1996). Ethical principles that students learn in the process of becoming a professional practitioner must be translated into everyday ethical comportment. Both narrative and community are important in learning the ethical and clinical distinctions that expert practitioners must develop (Benner et al., p. 232). Narratives form a critical function in shaping ethical decision making when expert practitioners relate stories to novice colleagues of "never again" experiences that they have worked through in their years of experience. This also indicates the role of community in shaping ethical decision making. Greenfield cites Engelhardt's (1996) description of a moral community:

Community is used to identify a body of men and women bound together by common moral traditions and/or practices around a shared vision of the good life, which allows them to collaborate as moral friends. Society is used to identify an association that compasses individuals who find themselves in diverse moral communities. (p. 7)

Novice practitioners, if isolated, have no context for learning how to translate rules they have learned in school to apply them to unique clinical situations. If they make an error, they may feel that they are alone and hide the mistake, for fear of losing their license. Novice practitioners need a community of ethical, expert practitioners to talk with, to hear their stories of how they translate ethical principles into practice.

Ethical Decision Making in the Professions

Weston (1997) points out that we tend to see ethical decision making in terms of opposites, like day and night, black and white, hard and soft. "But is it?" he asks (p. 52). Each side is often advocating for something that is important. When right conflicts with right, as it often does for healthcare practitioners, how do we decide? Weston's answer is that we try to integrate the conflicting values, so that we honor what is right in each of them. Arriving at this type of ethical understanding comes not from slavishly following rules but from challenging traditionally charted systems and maps that pretend that moral practitioners only need to follow rules. One way to begin to build this ethical understanding that integrates conflicting values is through exploring the experiences of expert practitioners as they make ethical decisions.

This brings us to reflect again on the language of ethical decision making. Weston (1997) points out that even the phrase "conflicts of values" sets us up to think in terms of polarization of values, making it sound as though we must choose (p. 59). He suggests that instead of focusing on conflicts, we think of them as reminders that values are complicated and that many ethical concerns must be addressed at once. Pellegrino states that "few issues are more relevant to contemporary society than the nature and ethics of the professions" (Pellegrino et al., 1991, p. viii). He notes that the ethical ground rules are changing dramatically. Greenfield's study suggests that one way of understanding the moral implications of today's healthcare system is as a paradigm shift that demands a rethinking of professional responsibilities and morality on the part of its practitioners. In this context, the professions have important power to shape culture, mores, and policy, creating integration of values and embodying the moral imagination that emanates from expert practice.

References

Benner, P., Tanner, C. A., & Chesla, C. A. (1996). *Expertise in nursing practice: Caring, clinical judgment, and ethics.* New York: Springer.

Benner, P., & Wrubel, J. (1989). *The primacy of caring: Stress and coping in health and illness.* Menlo Park, CA: Addison-Wesley.

Engelhardt, T. (1996). *The foundations of bioethics* (2nd ed.). New York: Oxford University Press.

Heidegger, M. (1962). *Being and time.* New York: Harper & Row.

Nodding, N. (1984). *Caring.* Berkeley: University of California.

Pellegrino, E. D., Veatch, R. M., & Langan, J. P. (1991). *Ethics, trust, and the professions: Philosophical and cultural aspects.* Washington, DC: Georgetown University Press.

Rich, A. (1978). *The dream of a common language: Poems, 1974–1977.* New York: W. W. Norton & Company.

Rubin, J. (1996). Impediments to the development of clinical knowledge and ethical judgment in critical care nursing. In P. Benner, C. A. Tanner, & C. A. Chesla. *Expertise in nursing practice: Caring, clinical judgment, and ethics.* New York: Springer.

Weston, A. (1997). *A practical companion to ethics.* New York: Oxford University Press.

6

Beyond the Individual

Healthcare Ethics in Diverse Societies

KATHRYN H. KAVANAGH

Twenty-first-century healthcare fuels new questioning about how we want to live and interact with others. While ethics in healthcare involves issues so interwoven into daily living that they are often taken for granted or overlooked, the literature on medical ethics and bioethics has historically emphasized extreme and overt situations—typically the margins of life and biomedical settings (see, for example, Kuhse, 2002). Everyday living with health or sickness and its interface with difference have been relatively neglected. In addition to those limitations, the ethical principles of Hippocratic and biomedical systems that are typically presented as the core of Western medical ethics fail to encompass alternatives to those traditions (Veatch, 1989). Furthermore, since the ethics literature traditionally assumes that European and European American culture defines moral development, the added bias of American individualism has resulted in a highly individualistic perspective that is insufficient in today's diverse society (Cortese, 1990).

A broader human discourse and understanding of social dynamics are needed to realistically explore alternative views of ethics. We must move beyond the individual to recognize and critically examine systems of oppression in and beyond the world of healthcare. In U.S. society, for instance, without identification and explication of phenomena such as race, class, and gender (including how these play out in healthcare), understanding of social realities influencing health status remains obscured. Without such an understanding, there is no way to change the unjust status quo. Ethical issues challenge every research, learning, and practice approach and effort in healthcare today. It is time that healthcare paid more attention to the phenomena of race, class, and gender.

The purpose of this anthropological study is to raise questions and explore ethical issues that surround research, learning, and approaches to practice in contemporary healthcare. Consistent with a critical perspective, extant literature is reviewed and the findings synthesized. This study asserts that, while Western ethical and moral systems reflect the privileging of individualism that shapes much of contemporary culture, it is highly significant that society is both more and differently diverse than in the past—and that it continues to diversify. At first glance, diversification may imply more numerous categories, but it can simultaneously be viewed as the dissolution of boundaries.

Recognition of differences (whether in terms of opportunity, lifeways, appearance, health status, or other characteristics) impacts both the social and political spheres. Political, social, and economic practices reflect cultural ideals that shape individual perspective and the experience of living. These ideals are embedded in language and expressed through cultural values and social norms as social comportment. The United States remains ideologically unresolved about being assimilationist (with goals of everyone conforming to a similar, dominant worldview) or pluralistic (welcoming differences). A tension is formed by ethics' conceptualization in terms of individuals that reflect western-European-based American values, while actual present-day society and social change imply new and unresolved concerns about health and healthcare in widely varied social and cultural contexts (e.g., Hoshino, 1995).

While the intellectual histories of the healthcare disciplines tend to emphasize individuals over society as a whole, people live in the world in fundamentally plural ways. Compared with American culture, most traditional and non-Western societies are far less invested in individuality and are instead more group oriented. Furthermore, ethical issues permeate societal relations, and health-related work is social in nature. Definitions of socially acceptable and unacceptable behavior and situations vary with context, including the differences between a legal and a moral context. Since diversity includes many types of difference, healthcare praxis may involve intervention with people whose ideals or actions do not conform to acceptable professional or personal moral standards. We make ethical decisions about interacting with, for instance, people and organizations whose objectives are met through dehumanizing means (Chambers, 2000). Focused as we are on individuals in healthcare ethics, however, when we observe "fallenness, averageness and inauthenticity" hardening into convention (Weiner, 2001, p. 51), the situation is likely to be viewed as outside our purview. This broader problem is typically left for others to deal with—presumably those others directly invested in the matter, or the people involved (who may be relatively powerless), or those charged with regulating society.

From a position of mindful social concern, this study argues that the reframing of such concealments in the everyday lifeworld must become the focus of healthcare ethics in order for new questions to emerge. Questions about understanding issues at the level of society and in diverse society are embedded throughout the study. Since many Americans do not engage politically beyond issues of personal interest, healthcare professionals may not feel obligated to attend to societal issues (such as immigration or social support programs) outside the context of a given professional or academic venue. It is precisely this issue of perspective and involvement that this study addresses. Health- and healthcare-related ethical issues are obfuscated by American individualism and a lack of concerted commitment to either the coexistence of diverse realities or assimilation into a shared worldview. Yet I assert that professionals in healthcare and the human sciences, as social beings, are ethically bound to respond to societal-level concerns.

Healthcare professionals are in positions that influence the views and actions of others. As personal selves, they exist within webs of interpretation that implicitly and explicitly acknowledge varied social orientations and conceptions of good and morality (Mulhall & Swift, 1996). In a society wrought with contradictions, do those in healthcare help people preserve their traditional health-related beliefs and behaviors, or do they help them adapt to change? I argue that neither stance is right or wrong, but that it is the healthcare professional's responsibility to think through her attitudes and positions toward such issues. The fact is that social interaction in healthcare contexts typically communicates perspective, even while superficially masking personal opinion with professional distancing. Accepting the premise that morality is to be found in the structure and organization of society rather than in human cognition (Cortese,

1990), anthropology's broad and critical stance allows the complexities of race, class, and gender (and how these shape and are shaped by personal and social interaction) to be revealed in healthcare contexts. Within that framework, it is helpful to inform and frame discussion of healthcare ethics and diversity in postmodern society with interpretive phenomenology.

Heidegger and Ethics in Postmodern Society: A Communitarian Perspective

Extrinsic ethical models focused on problems (betrayal, deception, rationed access, or harm, for example) fail to protect persons adequately in today's unprecedented and increasingly complex interface between society and healthcare. Codes of professional ethics suffice in value-free enterprise, but what professionals do in healthcare and the human sciences is not value free. Different peoples espouse different values; ethics reflect values. Only ontologically transformed views of ethics can contend with the interaction of human action and varied conceptions of good. Misinterpretation, misrepresentation, and nonrecognition instill deep injuries (Kavanagh, 2005). In physically diverse, multicultural, and economically stratified societies, potential harm includes social phenomena such as loss of dignity or agency at the aggregate as well as individual level (Guba & Lincoln, 1989).

The plurality of difference among humans is not brought routinely into ontological discussions, but Heidegger's "being with one another" (what psychologically is called intersubjectivity or ontologically called *Mitsein*) alludes to consideration of such plurality (Olafson, 1998). The capacity to understand the world we share with other people is a constituent element in our ontological constitution. Humans always already exist in the world with other humans. Socialization to healthcare-related disciplines may emphasize individualism in preference to more mechanical and disease-oriented perspectives but leave us attending to process only at the level of individual rights and responsibilities. We lack adequate ethical directives to fit today's critical and postcolonial sensibilities. The language of political correctness may further preclude understanding, as do long-held patterns of association that limit knowing others who seem significantly different from ourselves.

We are always both singular individuals and plural, simultaneously present and becoming, ever changing, always already becoming while "Being-towards-death" (Heidegger, 1962, p. 310). The days of illusory "one-way meaning" are over; possibilities of communal bonding and sharing invite our exploration (Gaillot, 1999, p. 17). We are not without values but rather face a bedazzling "multiplicity of meanings" (Heidegger, 1968, p. 71). There is always strong evidence of great differences in the values that exist. No single meaning—"given or produced, divine or ideological"—can be complete and fulfilling by itself (Jean-Luc Nancy in Gaillot, 1999, p. 94). It is in interpretive thinking and dialogue that multiple meanings in ethics can be opened and considered.

Because Heidegger's concept of *Dasein* as being-there shows that human being is essentially relational, it is important to note that the relation is not only to itself and other humans but also to both known and unknowable otherness (Hodge, 1995). Yet, while we long for authentic, reciprocal intersubjectivity, our worlds remain constituted of our individual (albeit culturally shared) referential contexts (Heidegger, 1962). Relationships among humans can be only external, existing as we do "side by side" *(nebeneinander)* (Olafson, 1998). We cannot crawl inside another's thinking, feeling, or experience, no matter how close we are. In healthcare, all "others" are interpreted through perspectives and social roles. It is in the co-disclosure of the shared world that issues of voice, reflexivity, identity, and understanding reveal themselves. Ethics, comprised of the study of morals and human duty, reflects responses to the presence of others dwelling in the world.

Heidegger insisted on embedding philosophy "back into the tradition out of which it emerges" (Hodge, 1995, p. 5). One wonders, then, whether Heidegger's failure to further develop his discussion of *Mitsein* (our being with others and "manyness") and *Fürsorge* (a word composed of *Sorge* [care] and *für* [for]) (Olafson, 1998), with understandable links between those, was not an artifact of cultural and linguistic constraint. It is the relationships *between* being with one another and caring about one another that are central to moral philosophy (Olafson, 1998). Hodge points out that it is unknown why Heidegger presumes that ontology is not ethics. In any case, in the politics of recognition, individualistic acknowledgment of others may occur only in terms of one's own being (for example, learning about others to understand ourselves). Society's commitment to individualization encourages that limited view as the norm.

Ethics and Social Categories: Why Concepts Such as Race, Class, and Gender *Matter*

The boundary is a limit that as mystery draws us by its very withdrawing.

John Diekelmann, 2005

From Herodotus on, Greek scholars turned their attention increasingly toward society. Typically they attempted to explain both physical and social evolution by the same basic principles. Alone, man was helpless to defend himself against stronger foes, so he sought strength in numbers. Such social cooperation could not be effective without communication, hence came language and technical inventions. This development could be seen in terms of survival, but given the abilities of the human mind to discern differences between unethical or antisocial acts and their socially acceptable counterparts, the latter certainly promised more peaceful and pleasurable states of mind (de Waal Malefijt, 1974). Aristotle, like Plato, emphasized the importance of society in an excellent human life: man was a social being, and his language and rational thinking served to further and better his social interactions.

In contrast, the 20th century trapped much thinking about health and healthcare in a cage of isolated rationality. The emphasis on reason sustained the Enlightenment's concern with rationality and the individual (Marshall & Koenig, 1996). Nineteenth-century thinkers generally followed their 18th-century predecessors in joining morality and intellect in a common progress to which reason appeared the keystone. As social and cultural differences came under closer scrutiny (a process aided greatly by imperialism and colonialism), science grappled with the amoral nature of the principle of natural selection. The doctrine of survival of the fittest raised serious problems for those who looked to civilization as a humanizing process. New concerns for societal roles of spiritual belief and religion were prompted by the notion that the weak were destined by natural selection to be ravaged and overcome by the strong. This prospect contradicted Western visions of civilized society as regulated by law, morality, and justice.

Avoidance of the ethical dilemma posed by natural selection led to denial that the social process of humankind was identical to the biological. Indeed, it was said, "in its ethical drive, the social was counterselective to the biological—the weak were protected, and rightly so"

(Voget, 1975, p. 223). Humankind was viewed as special—as outracing biological processes and evolving its own special social environments. This renovation of old religious issues as a moral and social force laid new foundations for the opposition of nature and nurture. It also brought with it the classificatory processes that represented scientific logical orderings and arrangements of phenomena through assignment to domains, taxonomies, paradigms, and trees.

The formation of general theory is the formation of categories. The pitting of those against each other in comparison and contrast is an essential aspect of rational thinking. Thus, cultural patterns disclose creation of identities, meanings of "otherness," ways of thinking, ideologies of hierarchy, and diverse ways of representing. Elaborate terminologies of differentiation and specialization promise mathematical precision and quantitative measurement to those invested in seeking statistical understanding and control. At the same time, categories, and the boundaries alleged to separate them, also become important when grappling with issues of reflexivity, incorporation of voices, and the ethics of rights and responsibilities (whether of the public as a collective or of various societal scales) in healthcare and health-related areas of concern.

Diversity and contradiction are now viewed essentially as human character, which poses ambiguities with regard to self-image and purpose (Voget, 1975). While moving beyond cultural ideals and preferences in assessing the relative value of perspective or behavior is laudable, it is also clear that absolute relativism (that is, the view that any behavior is acceptable as long as its perpetrator justifies it to himself) leads to social nihilism (de Waal Malefijt, 1974). Such a stance has limitations of applicability akin to those of idealized notions such as psychobiological intermingling of all peoples through ever-expanding conscious awareness (de Chardin, 1961).

In interpretive work, misinterpretation, like misrepresentation, "spreads in wider circles and takes on an authoritative character" (Heidegger, 1962, p. 212) so that failure to rectify transforms "an act of disclosing" into "an act of closing off" (Olafson, 1998, p. 38). Presuming concordance is reachable, to go beyond "a common understanding of what is said" (Heidegger, 1962, p. 212) to responsible ethical interpretation requires, minimally, the representation of multiple voices, the enhancement of moral discernment, and the promotion of social transformation (Christians, 2000). Focusing on general morality and our human "manyness," we need to understand healthcare ethics from a communitarian perspective, that is, one that is inclusive, democratic, and open to the claims of disempowered peoples (Sandercock, 1998).

Since examination of diversity and ethics is social in character, it is *not* limited to the subjectivity of personal viewpoint, the protection of individual autonomy, or the supposed neutrality aimed at protecting "free and equal rational beings legislating their own principles of conduct" (Root, 1993, p. 198). In fact, preoccupation with individual rights undermines exploration of the social, for culture is then viewed as something extraneous to the rational core human, or something that can be stripped away to reveal a universal being (Callahan, 1996). The notion of universality likewise precludes the deliberation of ethics as both cultural and contextualized, that is, the view that difference has meaning and significance. The generalization or universalization of ethics threatens reduction of the question "What is it to be human?" to a metaphysical fixity that would take priority over "a lived negotiation with being human" (Hodge, 1995, p. 27). However, even where there is agreement that morality is inherently social, meaningful dialogue across disciplines and peoples may be constrained in the name of so-called political correctness. Politics then becomes a substitute for an ethical system grounded in custom and community and represents a metaphysical "will to truth and identity" (Hodge, 1995, p. 21).

Societies are embodiments of institutions, practices, and structures that are recognized, at least internally, as legitimate (Christians, 2000). There can be no gathering of humans into ordered associations without "politics" designed to attend to and regulate the needs, desires, and interests of those committed to conserving the association (Outlaw, 1998). Subsequently, no community can persist across time without ascription to correctness in political life. The goal for overcoming the ensuing constraint is a critical consciousness that directs praxis and reflection in daily life toward awareness of conditions of sociopolitical control that may seem so natural as to go unquestioned (McLaren & Lankshear, 1994).

There are actually two important issues here: one is the extent to which social realities continue to reflect the "centrisms" (e.g., racism, sexism, classism or elitism, etc.) and the other is the question of how a decent society treats issues such as race, sex, and class (Wasserstrom, 1993). First, the human sciences are increasingly cognizant that the most debilitating impact of the social "centrisms" is not rooted in blatant discrimination against individuals but in support at population levels by institutionalized practices (Better, 2002). Even the most well-intended social policies and practices may have unforeseen results (Murray, 1993). We lack good ways to recognize such misguided practices, which are often subtle and may not be obviously connected with the negative outcomes they cause. However, we are moving toward understanding the implications of centrisms through interpretive research such as that in volumes 1 (Diekelmann, 2002) and 3 (Kavanagh & Knowlden, 2004) of this book series.

Second, in North American healthcare, the social origins of suffering and distress, including poverty and discrimination, are typically set aside in lieu of expanding biomedical interventions focused on signs and symptoms rather than causes (Kleinman, Das, & Lock, 1997) and on curing rather than healing. In a culture highly vested in the civil rights of individuals, ethical concerns more often focus on individual rights, autonomy, and justice than on social and cultural characteristics and plights. Thus, for example, medicine struggles to save extremely premature infants but rarely asks questions about other meanings of that struggle—such as the reasons for their premature births or the social consequences of their continued existence (Lock, 1996).

Even at the level of individuals, in a society focused on doing and producing, cultural issues around *being* often go unnoticed. We can "lose the sense of a domain that lies beyond the power and limits of the human" (Weiner, 2001, p. 164) and must rely on the revealing or unconcealing of those characterizations of being that we frame as ethical concerns. The practices of engendering community matter. Through shared understanding, we have the potential to settle differences or to experience public discourse oriented toward mutual understanding that respects communicative freedom to voice varying positions (Habermas, 1990). In this view of moral discernment, knowing is produced and disseminated through representation and discourse, while ideological hegemonies are consumed, resisted, and altered for various purposes. Since discourses are usually rooted in political, corporate, educational, media, or academic contexts (van Dijk, 1993), clinicians, educators, and researchers have a responsibility to understand the political contexts within which health-related issues are situated. Lack of such understanding can readily lead to our own writing, research, health policy decisions, and teaching becoming part of the "contradictory processes that at once challenge and articulate the cultural politics of race, racism and democracy" (Baker, 2001,

p. 116). Since power is seldom exercised in overt, observable ways (Peters, Marshall, & Fitzsimons, 2000), it is easy to become part of the problem by perpetuating systems of knowledge and power that are oppressive.

As researchers, writers, teachers, and clinicians, understanding the social and ethical nuances of our work is our first challenge. Effective and meaningful change hinges on the understanding of circumstances at the level of everyday lived experience, but not only at the individual level. It is this attention to the nature and practices of community that opens new possibilities for understanding. Understanding then discloses complex societal influences upon experience and makes way for meaningful intervention. For instance, small, local actions can help sustain cultural themes. A good example is found in the use of everyday indigenous narrative practices, for instance, to counter external storytelling practices that objectify and stigmatize specific ethnic groups. However, the potential of storytelling to effect change and produce new knowledge, as well as to maintain and explicate commonplace knowledge, is usually subdued, even ignored, in medical discourse (Dossa, 2002).

Understanding requires both thinking within a conceptual paradigm and exchanging properties of that paradigm, thereby disrupting it. The latter possibility, lending itself aptly to interpretive work, takes marginal ideas or images and attempts to disrupt the assumptive flow in which those ideas are contained. These cycles of interpretation, in which critique, interpretation, and understanding are explored continuously, extend discourses that foster new questions and understandings. Additionally, using deconstruction in juxtaposition with critical postmodern perspectives helps an interpreter think between and beyond the established categories. For example, it has been generally assumed that the driving force behind creation of technologies is the desire to meet universal human needs (Lock, 1996). Some theorists contend, on the other hand, that acceptance of such imagined consensus around the rationale of technological progress veils the interests of powerful elites and removes debate from the public sphere. Meanwhile, to presume that it is wholly power that serves as the standard is limiting, for it leaves intact the dominant modernist ideology of "progress" as an inherently rational pursuit in which culture makes no contribution (Lock, 1996). In sum, every perspective requires analysis of its own foundations and arguments as a way of navigating complex and changing phenomena (Diekelmann & Diekelmann, 2000). Examination of ethics and diversity in healthcare prompts questioning of power and hegemonic influence as well as of the interests being served by constructions of "otherness" in diverse societies.

Meanwhile, culture is always changing. It is the web of societal interaction and culture, in the context of ethics and healthcare, that grounds this chapter. The approach borrows from Heidegger the concept of *Fürsorge*, human beings caring about each other, with caring being central to our being with one another (Olafson, 1998). Such a "Being-with, like concern, is a *Being towards* entities encountered within-the-world" (Heidegger, 1962, p. 157). Heidegger refers to those entities toward which Dasein as Being-with comports itself as entities that are not objects of concern but rather of *solicitude* (Heidegger, 1962)—a more inclusive state of being uneasy of mind, disquiet, anxious, concerned, and caring (Oxford English Dictionary, 2002). Under the rubric of ethics, concerns around multivocal and cross-cultural representation, moral discernment, and resistance and empowerment are explored as they relate to healthcare and the human sciences today. Such exploration focuses, for the most part, on the study of social practices and processes and cultural politics in shaping differences rather than on the differences themselves (Foley & Moss, 2001). We must ask how we shape and are shaped by cultural values and social practices as well as how ethical stances shift from right to wrong according to the meanings and significances of social norms, events, and situations.

In recent decades, efforts to sensitize clinicians, teachers, and researchers to the significance of cultural meanings have made significant inroads in healthcare (e.g., Andrews & Boyle, 2003). People generally desire—for reasons of political correctness, if no other—to present themselves as culturally sensitive, knowledgeable, and skillful. However, we have an ethical responsibility to move beyond the mere avoidance of stereotyping and blatant ethnocentrism to being socially informed and involved. Commitment to that level of response requires understanding a configuration of diversity that involves an *amalgamation* of racialized ethnicity, class, and gender stratification (Marable, 2000).

Diversity, and the extent to which it does or does not exist as social fact in any given place and time, is culturally and socially constructed. Anthropology, involved as it is with the critique of civilization, is composed of four fields: cultural anthropology, linguistics, biological anthropology (human variation), and archaeology. These fields also come together in medical anthropology, making that discipline particularly well situated for examining links between diversity and health. While much work in ethics and healthcare is done from points of specialization, it is from a broad anthropological perspective that this study is conducted with the hope of prompting new questions about the interface of ethics and diversity. The following exegesis situates sameness and difference as a cultural challenge of identifying practices. It is human practice to create categories. Without those, there would be no similarities or differences to which to assign valuation. Such rankings and ideals are learned, via enculturation (being raised in a culture) or acculturation (learning a different culture), as properties of culture that may or may not be reflected upon and explored.

Sameness and Difference as Cultural Challenge

Understanding traditionally rests on three assumptions: human manifestations can be interpreted and are explainable in historical terms, different peoples and circumstances can be understood only by entering imaginatively into their specific points of view, and interpretation is always bound by one's own realities and horizons (Frank, 2000). Postmodern discourse, with its myriad images and dissolution of the established categories and identities linked to ideological positions of authority, opens possibilities for other views. For instance, exploring diversity today involves recognizing how modern societies contend with strong, media-dominated cultural influences that systematically produce a multitude of objectified cultural "others" associated with political and economic interests (Bok, 1998) and how neutrality gives way to either backlash toward or romanticizing of cultural groups or views that are far from neutral. Bias tends to be more subtle than in times past, and in the mélange of portrayals met on a daily basis, it can be difficult to recognize cultural struggles, particularly of stigmatized others, even when those others try to produce their own cultural images (Foley & Moss, 2001).

One of the products of any culture is the set of categories used in daily explanation, understanding, and interaction. Despite the reality of blurring where boundaries are said to be, categories such as race, ethnic group, class, and gender are used as if discrete. Yet we lack theories that adequately support the importance of, and demand respect for, difference in the development of humans and their societies. Respect alone is not enough; it is everyday lived experience that counts (Seidler, 1991). Yet, in everyday living, it is difficult to see the constructed nature of diversity and the complex processes underlying the categories used. While efforts are made in healthcare to minimize risks associated with labeling, stereotyping, prejudice, and discrimination, attending to social process more closely reveals old patterns of dichotomous categorization (Brodkin, 2001). Ideas about blackness are still constructed in relationship to whiteness, for instance, ideas about female in relationship to male, and being poor in relation to being wealthy. Whiteness, maleness, and wealth become invisible, despite functioning as the standards against which blackness, femaleness, and poverty are measured and become "other" or take on minority status. The goal of deconstructing ideas is to systematically displace such conceptual hierarchies as male/female, black/white, lower class/working class/middle class, and subjective/objective (Moss, 1998).

Further complicating the phenomena of commonly used categories is the fact of their interaction. Labels such as race, gender, and class are actually mutually constituted; they do not act alone (Lamphere, 2001). For example, men and women do not belong to the same class in the same way; they are defined differently (Lerner, 1997). Social scientists have explicated "whiteness," for instance, as dependent on class, gender, and sexual orientation as well as those phenotypic properties ascribed to race (see Kavanagh, 2005). Only with deconstruction can the alluring "naturalness" of those separate categories, and the power they hold in social relationships and discourse, be revealed.

Oppression has five faces: exploitation, marginalization, powerlessness, cultural imperialism, and violence (Peters, 1996). In a population as diverse as that of the United States, different peoples story those phenomena in different ways. Recognizing how difference works in society reveals and allows challenging of ideologies around, for example, the experiences of peoples marginalized in categories such as "mixed-race" (e.g., Feagin & McKinney, 2003), "non-white" (e.g., Fong, 2002), "disabled" (Frank, 2000), or "underclass" (Bigler, 1999)—along with untold others.

Culture and "Race": An Example of Social Fusing

There is no question that differences exist among humans, although ontologically, identity grants similarities as well as differences. As humans spread over the planet, adaptation to diverse climates and living conditions resulted in a profusion of complexions, colors, and shapes (Middleton, 2003). Stir those variations into gene pools and extract some isolated examples—and the myth of race is born. But the concept of "race" as a means of classifying people is both a recent phenomenon and peculiar to a specific time and place. Marco Polo (1254–1324), a medieval traveler from Venice, went from Italy to China and back, writing about diverse peoples he encountered but never using terms that corresponded to categories later known as "races" (Brace, 2002). Polo, like others of the time, traveled *on the ground*—something less often done today, especially over great distances, in our capacity to transport ourselves electronically or physically to any place on earth (and many in space, for that matter) while ignoring whatever lies between "here" and "there." Observing those peoples inhabiting the places between his origin and his destination, Polo saw the gradual differences that occur among peoples in situ. Such gradations—small genetic differences causing shades in coloring, for example—reflect a lack of authentic and categorically distinct "races" of people.

The concept of race was not used until science began scrutinizing biology at the same time that European societies were colonizing other parts of the globe. "Race is a category of biological classification, related to other taxonomic categories such as phylum, class, order, genus, and species" (de Waal Malefijt, 1974, p. 256). Phenotypic contrasts (that is, differences in appearance) fed categories, which in turn facilitated social processes based on the myth of distinct classifications. The Americas provide a prime example. The importation of slaves from West Africa by a European-based population resulted in a juxtaposition of people from three separate portions of the Old World: Africa, Europe, and Asia (Native Americans having migrated many centuries earlier from northeastern parts of Asia). With such apparent extremes, it was easy to overlook the gradations that remained elsewhere to belie the paradigm of race, which was reified through a collusion of scientific theory and economic interest. It is a measure of America's influence and the power of ideas that the concept of "race" that was essentialized in the settling of the Western Hemisphere is now being accepted uncritically in other parts of the world—China for example—where it did not previously exist (Brace, 2002).

"Race" has become a basis of identity, while focus on the individual has helped obscure its questionable origins. Over time, the notion of "race" has held up only as a *social* invention—not biological, despite its supposed conception in that area of study. There has never been agreement on how to categorize or number the biological evidence of "race": blood types, gene frequencies, or physical characteristics. Scientists have categorized humans into as few "races" as 2 and as many as 2,000 (Montagu, 1999). The notion of a "pure race" fails completely because there is such mixture of hair textures, eye colors, nose shapes, and lip structures that patterns last only until one looks beyond the immediate. In the absence of discrete categories, racial classifications are cultural constructs masquerading as biology (Marks, 1994).

Thus racial categories are historical phenomena that developed over time in societal contexts. As such and only as such, they are real. Now, however, mapping the human genome has specified how strikingly homogenous humans really are: the so-called racial groupings differ from one another only about once in a thousand subunits of the genome (Angler, 2000). Yet, for all this knowledge of how miniscule our biological differences are, "race" is still debated as if its supposed categories exist. But is it ethical to use "race," as has been done in medicine and nursing, as if it has biological meaning? As institutionalized as use of "race" is, change does not occur without concerted effort, and the lack of opposition to traditional uses of "race" both condones and perpetuates the practice.

Various interpretations of race have emerged out of a conflicted history of resistance, accommodation, integration, and transformation. From the days of slavery, colonialism, and forced assimilation to the days of "the colors of Benetton," "multicultural crayons," and issues of diversity in postcolonial society, political and economic relations have required the participation of diversified populations in the production and consumption of goods and services. The factual differences among such populations are less significant than the *meanings* ascribed to identity, affiliation, and both similarity and dissimilarity. The transformative powers of inclusion or exclusion adjust to appropriate cultural expressions of the "other" while holding that "other" at a nonthreatening distance in relation to the dominant body politic through dynamics of integration and marginalization. Healthcare holds itself aloof from this issue. The more deeply it burrows into a biological paradigm of race, the less responsibility it assumes for the social realities of those individuals it treats. Is that how we want to define health*care*?

The emergence of contemporary multiculturalisms and sociopolitical diversity must be understood in relation to 20th-century dominance of monoculturalism, which remained essentially unchallenged for the first half of the century (Goldberg, 1998). Given the United States' preoccupation with race for most of its opening centuries, it is not surprising that the United States has a history of ambiguous and often contradictory relationships with diversity and that the very term "diversity" often conjures notions of race.

Over several centuries, the diversity of migrating populations formed the foundation for multiple pluricultural colonial societies in which newcomers collided with indigenous peoples (Kunitz, 1989, 1994). Indigenous societies and their cultures not only experienced disease and abuse, but their peoples continue to suffer misinterpretation and misrepresentation. One small example (given that Native Americans are grouped officially by tribe, and tribes are popularly associated with chiefs) is that the concept of American tribal chiefdoms is an artifact of postmedieval European preconception and *not* an accurate depiction of the social organization of hundreds of diverse Native American societies (Kehoe, 2004). Colonial invaders interpreted what they saw with their old expectations and understandings. Ideas about categories (whether "races" or "tribes"), like other colonial vestiges, linger—tenacious and resistant to change.

We remain a confused society in which the concepts of race and ethnicity have evolved very differently. While race is a dynamic social construct with roots in the economics of slave labor and the ideological rationalization of exterminating indigenous others, ethnicity is a more recent concept. From the Greek *(ethnikos)*, "ethnic" refers to a cultural grouping that differs from that which dominates. There are no references to ethnicity prior to the late 19th and early 20th centuries, when the term surfaced as a means of differentiating those migrants "new" to America at the time and usually carried with it an implication of marginalization. Meanwhile, the racialization of some minority groups cast those as too "different" to assimilate (Marable, 2000). For example, although they are about 15% of the nation's juvenile population, African Americans aged 10 through 17 still account for more than 26% of juveniles in the criminal justice system (Better, 2002). While it has been known for a long time that so-called punitive corrections produce few positive outcomes, only now are some innovative programs (based on high-quality, personalized treatment programs in intimate settings) helping law-breaking youths to change in constructive ways (Warren, 2004). Missouri happens to be the leader in reconceptualizing juvenile corrections, while opponents of the approach insist such ideas would not work in *more diverse* California.

Humans are always already participating in identifying practices, and the meanings of similarity and diversity are continuously changing. Heritage is increasingly difficult to specify, but language, used as it is to grant both difference and similarity, continues to serve as a means of shaping meanings. As ridiculous as the formula sounds, analysts who strive to quantify ethnic heritage put golfer Tiger Woods at one-quarter Thai, one-quarter Chinese, one-quarter "white," an eighth Native American, and an eighth African American (Hall, 2001). He refers to himself as "Cablinasian," while typically being characterized in the media (particularly when his game is not at its best) as "African American." While the need to assign any categorical label reflects a reductionist Western proclivity for dissecting and classifying (Kavanagh, 2005), emphasis on a golfer's African American "eighth" surely suggests that the old "color line" has not dissolved completely.

We may no longer use "race" in the census to count five Blacks to equal three Whites, but obviously we are still counting in black and white and confusing race (biological differences that are presumed to be significant) with ethnicity and culture. We live in an epoch that valorizes similarities and differences, assigning great power to the categorical. It has long been known that language and labeling strongly affect behavior. Language both objectifies concepts and provides incentives to perpetuate them (Whorf, 1956). Surely we have an ethical responsibility to critique the impact of our thinking and practice.

Affirmative Action, Color Blindness, and Other Ethical Slippery Slopes

The use of categories continues to shape social relations. For example, "affirmative action," a formalized construct peculiar to the United States, denotes action taken to verify an established policy, such as fair practices during recruitment or employment (Arthur, 1993; Oxford English Dictionary, 2002). Based on the existence of notable differences, affirmative action continues to play an unsettling role in our present national debates about ethnic and racial relations. Initiated by John F. Kennedy in 1961, goals based on race and sex were used in hiring, promoting, and college admissions (Henslin, 2005). It is difficult to separate the results of the policy from economic booms and busts and the impact of increased numbers of women in the workplace, but affirmative action is viewed to have had a modest positive impact on diversity in schools and the workplace (Badgett & Hartmann, 1995; Reskin, 1998). Reaction to the policy, meanwhile, has been anything but modest.

While some say affirmative action levels the playing field of economic opportunity, others believe that prioritizing by race and sex reeks of reverse discrimination or unintended new forms of racism. Furthermore, affirmative action has led to widespread stigmatizing of those who benefit from it by suggesting that their hiring, promotion, or admission is *due to* their race or sex rather than merit (Henslin, 2005). In many parts of the world, meanwhile, the dictatorial character of antiracist ideology, presented as it has been as a moralistic and legalistic matter, has become a strong theme within the discourse of popular racism and a conservative sense of race, nation, and culture as rightfully one of kinship, blood, and ethnic identity (Gilroy, 1992). Confounded with those ideas are other people who resist the entire notion of classification put forth by both governments and academics and, decrying labeling people as "blacks" and "whites" and describing their relations based on that division a violation of basic logic and inevitably self-defeating in terms of "race relations," call for more sophisticated views of human interaction (Webster, 1992).

In 2003, in response to claims that underrepresented minorities were displacing qualified white applicants in college admissions, a ruling on affirmative action (following and upholding a 1996 amendment to the California state constitution that banned preferences to minorities and women in hiring, promotion, and college admissions) further complicated the situation with official ambiguity. The goal of racial diversity was laudable and minorities could be given an edge, the Supreme Court ruled, but that could occur only as the result of *individualized* review of applicants; automatic extra points for "difference" were unconstitutional (Henslin, 2005). The haziness—diversity is good but achieving it through quotas or automatic biases is not, in which case justice both demands and condemns affirmative action (Wilcox & Wilcox, 1997)—both tarnishes the idea of diversity and leaves educational officials, businesses, agencies, and society at large without real direction.

A new school of universalists has developed, meanwhile, based upon the notion that *any* recognition of unique status for racialized ethnic groups veers dangerously toward racial essentialism and separatism (Marable, 2000). Conservatives have denied difference by dismantling affirmative action programs, while liberals have promoted multiculturalism and ethnic diversity (Baker, 2001). Again, language has shaped and been shaped by classificatory ideals, and society remains frozen in the headlights of ambiguity and ambivalence.

Affirmative action has been used by both parties as a powerful political wedge. However, while affirmative action is often viewed as perilous with regard to school admissions, contracting, and employment, the public has reacted even less to the explicit creation of minority-majority districts that have helped nearly double the African American representation in Congress *while* creating what Supreme Court Justice Sandra Day O'Connor noted "bears an uncomfortable resemblance to political apartheid" (Baker, 2001, p. 110). These phenomena are ethical ramifications of "race" that are becoming so much a part of the American landscape that "politically correct" society generally no longer responds to the hegemonic manipulation.

In 1896 the Supreme Court ruled on *Plessy v. Ferguson,* making Jim Crow segregation the law of the land. A century later, the justices delivered similar watershed decisions with which they shepherded in a new, far less obvious, and apparently more benign era of race relations for the 21st century. The principle of a color-blind Constitution was used by the conservative bloc of the Supreme Court to challenge District Court desegregation orders, minority-majority voting districts, and federal affirmative action (Carr, 1997). The same principle mirrors the editorial positions of leading news publications grappling with the science and politics of race over the past decade. Although it is commendable when public discourse extends to such important issues, a profound problem remains with using arguments against the inanity of biological concepts of race to advance a color-blind thesis. Just as crediting Ashley Montagu with the concept that equating biological differences with race is *Man's most dangerous myth* (1952) in no way calls into question the ideal of a color-blind, meritocratic society, the rationale of the conservative bloc of the Supreme Court leaves American society with a profound ethical predicament. The situation serves as an exemplar of the accusation that agreement or "communion" can represent a complicity and complacency that is, in reality, the opposite of community but rather a withdrawal likened to a trancelike state (Nancy, 1997).

The problem with color-blindness is that there can be no identity or identifying practices without awareness of similarities and differences. Color blindness is but one kind of response to the categorical, even though it is an important one. The real issue, instead, is how similarities and differences are experienced or lived. No matter what is known about their being biological myths, everyday cultural categories of race continue to accrue social legitimacy and become encoded in practices and policies. If those phenomena are not recognized, made explicit, and dealt with, they have painful consequences for racially designated groups (Merry, 2001). While laws and policies rarely create racial categories, social rules governing such phenomena as immigration, naturalization, citizenship, political participation, sexual interaction, and access to healthcare have different meanings for differently racialized identities. Actual experience *matters,* and social categories and language shape how experience matters. Humans do not so much have histories as we live them, presented as we are with the past and present to shape the future of our possibilities.

Where do we go from here? We need to move beyond the categories and dynamics—not by avoiding them but by developing more inclusive ways of thinking and acting. The need is ever more apparent. It is highly unlikely that the constructed categories of white, black, Asian American, Latino, and Native American will be any more reliable in the future than they are now. Recognizing the increasingly unrealistic application of discrete categories (Root, 1992; Steinberg, 1989), the 2000 U.S. census allowed subjects to choose more than one "race," reflecting new assertiveness about mixed cultural heritage, biracial and multiracial identities, and various other hybridized validations. Twenty-five years from now the racial–ethnic mix in the United States will be dramatically different, in large part due to immigration. One of every 19 Americans is expected to have some Asian background and 1 of every 6, a Latino background (Henslin, 2005, based on *Statistical Abstract of the United States, 2002;* and Bernstein & Bergman, 2003). From any of the predominant ways of analyzing society—for instance, a conflict model (struggle for resources), a symbolic interactionist perspective (how groups might perceive one another differently as their relative proportions of the population change), or a functionalist view (seeing how each racial/ethnic group benefits, or doesn't)—it is clear that this shifting mix is one of the most significant events to occur in U.S. history. Whatever the ethical fallout will be, it is likely to be both substantial and insidious.

Policies of multiculturalism and pluralism support acknowledgment of racial and ethnic variation through citizenship education, antiracist ideology, and social action (Burbules & Torres, 2000). Minority groups maintain their separate identities while freely participating in national social institutions, such as education and politics. In authentically pluralistic societies, no one group is dominant. Switzerland provides such an example. Composed of four ethnic groups (French, Italians, Germans, and Romansh), each group has kept its own language and lives in relatively peaceful political and economic unity with none being a minority (Henslin, 2005). Can such a phenomenon occur in a much larger society or one with a history such as that of the United States? While biological differences dividing us are negligible, social implications of racial differences continue—and will continue—to demand attention. Ethics focused on individuals does nothing to either alleviate that or promote new understandings of it.

Although the knowledge of the Tuskegee experiment continues to have serious implications for health education and intervention programs, we are no longer the society that allowed African American men in Alabama in the 1930s to participate in an experiment so callous that it has gone down in history with those of the Nazis (Caplan, 1992). Nonetheless, the abstraction called equality, in which Americans often profess belief, can exist only if and when we figure out how to fairly reduce "racial" difference to the irrelevance it deserves (Cose, 2000). Meanwhile, we can dwell on why race is so important—or we can move on to other constructs, such as ethnicity, which itself becomes entangled in complex and racialized realities. Many theorists have proposed that the construction, deconstruction, and reconstruction of "race" as an intellectual device and social reality should lead to focusing on ethnicity and ethnicity-based principles of classification and organization (Webster, 1992). Yet, while such a change of stance may alleviate race's volatility in society and culture, it fails to address the invidious, continued impact of racism in everyday life.

For all of the unpleasantness of this socioethical quicksand, the ongoing raciation of ethno-nationalist conflicts and international variations in racial constructions (including the conventionally neglected configurations of whiteness) need to be addressed. "Race" still matters because the realities of racism continue to be reproduced (Donald & Rattansi, 1992; West, 1993). While political correctness is substantively withstood by the unpopularity, even illegality, of overt racism and other "isms," research demonstrates that discrimination in housing markets, for instance, continues to occur regularly, often in response to language and voice patterns linked with race. Speakers of Black English vernacular have significantly fewer opportunities to rent apartments than those who use White English, while the difference is most profound for women of color (Massey & Lundy, 2001). In sum, it remains paramount that diversity be understood as a nexus of social and discursive practices that perpetuate oppressive power relations between and among populations that some people with influence judge to be essentially different. Lived out on a day-to-day basis, an ethics that attends to practices of oppressing groups as well as individuals might offer new takes on the understanding of diversity and its role in healthcare.

More Ethical Quagmires: Ethnicity, Immigration, Class, and Gender

Contradiction sometimes seems an inherent aspect of diverse society—Heidegger's "restless to and fro." "Care becomes concern with the possibilities of seeing the 'world' merely as it *looks* while one tarries and takes a rest" (Heidegger, 1962, p. 216). Lest we be lulled into thinking race is society's major issue, or even that race operates in ethical seclusion, I return to my original premise that the ethics of responsible healthcare include not only the building of community but attention to the comingling of the many influences that provide problems through reification of difference.

In a culture that publicly supports violence as entertainment (Bok, 1998), speech codes and anti-hate/violence codes, which have spread through American schools and colleges, are argued against as thought control and violations of the constitutional amendment guaranteeing free speech. Yet, silencing people who oppose the presence of difference in society essentially promotes sameness, albeit through the silencing of criticism that is also often aimed at the double standards practiced by institutions. Many caution that recklessly large numbers, for example, of

Hispanic immigrants in the United States may lead to division of the country into two languages and two cultures (Grossman, 2004). Difference is demanded, even as it is rejected.

Advocates of linguistic assimilation (that is, of "English only" policies) note that European immigrants of a century ago typically lived in large enclaves such as Chicago's Polonia, New York's Little Italy, or San Francisco's Chinatown. Each city was a mosaic of ethnic villages adjoined by other ethnic communities. Over time, the offspring of those earlier immigrants generally dropped their original languages, acculturated (that is, while retaining some traditional ways, learned to get along in Euro-American culture), or even assimilated wholly into the English-speaking, European-based cultural mainstream. Public schools, during the great waves of European immigration between 1880 and 1920, were systems intended to facilitate the education of immigrants or their children for the mythical "melting pot" by trading ethnic uniqueness for preparation for industrial employment (B. M. Franklin, 2000). Today's schools are differently challenged to accept nearly all students, keep them longer, and send them into a very different job market.

While public schools were mass producing Americans, health problems blossomed in rapidly growing cities teeming with migrants from rural America and other countries. Hospitals mushroomed, while the overall societal response, swathed in reform, resulted in the Progressive Era with public programs centered on maternal and child health, protective codes, and the public health movement (Kavanagh, 2003). Biomedicine grew and flourished, specialized and diversified, medicalizing society and monopolizing healthcare until the bias of medical training against primary care and general practice, along with rising costs, led to a malpractice and insurance debacle (e.g., Good, 1998).

Meanwhile, American society also continued to enlarge and diversify, along with its health and healthcare problems. Cultural histories and ethnographic studies of the movements of populations (typically through study of immigration and other historical phenomena, such as political conquests) illuminate the many ways in which ethnic, racial, and gendered groups enter and transform societies (Nash, 2001). With varying degrees of representational accuracy, such studies relate directly to health and healthcare. For example, Ho's (2003) study of illness narratives of immigrant Chinese in New York City indicates that the dominant biomedical explanation of immigrant tuberculosis (58% of new cases of

TB in 1999) would benefit by being modified to look at *specific* migratory processes as risk factors. Gloss association of new immigrants with risk of disease is inaccurate and leads to negative stereotyping and racial discrimination. As is the case with other stigmatized conditions, blame and counterblame offer no safety from disease but seriously interfere with mobilizing work toward improved health—in addition to positive social interactions and adjustment.

Most healthcare researchers, faculty, and clinicians do not face an immediate or personal need to be knowledgeable about current patterns in migrant or ethnic relations. However, given the interface of healthcare with societal concerns about diversity, it is important that we stay informed. Ethics plays a larger role in some healthcare education programs than others, but few connect ethics and diversity in the context of social health or healthcare. Just as there exists in the West an undeniable lack of knowledge and appreciation for the contributions of other ways of knowing and living, there is also limited interest in health status beyond our borders. Only 15% of the world's population lives in industrially developed countries (the United States' share of that being 4.5%) (Watts, 2003). Previously, the ethical debate was between John Locke's theory (which strongly influenced American political and social life) that individuals must struggle on their own toward their own interests (Locke, 1690/ 1993) and Peter Singer's ideas about providing aid because people are not poor due to their nature and, therefore, we have obligations to assist populations toward industrialization (Kuhse, 2002). The question has now evolved in America into an irresolute ambivalence toward difference. Healthcare concerns are generally presented as having transitioned from being epidemiologically acute (infectious diseases) into conditions associated with chronicity, lifestyle, and aging. Poverty and national levels of industrialization or exploitation are typically left out of the equation. While such patterns do indeed represent much of society in industrialized society, they by no means represent more than a fraction of the world's population. Nor do they represent the millions of Americans who go to bed hungry at night—or do not have a bed to go to.

Despite possibilities for serious dialogue, it is difficult to refute that "the basic problems facing humanity continue to stem from its own disorganization, misdistribution of wealth, and prevailing relations of domination and economies of power and privilege" (Gaudiano & de Alba, 1994, p. 138). Throughout history, and in particular since the 1930s, those interested in social welfare in the United States have had to juggle political entanglements between private and public entities as well as balance attention between individual and societal issues. The pushes and pulls of our culture and language discourage attending to areas of concern beyond those most visible, powerful, and politically persuasive. In health and healthcare, those are embedded in biomedicine and the expectation that anyone partaking of the biomedical product will conform to that paradigm. In a society in which schools and programs are not competitive unless they offer credentials in ever less time and for fewer credits and dollars, education is increasingly compromised and "multicultural sensitivity" relegated to levels of political correctness that are inadequate for both understanding and quality care for individuals—to say nothing of diverse aggregates. Interaction is diluted to professional objectivity (including attentiveness to the issues around risk of litigation) and language limited to careful and defensive minimums. It is time to reconsider the ethics of healthcare and its teaching and practice.

The desire for an ethics becomes all the stronger as the open unknowing of human beings increases, no less than a hidden unknowing increases. A connection through ethics is all the more sought after where human beings have been handed over to a mass existence and can be brought to a reliable stability only through a collectivity and order of plans and action which are grounded in technical relations. (Heidegger, 1967, p. 349, as cited in Hodge, 1995, p. 99)

Until we find ways to broaden or otherwise transform our sphere of attention—in education, practice, and research—we will continue to be narrow in our social construction of medical knowledge, health needs, and ideas about ethical responsibility. I assert that perpetuating such a perspective does not do justice to our students, clients, and participants, or to humanity at large.

The United States of America remains the only industrialized country that does not provide guaranteed access to health services for all of its citizens (Davidoff, 1999). Meanwhile, the healthcare "safety net" presumed to catch the uninsured (of which the United States currently has more than 43 million) has been documented as being too costly to be feasible and as promoting negative experiences with, and overall avoidance of, healthcare (Becker, 2004). The fact that there is no official commitment to universal healthcare coverage in the United States means that health status will not change for the better without strong professional opinion, commitment, and involvement.

In addition to access issues, there are many other culture-based concerns in healthcare today. For example, AIDS education programs have failed to stop clients from practicing unsafe sex when cultural priorities dictate otherwise, which is often the situation for women who happen to be poor as well as at risk (Sobo, 1995). And across America, clinicians must contend with questions around "female circumcision" or genital cutting. If they are not dealing with such issues, it is more likely because professional healthcare is not viewed as a safe place to take such concerns than that there are no members of the community for whom the issue is a real and lived one (Gruenbaum, 2001). It is not easy to determine how biomedicine should participate in cultural practices when ideas about women's health and well-being vary greatly by culture. It is argued both that traditional genital cutting may have relatively few health effects (Obermeyer, 2003) and that it is ethically unsupportable because it is "irreversible reduction of a human capacity in the absence of meaningful consent" (Mackie, 2003, p. 135). Thus the complexity of measuring harm, something to which healthcare personnel are likely to attend to, obscures deeper ethical issues embedded in culture and cultural differences. Whatever the stance, the need for informed discourse is not alleviated by ignoring the issue. In a culture in which the self is put before society to such an extent that many Americans claim not to be "ethnic" or even to "have a culture" (Chávez & O'Donnell, 1998), there is a need to question courses, seminars, and literature that pertain to ethics but concern themselves with only legalistic matters and avoid those that muddy the waters—which may already seem uncomfortably deep at times—by including topics that are controversial, fly in the face of certainty, or call for narrative interpretation (Diekelmann & Diekelmann, 2000).

Cultural orientations differ widely in attitudes toward reproductive health and family planning as well as in utilization of the current technologies, although that should not obscure the fact that much of the earth's population still lacks reliable access to effective contraception. While knowledge is contested with regard to fertility regulation and family ideals, contraceptive and other health-related resources can be, and are, used by governments to manipulate land loss, political and military strife, and economic insecurity (Russell, Sobo, & Thompson, 2000). Among the many variables involved are traditional practices and relationships (e.g., spousal communication patterns), the genderization of reproduction as a "female" issue, lack of empowerment, and the way contraception is presented (since acceptability often depends on how aggressively it is promoted, and whether it is presented as "preventing" births or merely delaying them). Despite world population being one of the greatest challenges facing life today, many professional education programs include scant, if any, current information on global population issues, or discussion of the ethical interface between culture and technology. How ethically responsible is it that healthcare professionals deal primarily with individualized local concerns? Lacking are discussions of the money to be made in assisted reproduction (that is, the claim that "anyone can have a baby") (Franklin & Ragone, 1999) or biomedicine's rise to the challenge of keeping alive the tiniest preterm infant (which may cost hundreds of thousands of dollars—or more) to prove that it can be done, in a society in which resources for primary healthcare and health education remain inadequate.

Since 2001, ethnic diversity and immigration have confronted renewed turmoil in terms of stigma, homeland security, and terrorism. The trend toward tighter rein on the nation's borders is, in reality, much older and broader than recent events suggest. Overall, for more than a decade legislation has reflected a resurgence in anti-"illegal alien" sentiment in response to rising numbers (Chavez, 1997). Many programs addressing the social welfare of migrants through education and healthcare have been eliminated by the U.S. government (Nash, 2001). Immigrants are increasingly singled out and labeled, as with the issuing of new driving "certificates" (rather than licenses that can be used for identification purposes) (Barry, 2004) and the monitoring of immigrant status in healthcare clinics. Emphases on immigrant status often overshadow occupational and environmental health risks among, for example, farm workers, while agriculture is one of the most hazardous industries in the United States (Arcury & Quandt, 2004). In an ongoing struggle to balance issues such as road safety against federal immigration policy and homeland security, states are finding new ways to identify and label people with distinctions that may interfere with healthcare utilization as well as access. "Us" and "them" categories are being reified nationally even as globalism is professed to make the world "smaller." A useful alternative conceptualization views members of groups and societies as intersections or nexuses in networks of relationships that cumulatively constitute societies, nations, and a complex of countries (Ratliff, 1996). From a practical perspective, the "social nexus" view argues for interdependent responsibility.

Families are most at risk in the new scheme of things. Immigration policy between the mid-1960s and mid-1990s emphasized family reunification, but the highly restrictive 1996 Immigration Reform and Immigrant Responsibility Act ruled that spouses, parents, and children of a legal immigrant who are living in the United States without documentation must leave the country until they can get alien registration cards allowing them to become legal residents (Wheeler & Bernstein, 1996). Women often have a more difficult time than men in establishing a "paper trail," so they are generally the net losers in new rules stipulating that reentry will be barred according to the length of time they resided in the United States. California, a state with especially high numbers of immigrants, deprived legal as well as undocumented workers of education, healthcare, and other social benefits taken for granted by residents of other advanced industrialized societies (Nash, 2001). Not only do such policies further preclude the possibility of incorporating migrants as citizens in society at large but, while reducing the "brain-drain" (the lure of highly qualified people from other nations to the United States) to a trickle, today's workers must also contend with time-limited contracts, being without families, and lack of security in addition to severely limited access to healthcare. Until the ethics of social responsibility seeps deeply into American values, more inclusive and less punitive initiatives will continue to be vulnerable when budgets are cut. There may be more interest in communitarian views of social ethics today than in the past, but the issues are typically left to political domains (e.g., response to environmental disaster) and seldom become the fodder of discussion of everyday health situations in teaching, research, or practice contexts.

Mainstream globalization theories tend to ignore gender or to view it as peripheral to the core issues (Blackmore, 2000). (Globalization, as used here, denotes "the growing perceived spread of a capitalist world system and its integration with systems of trade, communication, transportation, patterns of urbanization, cultural influence, and migration throughout the world" [Gutiérrez & Kendall, 2000, p. 84]). However, myths such as that of the "male breadwinner" are being unmasked (Safa, 1996), while transnational networks are developing (for instance, between New York, Los Angeles, or Chicago and the Caribbean, Latin

America, the Philippines, or other low-wage countries) as people strive to maintain family ties and households. With changes in migration rules, men often lose their priority as providers while women enter marginal factory work or become domestic workers. In either case, many women interact with educated and professional women and are learning to politicize their concerns (Nash, 2001). Such community organizing and union building translates social disadvantages into political issues through which transformation and change, including that related to health, can transpire.

Many other societal issues outside the purview of immigration in the United States have ethical implications. For example, women and children, who are disproportionately the victims of domestic violence, continue to suffer from inadequate protection and a scarcity of shelters (Mwaria, 2001). When a Florida statute expanded child abuse to include drug-dependent newborns, many mothers were incarcerated. It has been argued that the law is sexist, racist, and classist in its effect of isolating poor women from other women, and that it reifies second-class citizen status by denying incarcerated women access to prenatal care and treatment for addictions (Whiteford, 1996). While no healthcare worker advocates that mothers give drugs to newborns, they may have reason to challenge the ethics involved in the ramifications of legislation.

It is not the intent of this study to thrust readers into despair and hopelessness with a litany of problems. There are many positive endeavors that could be sited—organizations providing basic care for needy populations, clinicians volunteering time, and increasing numbers of people engaged in service learning. People can and do make a difference—and they can learn to believe in and value that ability. The point is, however, that such efforts reflect the investment and sacrifice of committed individuals. Often, a significant contribution is so unusual as to be deemed newsworthy. The nation's global reputation is one of sociocentric aggression and consumerism; Von Dohlen (1997) uses the term "ethical hedonism" to describe the egoistic goal of avoiding pain and getting pleasure. The national policy is that healthcare is a privilege rather than a right, and ethics is presented in an atomistic model in which society is merely an aggregate of individuals who are essentially isolated and autonomous—connected only by physical location. Ethical systems grounded in the notion of beneficence often propose that action bringing the greatest benefit to the greatest number of people is the most ethical choice, but on the face of it, this position favors whatever views the majority holds; minority issues therefore clearly suffer. The focus on individual application aside, even with the "cause no harm" rule in place, which would merely safeguard the status quo of minority peoples, the model lacks any advocacy for parity or remediation (Ratliff, 1996). Only a communitarian view of ethics acknowledges that anything that impacts one group ultimately impacts the entire network and associated networks; in other words, "if one end of the social ship has sustained damage, passengers at the other end are unwise to dismiss it as 'their problem'" (Ratliff, 1996, p. 175). Healthcare educators, researchers, and practitioners are not going to resolve the world's problems—but they can make sure that the discourse is not allowed to stagnate or dwindle into individualistic concerns. What has become conventional discourse on ethics remains necessary, but it is not sufficient. Interpretive approaches can create new questions and take the project of ethics to both broader and higher reaches, and I would argue that interpretive inquirers have a responsibility to do so.

Class and Diversity: Ethical Implications for Health and Healthcare

Given that phenomena such as race, class, and gender do not operate in isolation, it is essential to examine each of these in light of their collective impact in systems of oppression in and beyond the world of healthcare. Democracy is diminished by the undoing of the historic balance between liberty (the full freedom to do as people please with their resources) and equality (economic opportunity ensuring a fair start in the pursuit of success) (W. Williams, 2004). Since these ideals pull in opposite directions, an imbalance seriously jeopardizes the chances of level playing fields. Evidence indicates that the United States has a long way to go before claims of being a meritocracy can be supported. Poorly funded and poorly provided education, for example, limits life chances, no matter what potential an individual is born with (Kozol, 1991).

It has been apparent for some time that the "American dream" can have nightmarish spin-offs. Ethnographies of serene white suburbs disclose residents sliding down the ranks of the social class ladder due to corporate downsizing, takeovers, or mergers. Images of mainstream middle-class American families and their lifestyles are neither homogeneous nor universally idealized. Privilege is an increasingly contested asset in confused racial and social class, gender, and other social identities (Moss, 1998). While 90% of people in the United States struggled, often in dead-end jobs, to maintain former standards of living, the other 10% experienced average incomes of more than $225,000 in 2000 (W. Williams, 2004). The average income for the former 90% has stagnated at $27,000 a year, but the latter 10% has experienced an income increase of nearly 90% since 1970. The gap between the "haves" and "have-nots" clearly continues to widen. Though they are still far short of fulfilling need, the number of shelter beds available to homeless persons in American cities has more than tripled since 1980 (Henslin, 2005).

Spiraling health costs and inadequate services have combined to make access to healthcare a major challenge for most Americans. Social and political policies related to immigration, housing, and the organization of labor are concurrent concerns (Mwaria, 2001). Since being economically poor is "synonymous with poor nutrition, poor healthcare, poor self-esteem, and poor educational and vocational opportunities" (Ramey & Ramey, 1995, p. 129), poverty is generally accepted as globally the most influential factor in the "web of contingencies" that results in vulnerability and risk for ill health (Stevens, Hall, & Meleis, 1992, p. 769). Because minority peoples are no longer systematically and blatantly denied access to healthcare, a shadow of complacency has allowed relegation of the issue to a back burner—or maybe a far closet. However, postures of nondiscrimination do not equate with access to quality care or (as cost containment becomes an ever more accepted goal) justification for the way resources are distributed. A large proportion of Americans are inadequately insured, but the same is true of an even larger proportion of members of minority groups. It is well documented that a century of urban epidemics in the United States—from tuberculosis to AIDS—has disproportionately affected African American communities (McBride, 1991).

On a global scale, the confluence of growing population, urbanization, migration, and economic change far outpaces investment in infrastructure and overwhelms local capacities to provide even basic services. "Never before in history have people gathered with such density; as a species prone to 'herd' diseases, the implicit danger is clear" (Gutiérrez & Kendall, 2000, p. 85). In light of well-being and health status, it has been proposed that the United States be described as two separate if intertwined societies: people of the inner city and everyone else (Singer,

2001). Neither minority oppression nor poverty is confined to inner cities, but the confounding of urban poverty with socially devalued ethnicity is a glaringly unhealthy combination. One cannot help but revisit Heidegger's lament over the "homelessness" brought about by the destruction of war and the economic necessity of moving away from the land into cities, while those who do not change, do not become homeless, "are more homeless than those who have been driven from their homeland" (Heidegger, 1966, p. 48). How often, and *how*, is the ethics of healthcare access and adequacy addressed in education, represented in research, or seriously queried in the clinical realm?

While household income is the best indicator of an infant's vulnerability to low birthrate and early mortality, as well as a strong indicator of older children's death rates from respiratory diseases and overt links between adequacy of nutrition and health (Pérez-Escamilla, Himmelgreen, & Ferris, 1996), federal cuts in food assistance programs are resulting in increased reporting of hunger and malnutrition from cities around the country (Becker, 2004). Women of color are at greater risk for HIV infection than any other group (Rowland, 2004). Patterns of high risk, which are often accompanied by high knowledge levels and/or low perception of risk, are threaded through complex social patterns of linguistic and social isolation, beliefs about male/female relations, and limited self-esteem and sexual assertiveness (Singer, 2001; Sobo, 1995). In sum, the contemporary healthcare scene is rife with ethical concerns—concerns that are socially patterned and interrelated.

Poor people in the United States and, in particular, members of ethnic and so-called racial minority groups, are relegated to areas where industrial pollution is the greatest and rates of morbidity and mortality associated with environmental concerns are highest (Baer, Singer, & Susser, 1997). Disproportionately high rates of infant mortality, low birth weight, diabetes, hypertension, cirrhosis, tuberculosis, substance abuse, immunodeficiency diseases, respiratory diseases, and sexually transmitted diseases have been documented many times over (e.g., Singer, 2001). Due to the emphasis in the United States on curative medical diagnosis and treatment rather than on healthcare, stratification and unequal access do not automatically imply better health status among the "haves" than the "have-nots." The reason is that high expenditures do not guarantee better health when so many of those expenditures are only indirectly related to health-promoting or curing practices. Basics, such as nutrition and sanitation, get left out of *medical* care costs. On the other hand, as Freund and McGuire (1995) point out, "the poor are not necessarily worse off for not being able to afford coronary by-pass surgery, Caesarian sections, and lots of tranquilizers" (p. 252). However, despite being less likely to be overmedicated or to undergo unnecessary surgery or lab tests, they *are* worse off for having minimal access to appropriate primary health education and care. Given that medicine is invested, by and large, in other interests, it is up to nursing and other fields to bring these ethical issues forth. Interpretive narrative and pedagogy could prove essential tools in accomplishing the task.

Standardization, Assimilation, Globalization, and Healthcare Ethics

Social change is the process through which beliefs and values (that is, culture) and behavioral norms, institutions, social relationships, and stratification systems (society) alter over time. Cultural ideals change slowly, while rates of change among cultural artifacts (technology and knowledge) vary with the complexity of societies, as inventiveness is associated with accumulated knowledge. Thus it is that, over the broad expanse of human history, social change occurs at an increasingly accelerated pace. Today modernization is a master process through which history unfolds. While governments, by definition, represent communities of interest and seem to become no more idealistic with time, much power today is in the hands of corporations and other nongovernmental interest groups (Kottak, 1999). Meanwhile, the deceptively open borders of globalization can be neither welcomed nor condemned uncritically.

It is not surprising that what is referred to as the homogenization (or the "McDonaldization") of society, that is, the increasing standardization of everyday life, occurs in the very face of unprecedented possibilities for variety. We find familiarity and comfort in predictable, controlled environments. We tolerate (even participate in) short, packaged, often computerized courses that teach the same ideas and answers to everyone, and bland, unanalyzed, often decontextualized and ahistorical bits of "Mc-News" (Ritzer, 1998). It is a new twist to the old adage that the more things change, the more they stay the same. In the midst of endless social revision, we pursue a sense of *home*.

With globalization comes tension between increased standardization and cultural homogeneity, on the one hand, and more fragmentation and local action on the other (Burbules & Torres, 2000). Consider the success of the global expansion of that familiar globalizing (albeit unabashedly culturally imperialistic) symbol, McDonald's. Given the tendency of humans to commit to foods as a matter of availability, social meaning, and familiarity, how can an American fast-food restaurant with a limited menu succeed internationally? The menu changes little cross-culturally except for some provision for local custom and beliefs—Hindus avoid beef and Muslims avoid pork, so, for example, India's McDonald's restaurants add vegetable McNuggets and a mutton-based Maharaja Mac (Watson, 1997). In the globalization of vascular peril, fries are universally accepted—but so are high standards of cleanliness of the kitchens and toilets, which has been noted to spark a hygiene movement among competing eateries.

Although McDonald's certainly spreads an air of homogeneity, it also represents opportunity and change in places where people strive to modernize. Moreover, its popularity hints at fundamental patterns in the conduct of daily life (Mintz, 1997). For all of their sameness, McDonald's restaurants serve different functions in different contexts. Each is half owned by a local manager who works hard to be an integral part of the community. In China, Aunt and Uncle McDonald record children's names and birthdays, send them cards, and visit them at school (Yan, 1997)—a move calculated to win long-term customer loyalty. In varied settings, McDonald's restaurants have been studied as sites of social gathering and exchange for many interest groups: women, elders, workers, teens, students, and so on (Schlosser, 2002).

McDonald's aside, food supply has become a major source of corporate cash flow, economic leverage, and currency—in short, a weapon of power and international politics (Vellema & Jansen, 2004). By the year 2050, the world's population is likely to exceed nine billion, while even now only 15% of the planet's soil can be described as having escaped degradation that reduces productivity (Millstone & Lang, 2003). An astounding 97% of the anticipated population growth will take place in developing countries where conditions are scarcely improved over a century ago—or may be worse, as in Zimbabwe, where the average life expectancy has plummeted from nearly 70 to 38 years because of AIDS (Iyer, 2000).

Current data provide chilling evidence of escalating AIDS infection rates and subsequent death tolls worldwide (Behrman, 2004; Levenson, 2004). Complicit in this devastation are politicians and religious leaders with moralistic views of HIV/AIDS. Despite the impact of immunosuppressant disease on the American healthcare front in recent years, from an ethical perspective, Behrman (2004), in the subtitle of his book, suggests far deeper implications: *How the U.S. Has Slept Through the Global AIDS Pandemic, the Greatest Humanitarian Catastrophe of Our Time.* The author concludes that the United States' failure to lead the fight against AIDS in Africa is "inglorious," while his conservative prose masks the charge of "racist."

Meanwhile, relationships between multinational corporations and the elites of the least industrialized countries barter access to raw materials, labor, and markets (Sklair, 2001). It is no secret that those elites often maintain privileged lifestyles and are able to purchase advanced weaponry that can be used to dominate and oppress their own people as well as maintain a modicum of political stability. Much of the world today is comprised of series of shiny high-rise downtowns surrounded by expanses of relative poverty (Iyer, 2000). A conglomeration of media industries contributes to the United States' hegemony in the creation of media icons. "Outsourcing" has become an everyday word. Such trends show no evidence of slowing, although they continue to transform in response to economic stimuli. But these are complicated stories, and there is no insular, sufficient version. Moving manufacturing to less industrialized nations brings money and jobs to those nations, despite both workers and other resources being cheaply bought, most of the profit returning to the industrialized nation, and only compromised opportunities to develop skills and a capital base (Kottak, 1999). Thus, in the era of de- and postcolonization, the world faces the pros and cons, risks and benefits, and overall ambiguities of neocolonialism (e.g., Haasoun, 2004; Smith, 2001).

We understand little about how globalization of capital is shaping diversity and health status. Majority populations hold the power, whether or not they numerically surpass others. Members of such categories have cultural privileges that most take for granted and many choose not to acknowledge. By definition, minority populations have less power and are *different.* They are, consequently, also likely to have a heightened sense of identity. What happens to cultural identities and "difference" as transnational corporations disperse production processes and require personnel to be more mobile (Lamphere, 2001)? An international wage labor force migrating far from their homes of origin, often at great cost to families and personal lives, changes health needs.

As multicultural human beings and planetary networks cross and transcend borders, other social forces fashion new divisions and aggravate old ones (Iyer, 2000); the more internationalism there is, the more nationalism there will be. Fewer wars take place today across borders than within them, and the number of countries on the planet more than tripled in the 20th century (Iyer, 2000; Levin, 1993). There are weighty ethical implications in the fact that, although we know more than ever about promoting health, and in the West remain preoccupied with diagnosis and treatment of chronic lifestyle-related problems, healthcare is—and is projected to be—increasingly oriented toward treatment and rehabilitation of largely preventable trauma (Albrecht & Verbrugge, 2000).

The globalization of production increasingly includes high-tech electronics that produce a vaguely understood "digital divide" and new meanings to "have" and "have-not" categories of humans. Even as healthcare is being telemedicalized, more indigenous, ethnic, and other distinct groups around the world strive to control their own media resources (radio stations, local television programming, and video) (Lamphere, 2001). Rapid development of biotechnology has reshaped the global market in reproductive medicine, genetics, and medical approaches to disease (e.g., Pilnick, 2002). Despite new literature on reproductive technologies and studies focusing on issues of race, gender, and class (for instance, Rapp, 1999; and Franklin & Ragone, 1999), little is understood about how assumptions about race, gender, and sexual orientation shape medical research, treatment possibilities, and access to care. We must seek ways to work ethically to maximize culturally acceptable opportunities for healthcare and, in particular, primary healthcare, health promotion, and disease prevention.

Bioethics, Medical Ethics, and Diversity in Healthcare: Cultural Studies

Against the backdrop presented in the preceding sections, I have drawn from the literatures of both bioethics and medical ethics for this section (anthropologists generally prefer the construct "medical ethics" due to its broader applicability across cultures). Medical ethics, being about the cultural construction of morality, manifests itself in beliefs and practices about health, illness, disease, curing, and healing. That description is broader than the conventional understanding of bioethics, which tends to be more specific to issues associated with the development and application of biomedical technology. Medical ethics generally extends to the lived experience of human suffering in the context of both disease (biological dysfunction) and illness (the meaning and experience of sickness), the moral discourse of healers and patients, the development and use of healing modalities, the professional organization of practitioners, and the social and economic regulation of both medical (curing) and healing environments (Muller, 1994).

While it is accepted that moral and ethical systems prosper or fail within specific cultural and historical contexts (Cortese, 1990), the exploration of medical ethics as a cultural phenomenon has been slow in coming (Armstrong & Humphrey, 1994). Intense technological change and the events that prompted creation of the field of bioethics—selection of patients for chronic dialysis in the early 1960s; the first heart transplants in the late 1960s; and disclosure in the 1970s of the Tuskegee, Willowbrook, and other experiments involving deceit, coercion, or excessive risk to participants (Marshall & Koenig, 1996)—seem farther in the past than they actually are. Various philosophical and theological analyses were applied, typically with prescriptive results (that is, what *ought* to be) to medical phenomena (Jonsen, 1994) while healthcare only halfheartedly commenced serious exploration of its own ethical milieu. The result has been a conspicuous dependence on principles, which have been questioned in terms of applicability only when and where bioethics and medical ethics come together (Davis & Koenig, 1996)—that is, when it becomes obvious that the principles do not work in some circumstances or for some peoples.

The fact that ethics is culturally situated and socially defined is more widely accepted by healthcare personnel and scholars today than in the past. Cultural differences in caring and healing beliefs and practices are replete with moral and ethical overtones (e.g., Culhane-Pera, Vawter, Xiong, Babbitt, & Solberg, 2003; Goldberg & Remy-St. Louis, 1998; and Green, 1999; plus many others). Moreover, entire new fields of culture-related concern have been generated in recent decades in response to advanced medical knowledge and biotechnology. Those most visible in the literature have been cultural issues in disclosure of diagnosis and prognosis (e.g., Orona, Koenig, & Davis, 1994); the role of families in making medical decisions (Hoshino, 1995); self-care (Lipson & Steiger, 1996); cultural responses to withholding or withdrawing treatment or care of terminally ill patients (Marshall & Koenig, 1996); and cultural questions around death with dignity, physician-assisted suicide, and euthanasia (e.g., Hillyard & Dombrink, 2001). For the most part, close examination across cultures of patient self-determination (Lynn & Teno, 1993), meanings and impact of autonomy (e.g., Elliott, 2001), living wills (Emanuel, Barry, Stoeckle, Ettleson, & Emanuel, 1991), and formal advance care directives as potential tools of empowerment (Murphy et al., 1996) has generated far more questions than answers. Knowledgeable practitioners increasingly recognize that collectivism (rather than individualism) is prioritized by many—probably most—peoples, and that the acceptability of candid discussion of diagnosis, prognosis, or end-of-life decisions cannot be assumed (Marshall, Koenig, Barnes, & Davis, 1998).

Concerns about communication style, cultural understanding, and varied ways of knowing are increasingly acknowledged in clinical ethics consultations (Orr, Marshall, & Osborn, 1995). Work on medical compliance as a problematic concept is closely allied (Roberson, 1992; Trostle, 1988). Threaded throughout cross-cultural aspects of bioethics and medical ethics are concerns about genetics, rising costs in healthcare, allocation of scarce resources, and movement toward healthcare reform through managed care and managed competition (Marshall & Koenig, 1996). Aside from issues of excessive expenditure and unwanted side effects, until recently there has been little resistance to the development and application of medical technology. Such supposition is now being challenged in the dominant culture (e.g., Diekelmann, 2002) as well as by other peoples. The characterization of suffering as culturally constructed (for instance, in North America, efforts to reduce suffering have traditionally focused on control and repair of individual bodies) has profound influence on the discourse associated with application of biomedical technologies (Kleinman, Das, & Lock, 1997). However, so has conceptualization of suffering as the *experience* of individuals. Medical ethics and bioethics are in some ways coming together, yet, as long as the focus remains on the individual, even together they will fail to deal with major issues of health and sickness facing humankind today.

That transplantation is an ethical netherworld is indicated by research on the sale of body parts (Monaghan, 2000; Roueche, 2001). Interestingly, the ethical aura around transplantation seems to have been studied more by those outside medicine than within (Kavanagh, 2002). Questions are emerging about the very nature of being human and about embodiment and personhood. Evidence suggests that such concerns are not only culturally oriented but, at least for some peoples, confounded with ideas about suffering and quality of life (Sloan, 2002). For instance, although a smaller proportion of African Americans than European Americans has access to transplantation, African Americans faced with end-stage kidney disease are more likely to turn down offers of kidneys from living, related potential donors (Gordon, 2001). Often such differences in decision making result from variations in moral understanding of concepts such as suffering. Another example of significant cultural variation is that, while law in the United States has codified "brain death," which allows the harvesting of viable organs, the concept has never been accepted in Japan, where (despite high levels of technological sophistication) organ transplantation seldom occurs due to different ideas about "whole brain death" (Lock, 1996).

The geneticization of medicine and society (Finkler, 2000) is blurring boundaries between health and disease. New ethical issues emerge around technologies and their integration into medical treatment and healthcare. With preventative medicine a cornerstone of public health, some people maintain that primary care settings are ideal locations for genetic screening and testing programs that would have to be large scale and widespread to be cost effective. Feasibility issues aside, the ethical implications of such work demand careful exploration. Reducing societies to individuals, and individuals to their genes, risks being unable to put them back together again in ways that allow us to understand interactions between genes and environments, individuals, and societies (Ramsay, 1994). Furthermore, historical context has always shaped what is thought to be genetic—poverty, intelligence, and aggression, for example. Genetic labels provide solutions that reflect and reinforce particular social and political environments. Why, for instance, is a genetic basis for human homosexuality being sought without comparable programs focused on less contentiously viewed traits, such as altruism (Pilnick, 2002)? It is presumptuous to think we are immune to what reductionism and biological determinism did in the form of eugenics in the past (Duster, 2003).

While American society's "technological imperative" pushes for the use and application of whatever is known and available, genetics must be carefully considered in social context (Cunningham-Burley & Kerr, 1999). Much current genetic knowledge is limited to monogenic disorders in which genetic factors are fairly clear. Decisions about testing and intervention may have unanticipated ramifications in the future when it is highly likely that genetic evidence will be more dependent on social and environmental variables, making any attempt to separate nature and nurture overtly spurious (Pilnick, 2002). Where are our discussions about the ethics of these situations—and of rethinking in that area?

Biomedicine has achieved a position of prominence in the healthcare systems of "advanced" societies and become nearly a monopoly in the United States, but it has never been the only mode of healthcare open to sick people (Cant & Sharma, 2000). That reality is often not apparent when examining curricula of healthcare programs or the findings of healthcare research, and there are many examples of its absence in clinical practice. "Alternative" health practices and systems seem novel to many today (despite some of them having been around for thousands of years), but there is at least more awareness of other ways of health-related thinking and practicing. Nonetheless, the terms "alternative" or "complementary" clearly illustrate the strength of the normative (that is, biomedical) gold standard against which every thing else is weighed. Language, for all of its transience and vulnerability to erosion (Heidegger, 1957, 1962), speaks volumes.

The other term currently encountered with more regularity is "integrative," which implies potential for a coming together of various interpretations of health promotion and care as "a collaborative, multidisciplinary approach that requires the application of the best options from different healing systems" (Adler, 2002, p. 413). The 1960s and '70s witnessed a concerted effort to explore varied healers' belief and practice systems and possibilities of integrating indigenous health beliefs and practices with biomedicine (see, for example, Landy, 1977). However, increasing medicalization (Conrad & Schneider, 1992) and concomitant medicocentrism have demonstrated limited tolerance for pluralistic views of healthcare. (For a telling example, see Fadiman, 1999, which presents the story of the juxtaposition of biomedical views of epilepsy with those of Hmong refugees—and attendant ethical dilemmas).

There is relatively little discussion today of integrating actual indigenous healing ways with biomedicine, despite considerable borrowing of techniques, procedures, and pharmacopeias. There are also few concerted challenges to biomedicine's presumptive right to subsume healing techniques or medicines from other paradigms, or, for that matter, challenges to views of ethics other than that dominating in the Anglo-American West. Other theories of ethics are known and have been well documented (see, especially, Veatch, 1989), but ethics reflects cultural worldviews, and as long as those are focused on individuality and norms established by the dominant paradigms and professions, other interpretations remain minimally explored.

Despite serious obstacles to integration of approaches to health, there is today far more attention to holism, a concept that runs counter to scientific values of objectivism, reductionism, and positivism. However, J. Diekelmann (2005) points out that science ensnares itself in its own shallow tautology by attempting to access and delimit objects of study that are not in reality either accessible or "graspable." At first take, it seems that the movement toward holistic thinking presents a successful countering to science, but at the same time, there is significant concern that the application of holism to health in "the holistic health paradigm" (as if there is one and it can be clearly delineated) will be subsumed by biomedicine in the process of legitimizing it (Baer, 2002). That turn of events is likely to diminish healing to the simpler level of curing (e.g., Williams, 1998), with reassertion of a general acceptance of biomedicine having the final word. Similarly, it seems that ethical issues involving intellectual property rights have scarcely begun to be acknowledged in healthcare (e.g., Greaves, 1994). Members of most clinically focused disciplines agree that what happens to patients (however individually or collectively that role is defined) is paramount, but there are issues around sources and ownership, reciprocity, and compensation for knowledge and resources originating with other peoples.

So much of the work in ethics and healthcare is medicocentric that potential discourse from other views is greatly constrained. For instance, the conventional separation between mind and body that characterizes Western biomedicine's version of Cartesian dualism generally has far less meaning to or influence among traditional non-Western peoples (Weiner, 2001)—a fact rarely noted in the West. Shaped as our healthcare thinking and interventions are by the schism of mind and body, the mind (and by extension its energies) eludes empirical examination and remains in large part unacknowledged and unexplored (Micozzi, 2001, 2002). Are there not ethical implications to aligning ourselves with biologically based medical research when concepts, rooted in other cultures but suggesting strong medical significance (such as those underlying much of the traditional Chinese and Ayurvedic paradigms), are studied only from Western perspectives? Medicocentrism can blind us to important knowledge, for example, that herbal medicine does not merely symbolize botanical commodities but ways of knowing.

In sum, the ethics of healthcare practice, being in practice *medical* ethics, is seldom examined in ways that elucidate either its contextualization within culturally embedded moral systems or the pluralistic character of ethical issues. Lack of attention to what has been referred to as "everyday ethical comportment" and conflict between principle-oriented ethics and actual care is acknowledged (Benner, 1991, p. 1). Yet, despite stories of practice and struggle being central to moral struggles, they are seldom emphasized in healthcare scholarship (Kleinman, 1988, 1995)—and even less often from social or cultural perspectives.

Despite such gaps, by the mid-1990s it was apparent that more ethicists were attending to the hermeneutic nature of clinical medicine (Good, 1998; Marshall & Koenig, 1996). There has been a move toward contextualized and meaning-centered work with open recognition of its interpretive basis and the sensitivity such approaches lend to the perplexing reality of moral conflicts. Discursive space has opened where topics generally forbidden in biomedicine, such as the meaning of suffering or dying, or the experience of iatrogenic phenomena, can be explored. While the histories of technology and medicine have traditionally been couched as heroic tales, actual experience in providing healthcare or practicing medicine is now being examined. For instance, Davis-Floyd and St. John (1998) examine the transformation of medical practices of American physicians who shifted from technocratic approaches to holism to offer more effective care. In another example, ethics-focused, ethnography-based, culture-specific clinical stories of Hmong families and Western providers both argue for and provide suggestions for culturally competent healthcare (Culhane-Pera et al., 2003).

Peoples of many perspectives are debating issues around the body and technology—and everything else related to health from scientific accuracy to political interests and issues around suffering (Lock, 1996). It is increasingly apparent that, like cultural beliefs and practices in general, ideas about healthcare morality and ethics cannot be represented by a single worldview. Culture is fluid, dynamic, and negotiable. Many healthcare settings today are either multicultural or are at least influenced by ideas and identities from diverse origins. Ethical ways of knowing are as diverse as humankind; they deserve the opportunity to be explored and critiqued. While commitment to more humanistic and communitarian perspectives would broaden the views that, in their inadequacy, threaten to stultify healthcare today, moving beyond those will require new ways—such as those of narrative interpretation—and commitment to exploring more extensive, inclusive, and transformative aspects of social discourse.

Conclusions: Vulnerability, Liminality, Possibility, and the Rethinking of Ethical Comportment

"Oh, send him somewhere where they will teach him to think for himself!" Mrs. Shelley answered: "Teach him to think for himself? Oh, my God, teach him rather to think like other people!"

Matthew Arnold, Essays in Criticism

Interpretive phenomenology makes possible ways of rethinking ethics and ethical comportment. Heidegger spoke of resoluteness pushing us into "a caring *Mitsein* with others" (1962, p. 345). It is the disclosure of that determination in the context of what is *"possible at the time"* (Heidegger, 1962, p. 345) that allows revealing and understanding, for *"[r]esoluteness is only that authenticity which, in care, is the object of care, and which is possible as care—the authenticity of care itself"* (Heidegger, 1962, p. 348). We have to question the strength of our commitment to *ethical* health-related care and caring today. In an age of specialization, it is easy to interpret health needs and healthcare in narrow and provincial terms. Hence, this interpretive study has argued for expanding our models of ethics and ways of exploring as well as for bringing more interpretive work into both bioethics and medical ethics. We contend abstractly with globalization but we are far from having or knowing a global civic culture (Parker, Ninomiya, & Cogan, 1999); never before have so many people been surrounded by so much that is alien to them—customs, languages, neighborhoods, technology (Iyer, 2000)—so much "homelessness" (Hodge, 1995), and never before have both massive conglomerates and local interest groups been so important (Kottak, 1999).

In an age when it is easier than ever before to affect entire populations, we are more dependent than ever on socially considered ethical decisions. How do we understand the implications for health in a world challenged by discontinuity and multiplicity (McCarthy & Dimityriades, 2000), if not through ethical and interpretive study? We need to find ways to share these concerns with others, to develop meaningful conversations, and to prevent such discourse getting lost in the daily shuffle of localized concerns. It is time for interpretive practices to help develop communitarian models of ethics that will respond to problems embedded in race, class, and gender and reveal issues around access to care, quality and congruence of care, paternalism, consent, and concern for the whole person and for whole groups. We need multimethod studies (and funding for those) that will deal with social issues, forums at meetings and institutes that support discourse, and strong commitment to broadening healthcare's ethical horizons.

In the United States, while positive change has come about at the local level through confrontation of exclusionary effects of health institutions, inclusion neither equates with fairness nor reflects concurrent political agenda. International issues aside, even within the United States there is evidence of many complex and vague interactions among health and the differential distribution of resources, including healthcare. The health status of African Americans is generally improved, for example, as is reflected in increased life expectancy, a decrease in the prevalence of disease, and a shift from infectious to chronic disease as the principal cause of death. Yet, in comparison to the health of European Americans, it is obvious that significant disparities in health status persist. Closer examination implicates the interaction of the socioeconomic situation with lifestyle and cultural traits and genetic differences (Mullings, 1989). Where is the discussion of implications for social transformation in the ethics literature? Lack of consensus over goals does not justify lack of discourse.

Working in healthcare today requires a critical and vigilant stance that will ensure ethical development that can put in perspective those representations of myriad diverse others that our society and the rest of the world continue to produce (Bok, 1998). Diversity is in no way limited to ethnicity, "race," gender, or class. It is a confusing fusing of all of those and more. What do we do about it from an ethical standpoint? While many social objectives today focus on flexibility, adaptability, and strategies for coexistence with others in diverse public spaces, other objectives counter those. With democracy increasingly defined in economic rather than sociopolitical terms (Apple, 2000), the commoditization of education, healthcare, and research reflects the dialectic between local and more global interests (Morrow & Torres, 2000). If "all interpretation is grounded on understanding" (Heidegger, 1962, p. 195), the thinking, dwelling, and attending to ethics that is essential to meaningful and significant interpretation can be easily lost in the demands to do more with less time and fewer resources. Ethical understandings are not so much determined as they are part of that way of being together or being-*with* that is neither conclusively positive nor negative but part of co-occurrence of meanings, possibilities, and openness (J. Diekelmann, 2005; Nancy, 1997). Solutions are not the immediate goal; understandings are.

Other approaches to ethics risk concessions that benefit no one and churn the wheels of the status quo rather than encouraging new understandings and criteria for comportment as well as developing possibilities perhaps still unimagined. Prioritizing interpretive thinking—which is a proceeding (a way) rather than a procedure (a work)—lets what has come before show itself in all of our created polarities and differences, technologisms, and compromises of humanity to reveal the limitations of the subject–object paradigm of outdated Greco-European metaphysics (J. Diekelmann, 2005).

Awareness of the cultural images we consume and project is an ideal starting place for increasing attention to health-related ethical issues. Cultural texts and objectifying discourses must be read politically to see how they are rhetorically and narratively produced and to discern counterhegemonic messages—all the while realizing that content is less vital to learning than are conversations (Diekelmann, 2001). As educators, researchers, and practitioners, we must learn to understand how we consume and produce cultural representations and what their ethical ramifications are in the interpretation of health. Practices such as attending to everyday language are an ongoing part of transforming discourse. We should be exploring the experiences of immigrant and other distinct communities. We should also be asking students, patients, and coworkers to critique materials and procedures in clinical, educational, or research settings in terms of personal and family identity. The bottom line is a need to increase recognition and critique of cultural metaphors, imagery, and paradigms so that their ethical reverberations—however convoluted—can be revealed and explored.

A simple, practical starting place for culturally responsive, ethically sensitive healthcare is the implementation and critique of models such as that explicated by Vawter, Culhane-Pera, Babbitt, Xiong, and Solberg (2003). The transformation from ethnocentric cross-cultural relationships to those that are ethnorelative involves keeping open and problematic ethical conflicts and challenges to professional integrity. Questions must be asked about relationships between care and outcomes. For example, how might treatment plans (whatever their biomedical, alternative, or indigenous sources) respect or disrespect patients, pose health risks or benefits, and serve health-related and other agenda?

The range of possible responses to ethical conflicts encumbered by social complications such as race, ethnicity, class, or gender—as virtually all of them are—is far wider than is typically formulated by principle-based ethical models. Serious ethical conflict occurs when people view others' "values as not only different, but wrong or extremely offensive, and therefore are unable to accommodate them" (Jecker, Carrese, & Pearlman, 1995, p. 12). Sometimes a case-by-case approach is indicated, using some agreed-upon procedure for negotiation. Sometimes a broadened perspective and awareness of the impact of social dynamics such as those discussed in this study can lead to amelioration of the power differentials that fuel conflict. We need to question whether resistance to compromise is rooted in actual unethical comportment or in interpretations founded in lack of understanding and knowledge. It takes an expansive and informed perspective to be aware of the range of possible responses to ethical conflicts. More often than not, when dealing with significant differences (whether cultural, economic, gender, or otherwise), prioritizing the preservation of patient–provider (whether medical or healing practitioner) relationships leads to the development of trust. On the other hand, prioritizing patients' physical health, personal moral beliefs, or professional interests over the context of the situation is likely to result in responses that include overriding wishes of the patient, family, or community and refused intervention (Vawter et al., 2003).

Emphasis on a more communitarian approach to healthcare ethics can be used in discussion and determination of healthcare needs of any group. It becomes easier all the time to supplement academic texts effectively with autobiographical, fictional, and other popular materials to juxtapose with scientific and media representations (see Foley & Moss, 2001, for suggestions). Materials composed by persons with significantly different viewpoints contain cues to the moral and ethical underpinnings of those views. The use of works from multiple approaches conveys the idea that scientific texts and voices are not necessarily superior to nonscientific or nonacademic texts. It also supports active collection and representation of dissenting voices of stigmatized others. Small oral and life history projects, as well as the careful use of materials explicitly organized to misrepresent others, work well. A class might be assigned to study, for instance, the various interpretations of tuberculosis among ethnic groups in a given community; such explanatory models generally vary far more than is expected. Or ideas about illness etiologies rooted in social disharmonies or the supranatural or supernatural world could be explored with respect and presented for discussion in ways that preclude the offhand trivialization of such views. Dialogue involving the sharing of viewpoints and working through of narrow, dichotomous ways of thinking is vital. Such deconstructions reveal ethical and social implications, however convoluted, at all levels.

Discussion of ethical objectives is integral: in light of health, healthcare, and diversity today, are the basic goals inclusivity, empowerment, fairness, social justice, equality, pluralism, or something else? Saying that we want to ensure that people get what they deserve is not enough; what, exactly, is deserved (Rachels, 1993)? On what levels (individual to global) are we to be ethically concerned, and on what levels are our voices heard? Is it the same or different for others' voices? At the very least, we can prompt thinking that leads to new and better questions: for instance, how do scholars write about the needs of people when many people do not trust themselves, their stories, or their communities to academics (and in particular, *white* academics)? Who owns the rights to an interview when it has been transcribed, or a cultural story or healing technique for which payment has been rendered? How does one deal with "race" in inquiry/teaching/practice when the concept is both an unstable fiction and a potentially ruthless manipulator of real-life experience? What ethical issues are hidden within cultural differences in research, teaching, and practice? How does culture influence the attitudes we take with respect to human suffering, given the fact, for instance, that by age 11 the average American child has watched 8,000 murders on television (Bok, 1998; Video violence, 2004)?

Obstacles to effective change are generally more basic than the level at which they are examined. A fundamental tenet of empowerment is that all involved have the ability to meet their own needs, to solve their own problems, to mobilize the resources necessary to feel in control of their own lives. How people prioritize and do those things vary widely; only participatory collaboration supports potential for authentic dialogue and discourse. By exploring the ethical aspects of health and healthcare in the context of society we can advocate for and empower diverse others.

The world continues to change. It is both smaller and larger, more interconnected and with larger gaps, more overt and more covert, more personal and more impersonal. We have every reason to believe that yet unimagined ethical issues will reveal themselves over time. We must be ready to meet them, for they will, without a doubt, involve health and healthcare. "What else is care about, if not in connection with bringing human beings back into their essence? What does it mean except that human beings should become human?" (Heidegger, 1967, p. 317, as cited by Hodge, 1995, p. 89). Heidegger seems to have had in mind "caring for" *(Fürsorge)* as a manner of interacting with other people (Olafson, 1998), but in our "side-by-side-ness," we cannot seek to understand, collaborate in, or transform what we fail to question and explore. Our questioning will be forever incomplete and insufficient if we fail to move beyond the individual.

References

Adler, S. R. (2002). Integrative medicine and culture: Toward an anthropology of CAM. *Medical Anthropology Quarterly, 16*(4), 412–414.

Albrecht, G. L., & Verbrugge, L. M. (2000). The global emergence of disability. In G. L. Albrecht, R. Fitzpatrick, & S. C. Scrimshaw (Eds.), *Handbook of social studies in health and medicine* (pp. 293–307). London: Sage.

Andrews, M. M., & Boyle, J. S. (Eds.). (2003). *Transcultural concepts in nursing care* (4th ed.).Philadelphia: Lippincott Williams & Wilkins.

Angler, N. (2000, August 22). Do races differ? Not really, DNA shows. *New York Times,* B1–2.

Apple, M. W. (2000). Between neoliberalism and neoconservatism: Education and conservatism in a global context. In N. C. Burbules & C. A. Torres (Eds.)., *Globalization and education: Critical perspectives* (pp. 57–77). London: Routledge.

Arcury, T. A., & Quandt, S. A. (2004, September). Occupational health risks among farmworkers. *Anthropology News, 45*(6), 34–35.

Armstrong, D., & Humphrey, C. (1994). Health care, sociology, and medical ethics. In R. Gillon (Ed.), *Principles of health care ethics* (pp. 855–860). Chichester, England: John Wiley and Sons.

Arthur, J. (Ed.). (1993). Affirmative action in universities: *Regents of the University of California v. Bakke.* In J. Arthur (Ed.), *Morality and moral controversies* (3rd ed., pp. 531–535). Englewood Cliffs, NJ: Prentice-Hall.

Badgett, M. V. L., & Hartmann, H. (1995). The effectiveness of equal employment opportunity policies. In Margaret C. Simms (Ed.), *Economic perspectives in affirmative action* (pp. 55–83). Washington, DC: Joint Center for Political and Economic Studies.

Baer, H. A. (2002). The growing interest of biomedicine in complementary and alternative medicine: A critical perspective. *Medical Anthropology Quarterly, 16*(4), 403–405.

Baer, H., Singer, M., & Susser, I. (1997). *Medical anthropology and the world system: A critical perspective.* Westport, CT: Bergin and Garvey.

Baker, L. D. (2001). The color-blind bind. In I. Susser & T. C. Patterson (Eds.), *Cultural diversity in the United States* (pp. 103–119). Malden, MA: Blackwell.

Barry, E. (2004, July 29). Tennessee limits who is eligible for a driver's license. *The Baltimore Sun,* p. 15A.

Becker, G. (2004). Deadly inequality in the health care "safety net": Uninsured ethnic minorities' struggle to live with life-threatening illnesses. *Medical Anthropology Quarterly, 18*(2), 258–275.

Behrman, G. (2004). *The invisible people: How the U.S. has slept through the global AIDS pandemic, the greatest humanitarian catastrophe of our time.* New York: Free Press.

Benner, P. (1991). The role of experience, narrative, and community in skilled ethical comportment. *Advances in Nursing Science, 14*(2), 1–21.

Bernstein, R., & Bergman, M. (2003, June 18). Hispanic population reaches all-time high of 38.8 million, new Census Bureau estimates show. *U.S. Department of Commerce News.*

Better, S. (2002). *Institutional racism: A primer on theory and strategies for social change.* Chicago: Burnham.

Bigler, E. (1999). *American conversations: Puerto Ricans, white ethnics, and multicultural education.* Philadelphia: Temple University Press.

Blackmore, J. (2000). Globalization: A useful concept for feminists rethinking theory and strategies in education? In N. C. Burbules & C. A. Torres (Eds.), *Globalization and education: Critical perspectives* (pp. 133–155). London: Routledge.

Bok, S. (1998). *Mayhem: Violence as public entertainment.* Reading, MA: Addison-Wesley.

Brace, C. L. (2002). The concept of race in physical anthropology. In P. N. Peregrine, C. R. Ember, & M. Ember (Eds.), *Physical anthropology: Original readings in method and practice* (pp. 239–253). Upper Saddle River, NJ: Pearson Education.

Brodkin, K. (2001). Diversity in anthropological theory. In I. Susser & T. C. Patterson (Eds.), *Cultural diversity in the United States* (pp. 365–388). Malden, MA: Blackwell.

Burbules, N. C., & Torres, C. A. (2000). Globalization and education: An introduction. In N. C. Burbules & C.A. Torres (Eds.), *Globalization and education: Critical perspectives* (pp. 1–26). London: Routledge.

Callahan, D. (1996). Can the moral commons survive autonomy? *Hastings Center Report, 26*(6), 41–42.

Cant, S., & Sharma, U. (2000). Alternative health systems and practices. In G. L. Albrecht, R. Fitzpatrick, & S. C. Scrimshaw (Eds.), *The handbook of social studies in health and medicine* (pp. 426–439). London: Sage.

Caplan, A. L. (1992). When evil intrudes. *Hastings Center Report, 22*(6), 29–32.

Carr, L. G. (1997). *"Color-blind" racism.* Thousand Oaks, CA: Sage.

Chambers, E. (2000). Applied ethnography. In N. K. Denzin & Y. S. Lincoln (Eds.), *Handbook of qualitative research* (2nd ed., pp. 851–869). Thousand Oaks, CA: Sage.

Chavez, L. R. (1997). Immigrant reform and nativism: The nationalist response to the transnationalist challenge. In J. F. Perrea (Ed.), *Immigrants out! The new nativism* and the anti–immigrant impulse in the United States (pp. 61–77). New York: New York University Press.

Chávez, R. C., & O'Donnell, J. (1998). *Speaking the unpleasant: The politics of (non)engagement in multicultural education terrain.* Albany: State University of New York Press.

Christians, C. G. (2000). Ethics and politics in qualitative research. In N. K. Denzin & Y. S. Lincoln (Eds.), *Handbook of qualitative research* (2nd ed., pp. 133–155). Thousand Oaks, CA: Sage.

Conrad, P., & Schneider, J. W. (1992). *Deviance and medicalization: From badness to sickness.* Philadelphia: Temple University Press.

Cortese, A. (1990). *Ethnic ethics: The restructuring of moral theory.* Albany: State University of New York Press.

Cose, E. (2000, September 18). What's white anyway? *Newsweek,* 64–65.

Culhane-Pera, K. A., Vawter, D. E., Xiong, P., Babbitt, B., & Solberg, M. M. (2003). *Healing by heart: Clinical and ethical case stories of Hmong families and Western providers.* Nashville, TN: Vanderbilt University Press.

Cunningham-Burley, S., & Kerr, A. (1999). Defining the "social:" Towards an understanding of scientific and medical discourses on the social aspects of the new human genetics. *Sociology of Health and Illness, 21*(5), 647–668.

Davidoff, F. (1999, April 20). Health care: A constitutional right—the 28th amendment. *Annals of Internal Medicine, 130*(8), 692–694.

Davis, A. J., & Koenig, B. A. (1996). A question of policy: Bioethics in a multicultural society. *Nursing Policy Forum, 2*(1), 6–11.

Davis-Floyd, R., & St. John, G. (1998). *From doctor to healer: The transformative journey.* New Brunswick, NJ: Rutgers University Press.

De Chardin, P. T. (1961). *The phenomenon of man* (B. Wall, Trans.). New York: Harper and Row. (Original work published 1955)

De Waal Malefijt, A. (1974). *Images of man: A history of anthropological thought.* New York: Alfred A. Knopf.

Diekelmann, J. (2005). The retrieval of method: The method of retrieval. In P. Ironside (Ed.), *Beyond method.* Madison: University of Wisconsin Press.

Diekelmann, N. L. (2001). Narrative pedagogy: Heidegerrian hermeneutical analyses of the lived experiences of students, teachers and clinicians. *Advances in Nursing Science 23*(3), 53–71.

Diekelmann, N. L. (Ed.). (2002). *First, do no harm: Power, oppression, and violence in healthcare.* Madison: University of Wisconsin Press.

Diekelmann, N., & Diekelmann, J. (2000). Learning ethics in nursing and genetics: Narrative pedagogy and the grounding of values. *Journal of Pediatric Nursing 15*(4), 226–231.

Donald, J., & Rattansi, A. (Ed.). (1992). *"Race," culture and difference.* London: Sage.

Dossa, P. (2002). Narrative mediation of conventional and new "mental health" paradigms: Reading the stories of immigrant Iranian women. *Medical Anthropology Quarterly, 16*(3), 341–359.

Duster, T. (2003). *Backdoor to eugenics.* London: Routledge.

Elliott, A. C. (2001). Health care ethics: Cultural relativity of autonomy. *Journal of Transcultural Nursing, 12*(4), 326–330.

Emanuel, L. L., Barry, M. H., Stoeckle, J. D., Ettleson, L. M., & Emanuel, E. J. (1991). Advance directives for medical care—A case for greater use. *New England Journal of Medicine, 324*(13), 889–895.

Fadiman, A. (1999). *The spirit catches you and you fall down: A Hmong child, her American doctors, and the collision of two cultures.* New York: The Noonday Press, Farrar, Straus and Giroux.

Feagin, J. R., & McKinney, K. D. (2003). *The many costs of racism.* Lanham, MD: Rowman & Littlefield.

Finkler, K. (2000). *Experiencing the new genetics: Family and kinship on the medical frontier.* Philadelphia: University of Pennsylvania Press.

Foley, D., & Moss, K. (2001). Studying U.S. cultural diversity: Some non-essentializing perspectives. In I. Susser & T. C. Patterson (Eds.), *Cultural diversity in the United States* (pp. 343–364). Malden, MA: Blackwell.

Fong, T. P. (2002). *The contemporary Asian American experience: Beyond the model minority.* Upper Saddle River, NJ: Prentice Hall.

Frank, G. (2000). *Venus on wheels: Two decades of dialogue on disability, biography, and being female in America.* Berkeley: University of California Press.

Franklin, B. M. (Ed.). (2000). *Curriculum and consequence: Herbert M. Kliebard and the promise of schooling.* New York: Teachers College Press.

Franklin, S., & Ragone, H. (Eds.). (1999). *Reproducing reproduction: Kinship, power and technological innovation.* Philadelphia: University of Pennsylvania Press.

Freund, P. E. S., & McGuire, M. B. (1995). *Health, illness, and the social body: A critical sociology.* Englewood Cliffs, NJ: Prentice Hall.

Gaillot, M. (1999). *Multiple meanings: Techno—an artistic and political laboratory of the present* (W. Niesluchowski, Trans.). Paris: Éditions Dis Voir.

Gaudiano, E. G., & de Alba, A. (1994). Freire—present and future possibilities (Adriana Hernández, Trans.). In P. L. McLaren & C. Lankshear (Eds.), *Politics of liberation: Paths from Freire* (pp. 123–141). New York: Routledge.

Gilroy, P. (1992). The end of antiracism. In James Donald & Ali Rattansi (Eds.), *"Race," culture, and difference* (pp. 49–61). London: Sage and The Open University.

Goldberg, D. T. (1998). Introduction: Multicultural conditions. In David T. Goldberg (Ed.), *Multiculturalism: A critical reader* (pp. 1–41). Oxford, England: Blackwell.

Goldberg, M. A., & Remy-St. Louis, G. (1998). Understanding and treating pain in ethically diverse patients. *Journal of Clinical Psychology in Medical Settings, 5*(3), 343–356.

Good, M.-J. D. (1998). *American medicine: The quest for competence.* Berkeley: University of California Press.

Gordon, E. J. (2001). "They don't have to suffer for me:" Why dialysis patients refuse offers of living donor kidneys. *Medical Anthropology Quarterly, 15*(2), 245–267.

Greaves, T. (Ed.). (1994). *Intellectual property rights for indigenous peoples: A source book.* Oklahoma City, OK: Society for Applied Anthropology.

Green, E. C. (1999). *Indigenous theories of contagious disease.* Walnut Creek, CA: AltaMira Press.

Grossman, R. (2004, July 6). A nation divided by language? *The Baltimore Sun,* p. 4A.

Gruenbaum, W. (2001). *The female circumcision controversy: An anthropological perspective.* Philadelphia: University of Pennsylvania Press.

Guba, E. G., & Lincoln, Y. S. (1989). Ethics and politics: The twin failures of positivist science. In E. G. Guba & Y. S. Lincoln (Eds.), *Fourth generation evaluation* (pp. 117–141). Newbury Park, CA: Sage.

Gutiérrez, E. C. Z., & Kendall, C. (2000). The globalization of health and disease: The health transition and global change. In G. L. Albrecht, R. Fitzpatrick, & S. C.

Scrimshaw (Eds.), *The handbook of social studies in health and medicine* (pp. 85–99). London: Sage.

Haasoun, R. (2004, September). Impact of U.S. occupation in the Middle East on Arab Americans. *Anthropology News, 45*(6), 18–19.

Habermas, J. (1990). *Moral consciousness and communicative action* (C. Lenhardt & S. W. Nicholson, Trans.). Cambridge, MA: MIT Press.

Hall, R. E. (2001, April). The Tiger Woods phenomenon: A note on biracial identity. *The Social Science Journal, 38*(2), 333–337.

Heidegger, M. (1957). *Der Satz vom Grund.* Pfullingen, Germany: Neske.

Heidegger, M. (1962). *Being and time* (J. Macquarrie & E. Robinson, Trans.). New York: Harper & Row. (Original work published 1927)

Heidegger, M. (1966). *Discourse on thinking* (J. Anderson & E. H. Freund, Trans.). New York: Harper & Row.

Heidegger, M. (1967). *Wegmarken.* Frankfurt am Main, Germany: Klostermann.

Heidegger, M. (1968). *What is called thinking* (F. D. Wiech & J. G. Gray, Trans.). New York: Harper & Row.

Henslin, J. M. (2005). *Sociology: A down-to-earth approach* (7th ed.). Boston: Pearson.

Hillyard, D., & Dombrink, J. (2001). *Dying right: The death with dignity movement.* New York: Routledge.

Ho, M.-J. (2003). Migratory journeys and tuberculosis risk. *Medical Anthropology Quarterly, 17*(4), 442–458.

Hodge, J. (1995). *Heidegger and ethics.* London: Routledge.

Hoshino, K. (1995). Autonomous decision making and Japanese tradition. *Cambridge Quarterly of Healthcare Ethics, 4,* 71–74.

Iyer, P. (2000, May 22). Are we coming apart or together? *Time,* 114–115.

Jecker, N. S., Carrese, J. A., & Pearlman, R. A. (1995). Caring for patients in cross-cultural settings. *Hastings Center Report, 25,* 6–14.

Jonsen, A. (1991). American moralism and the origin of bioethics in the United States. *Journal of Medicine and Philosophy, 16,* 113–130.

Jonsen, A. (1994). Clinical ethics and the four principles. In R. Gillon (Ed.), *Principles of health care ethics* (pp. 13–21). Chichester, England: John Wiley and Sons.

Kavanagh, K. H. (2002). Neither here nor there: The story of a health professional's experience with getting care and needing caring. In N. L. Diekelmann (Ed.), *First do no harm: Power, oppression, and violence in healthcare* (pp. 49–117). Madison: University of Wisconsin Press.

Kavanagh, K. H. (2003). Mirrors: A cultural and historical interpretation of nursing's pedagogies. In N. L. Diekelmann (Ed.), *Teaching the practitioners of care: New pedagogies for the health professions* (pp. 59–153). Madison: University of Wisconsin Press.

Kavanagh, K. H. (2005). Representing: Interpretive scholarship's consummate challenge. In P. M. Ironside (Ed.), *Beyond method.* Madison: University of Wisconsin Press.

Kavanagh, K. H., & Knowlden, V. (Eds.). (2004). *Many voices: Toward caring culture in healthcare and healing.* Madison: University of Wisconsin Press.

Kehoe, A. B. (2004, April). When theoretical models trump empirical validity, real people suffer: Why anthropologists should abandon the term "chiefdom." *Anthropology News,* 10.

Kleinman, A. (1988). *The illness narratives.* New York: Basic Books.

Kleinman, A. (1995). *Writing at the margin: Discourse between anthropology and medicine.* Berkeley: University of California Press.

Kleinman, A., Das, V., & Lock, M. (Eds.). (1997). *Social suffering.* Berkeley: University of California Press.

Kottak, C. P. (1999). *Mirror for humanity: A concise introduction to cultural anthropology* (2nd ed.). Boston: McGraw-Hill College.

Kozol, J. (1991). *Savage inequalities: Children in America's schools.* New York: Crown.

Kuhse, H. (Ed.). (2002). *Unsanctifying human life: Essays on ethics [by] Peter Singer.* Oxford, England: Blackwell.

Kunitz, S. J. (1989). *Disease change and the role of medicine: The Navajo experience.* Berkeley: University of California Press.

Kunitz, S. J. (1994). *Disease and social diversity: The European impact on the health of non-Europeans.* New York: Oxford University Press.

Lamphere, L. (2001). Afterword: Understanding U.S. diversity—Where do we go from here? In Susser & T. C. Patterson (Eds.), *Cultural diversity in the United States* (pp. 457–464). Malden, MA: Blackwell.

Landy, D. (Ed.). (1977). *Culture, disease and healing: Studies in medical anthropology.* New York: Macmillan.

Lerner, G. (1997). *Why history matters: Life and thought.* New York: Oxford University Press.

Levenson, J. (2004). *The secret epidemic: The story of AIDS and Black America.* New York: Pantheon/Random House.

Levin, M. D. (Ed.). (1993). *Ethnicity and aboriginality: Case studies in ethnonationalism.* Toronto: University of Toronto Press.

Lipson, J. G., & Steiger, N. J. (1996). *Self care nursing in a multicultural context.* Newbury Park, CA: Sage.

Lock, M. (1996). Displacing suffering: The reconstruction of death in North America and Japan. *Daedalus, 125*(1), 207–245.

Locke, J. (1993). The state of nature and the right to property. In J. Arthur (Ed.), *Morality and moral controversies* (3rd ed., pp. 85–92). Englewood Cliffs, NJ: Prentice-Hall. (Original work published 1690)

Lynn, J., & Teno, J. M. (1993). After the patient self-determination act: The need for empirical research on formal advance directives. *Hastings Center Report, 23*(1), 20–24.

Mackie, G. (2003). Female genital cutting: A harmless practice? *Medical Anthropology Quarterly, 17*(2), 135–158.

Marable, M. (2000, January 25). We need new and critical study of race and ethnicity. *The Chronicle of Higher Education,* pp. B4–B7.

Marks, J. (1994, December). Black, white, other. *Natural History,* 32–35.

Marshall, P. A., & Koenig, B. A. (1996). Bioethics in anthropology: Perspectives on culture, medicine, and morality. In C. F. Sargent & T. M. Johnson (Eds.), *Medical anthropology: Contemporary method and theory* (pp. 349–373). Westport, CT: Praeger Press.

Marshall, P. A., Koenig, B. A., Barnes, D. M., & Davis, A. J. (1998). Multiculturalism, bioethics, and end-of-life care: Case narratives of Latino cancer patients. In J. F. Monagle & D. C. Thomasma (Eds.), *Health care ethics: Critical issues for the 21st century* (pp. 421–431). Gaithersburg, MD: Aspen.

Massey, D. S., & Lundy, G. (2001). Use of Black English and racial discrimination in urban housing markets: New methods and findings. *Urban Affairs Review, 36,* 451–468.

McBride, D. (1991). *From TB to AIDS: Epidemics among urban Blacks since 1900.* Albany: State University of New York Press.

McCarthy, C., & Dimityriades, G. (2000). Globalizing pedagogies: Power, resentment, and the re-narration of difference. In N. C. Burbules & C. A. Torres (Eds.), *Globalization and education: Critical perspectives* (pp. 187–204). London: Routledge.

McLaren, P. L., & Lankshear, C. (Eds.). (1994). *Politics of liberation: Paths from Freire.* New York: Routledge.

Merry, S. E. (2001). Racialized identities and the law. In I. Susser & T. C. Patterson (Eds.), *Cultural diversity in the United States* (pp. 120–139). Malden, MA: Blackwell.

Micozzi, M. S. (2001). *Fundamentals of complementary and alternative medicine* (2nd ed.). New York: Churchill Livingstone.

Micozzi, M. S. (2002). Culture, anthropology, and the return of "complementary medicine." *Anthropology Quarterly, 16*(4), 398–403.

Middleton, D. R. (2003). *The challenge of human diversity: Mirrors, bridges, and chasms* (2nd ed.). Prospect Heights, IL: Waveland Press.

Millstone, E., & Lang, T. (2003). *The Penguin atlas of food.* New York: Penguin.

Mintz, S. W. (1997). Swallowing modernity. In J. Watson (Ed.), *Golden arches east: McDonald's in East Asia* (pp. 183–200). Stanford, CA: Stanford University Press.

Monaghan, P. (2000, October 6). Scholarly watchdogs for an ethical netherworld. *The Chronicle of Higher Education,* pp. A23–A24.

Montagu, M. F. A. (1952). *Man's most dangerous myth: The fallacy of race.* New York: Harper Brothers. (Original work published 1942)

Montagu, M. F. A. (1999). *Race and IQ: Expanded edition.* New York: Oxford University Press.

Morrow, R. A., & Torres, C. A. (2000). The state, globalization, and educational policy. In N. C. Burbules & C. A. Torres (Eds.), *Globalization and education: Critical perspectives* (pp. 27–56). London: Routledge.

Moss, K. (1998). *Interrogating images: Poor Whites and the paradox of privilege.* Doctoral dissertation, University of Texas at Austin.

Mulhall, S., & Swift, A. (1996). *Liberals and communitarians* (2nd ed.). Oxford, England: Blackwell.

Muller, J. H. (1994). Anthropology, bioethics, and medicine: A provocative trilogy. *Medical Anthropology Quarterly, 8*(4), 448–467.

Mullings, L. (1989). Inequality and African-American health status: Policies and prospects. In W. VanHorne (Ed.), *Race: Twentieth-century dilemmas—Twenty-first-century prognoses* (pp. 154–182). Madison: University of Wisconsin Institute on Race and Ethnicity.

Murphy, S. T., Palmer, J. M., Azen, S., Frank, G., Michel, V., & Blackhall, L. J. (1996). Ethnicity and advance care directives. *Journal of Law, Medicine and Ethics, 24,* 108–117.

Murray, C. (1993). Affirmative racism. In J. Arthur (Ed.), *Morality and moral controversies* (3rd ed., pp. 523–531). Englewood Cliffs, NJ: Prentice Hall.

Mwaria, C. (2001). Diversity in the context of health and illness. In I. Susser & T. C. Patterson (Eds.), *Cultural diversity in the United States* (pp. 57–75). Malden, MA: Blackwell.

Nancy, J.-L. (1997). *The gravity of thought* (F. Raffoul & G. Recco, Trans.). Highlands, NJ: Humanities Press.

Nash, J. (2001). Labor struggles: Gender, ethnicity, and the new migration. In I. Susser & T. C. Patterson (Eds.), *Cultural diversity in the United States* (pp. 206–228). Malden, MA: Blackwell.

Obermeyer, C. M. (2003). The health consequences of female circumcision: Science, advocacy, and standards of evidence. *Medical Anthropology Quarterly, 17*(3), 394–412.

Olafson, F. A. (1998). *Heidegger and the ground of ethics: A study of Mitsein*. Cambridge, England: Cambridge University Press.

Orona, C. J., Koenig, B. A., & Davis, A. J. (1994). Cultural aspects of nondisclosure. *Cambridge Quarterly of Healthcare Ethics, 3*, 338–346.

Orr, R. D., Marshall, P. A., & Osborn, J. (1995, February). Cross-cultural considerations in clinical ethics consultations. *Archives of Family Medicine, 4,* 159–164.

Outlaw, L., Jr. (1998). "Multiculturalism," citizenship, education, and American liberal democracy. In C. Willett (Ed.), *Theorizing multiculturalism: A guide to the current debate* (pp. 382–397). Oxford, England: Blackwell.

Oxford English Dictionary. (2002). CD-ROM Version 3.00. Oxford, England: Oxford University Press.

Parker, W. C., Ninomiya, A., & Cogan, J. (1999). Educating world citizens: Toward multinational curriculum development. *American Educational Research Journal, 36*(2), 117–145.

Pérez-Escamilla, R., Himmelgreen, D., & Ferris, A. (1996). *The food and nutrition situation of inner-city Latino preschoolers in Hartford: A preliminary needs assessment.* Hartford: University of Connecticut and the Hispanic Health Council.

Peters, M. (1996). *Poststructuralism, politics, and education*. Westport, CT: Bergin & Garvey.

Peters, M., Marshall, J., & Fitzsimons, P. (2000). Managerialism and educational policy in a global context: Foucault, neoliberalism, and the doctrine of self-management. In N. C. Burbules & C. A. Torres (Eds.), *Globalization and education: Critical perspectives* (pp. 109–132). London: Routledge.

Pilnick, A. (2002). *Genetics and society: An introduction*. Buckingham, England: Open Press.

Rachels, J. (1993). What people deserve. In J. Arthur (Ed.), *Morality and moral controversies* (3rd ed., pp. 505–514). Englewood Cliffs, NJ: Prentice Hall.

Ramey, C. T., & Ramey, S. L. (1995). Successful early interventions for children at high risk for failure in school. In G. J. Demko & M. C. Jackson (Eds.), *Populations at risk in America: Vulnerable groups at the end of the twentieth century.* Boulder, CO: Westview Press.

Ramsay, M. (1994). Genetic reductionism and medical genetic practice. In A. Clarke (Ed.), *Genetic counseling: Practice and principles.* London: Routledge.

Rapp, R. (1999). *Testing women, testing the fetus: The social impact of amniocentesis in America.* New York: Routledge.

Ratliff, S. S. (1996). The multicultural challenge to health care. In M. C. Juliá (Ed.), *Multicultural awareness in the health care professions* (pp. 164–181). Needham Heights, MA: Simon & Schuster.

Reskin, B. F. (1998). *The realities of affirmative action in employment.* Washington, DC: American Sociological Association.

Ritzer, G. (1998). *The McDonaldization thesis: Explorations and extensions.* Thousand Oaks, CA: Sage.

Roberson, M. H. B. (1992). The meaning of compliance: Patient perspectives. *Qualitative Health Research, 2*(1), 7–26.

Root, M. (1993). *Philosophy of social science: The methods, ideals, and politics of social inquiry.* Oxford, England: Blackwell.

Root, M. P. P. (1992). *Racially mixed people in America.* Newbury Park, CA: Sage.

Rouche, A. (2001, December). Policy monitor: Is selling your kidney a right? *Anthropology News,* 25.

Rowland, D. (2004). *The boundaries of her body: A shocking history of women's rights in America.* New York: Sourcebooks.

Russell, A., Sobo, E. J., & Thompson, M. S. (Eds.). (2000). *Contraception across cultures: Technologies, choices, constraints.* New York: Berg.

Safa, H. I. (1996). *The myth of the male breadwinner.* Boulder, CO: Westview Press.

Sandercock, L. (1998). Framing insurgent historiographies for planning. In L. Sandercock (Ed.), *Masking the invisible visible: A multicultural planning history* (pp. 1–33). Berkeley: University of California Press.

Schlosser, E. (2002). *Fast-food nation.* New York: HarperCollins.

Seidler, V. J. (1991). *The moral limits of modernity: Love, inequality and oppression.* New York: St. Martin's Press.

Singer, M. (2001). Health, disease, and social inequality. In I. Susser & T. C. Patterson (Eds.), *Cultural diversity in the United States* (pp. 76–100). Malden, MA: Blackwell.

Sklair, L. (2001). *Globalization: Capitalism and its alternatives* (3rd ed.). New York: Oxford University Press.

Sloan, R. S. (2002). Living a life-sustained-by-medical-technology: Dialysis is killing *me.* In N. L. Diekelmann (Ed.), *First do no harm: Power, oppression, and violence in healthcare* (pp.118–163). Madison: University of Wisconsin Press.

Smith, S. C. (2001). The making of a neo-colony? Anglo-Kuwaiti relations in the era of decolonization. *Middle Eastern Studies,* 37(1), 159–173.

Sobo, E. J. (1995). *Choosing unsafe sex: AIDS-risk denial among disadvantaged women.* Philadelphia: University of Pennsylvania Press.

Statistical Abstract of the United States. (2002). Washington, DC: Bureau of the Census.

Steinberg, S. (1989). *The ethnic myth: Race, ethnicity, and class in America.* Boston: Beacon.

Stevens, P. E., Hall, J. M., & Meleis, A. I. (1992). Examining vulnerability of women clerical workers from five ethnic–racial groups. *Western Journal of Nursing Research, 14,* 769.

Trostle, J. A. (1988). Medical compliance as an ideology. *Social Science and Medicine,* 27(12), 1299–1308.

Van Dijk, T. A. (1993). *Elite discourse and racism.* Newbury Park, CA: Sage.

Vawter, D. E., Culhane-Pera, K. A., Babbitt, B., Xiong, P., & Solberg, M. M. (2003). A model for culturally responsive health care. In K. A. Culhane-Pera, et al. (Eds.), *Healing by heart: Clinical and ethical case studies of Hmong families and Western providers* (pp. 297–356). Nashville, TN: Vanderbilt University Press.

Veatch, R. M. (Ed.). (1989). *Cross-cultural perspectives in medical ethics: Readings.* Boston: Jones and Bartlett.

Vellema, S., & Jansen, K. (Eds.). (2004). *Agribusiness and society: Corporate responses to Environmentalism, market opportunities, and public regulation.* New York: Zed Books.

Video violence. (2004, July 11). *Parade Magazine,* p. 18.

Voget, F. W. (1975). *A history of ethnology.* New York: Holt, Rinehart and Winston.

Von Dohlen, R. F. (1997). *Culture war and ethical theory.* Lanham, MD: University Press of America.

Warren, J. (2004, July 18). Mo.'s homey juvenile prison system a success: Focus on treatment in an intimate setting helps youth change. *The Baltimore Sun,* p. 9A.

Wasserstrom, R. A. (1993). On racism and sexism: Realities and ideals. In J. Arthur (Ed.), *Morality and moral controversies* (3rd ed., pp. 453–467). Englewood Cliffs, NJ: Prentice Hall.

Watson, J. (Ed.). (1997). Introduction: Transnationalism, localization, and fast foods in East Asia (pp. 1–38). In J. Watson (Ed.), *Golden arches east: McDonald's in East Asia.* Stanford, CA: Stanford University Press.

Watts, S. (2003). *Disease and medicine in world history.* New York: Routledge.

Webster, Y. O. (1992). *The racialization of America.* New York: St. Martin's Press.

Weiner, J. F. (2001). *Tree leaf talk: A Heidegerrian anthropology.* Oxford, England: Oxford University Press.

West, C. (1993). *Race matters.* Boston: Beacon Press.

Wheeler, C., & Bernstein, J. (1996). New laws fundamentally revise immigrant access to government programs: A review of the changes. In National Law Immigration Center, *Immigrants and the '96 welfare law: A resource manual* (pp. 1–28). Los Angeles: National Immigrantion Law Center.

Whiteford, L. (1996). Political economy, gender, and the social production of health and illness. In C. Sargent & C. Brettell (Eds.), *Gender and health: An international perspective* (pp. 242–259). Upper Saddle River, NJ: Prentice Hall.

Whorf, B. L. (Ed.). (1956). *Language, thought and reality: Selected writing of Benjamin Lee Whorf.* Cambridge, MA: MIT Press.

Wilcox, D. M., & Wilcox, W. H. (1997). *Applied ethics in American society.* Fort Worth, TX: Harcourt Brace.

Williams, A. (1998). Therapeutic landscapes in holistic medicine. *Social Science and Medicine, 46*(9), 1193–1203.

Williams, W. (2004, July 6). Two Americas. *The Baltimore Sun*, p. 11A.

Yan, Y. (1997). McDonald's in Beijing: The localization of Americana. In J. Watson (Ed.), *Golden arches east: McDonald's in East Asia* (pp. 39–76). Stanford, CA: Stanford University Press.

Community, Caring, and the Double Bind

In Ancient Greece, Socrates, Plato, and Aristotle realized that the individual cannot be understood apart from society. Socrates chose to die rather than live without the daily social interaction of his philosophical dialogues. Plato considered the pursuit of a just society to be a necessary pursuit of a just individual. Aristotle thought it pointless to consider the ideal of human excellence in isolation from society, since humans are social beings; he therefore defined the best human life in terms of social interaction and moral virtue.

Centuries later, from his cell in a Birmingham jail, Martin Luther King, Jr. (1963) wrote: "We are caught in an inescapable network of mutuality, tied in a single garment of destiny. Whatever affects one directly affects all indirectly" (pp. 1–2). King penned these words to justify his involvement in Birmingham's civil rights activities. But he also wrote them to warn those who mistakenly thought that some groups can remain unaffected by other groups and that individuals can stand apart from their community.

Heidegger's (1996) use of the term "destiny" echoes that of King's. He states that Da-sein's existence as being-in-the-world, always intertwined with being-with others, is "determined as *destiny*." This destiny, Heidegger says, "is not composed of individual fates, nor can being-with-one-another be conceived of as the mutual occurrence of several subjects. These fates are already guided beforehand in being-with-one-another in the same world and in the resoluteness for definite possibilities" (p. 352). Even though, as Kavanagh points out, we cannot ever know as another knows, experience as another experiences, our very understanding of ourselves is always in terms of being-with, in other words, in terms of our community. Da-sein in its essence is always being-in-the-world and being-with others: *Mitda-sein*. We experience our world and our possibilities *with* those in that same world.

Heidegger (1996) insists that even when we attempt to turn away from others, or when we are feeling alone despite the presence of others, these very acts and experiences are possible only because Da-sein is already being-with. Being-with-others "belongs to the being of Da-sein. . . . As being-with, Da-sein 'is' essentially for the sake of others" (pp. 115–116). We cannot isolate ourselves from others even if we wish. Being a member of a community, being *with*, is an essential part of our existence. We relate to others in our world in varying modes of *concern*, but Heidegger observes that each of us as Da-sein lives "initially and, for the most part, . . . in the deficient modes of concern. Being for-, against-, and without-one-another, passing-one-another-by, not-mattering-to-one-another"—these are modes of concern, even though deficient, because we experience them differently than we would the being-together with arbitrary things to which we were indifferent (p. 114).

Even when Da-sein is in a positive mode of concern, though, that concern can take either the form of domination or of liberation. The dominating form of concern can be seen in many of the current practices Kavanagh identifies. In defining healing in terms of *medicine*, healthcare practitioners may cure a person's physical ills while promoting their own practices and assumptions as the preferred or only approach. If a practitioner treats a person's immediate condition without attention to the underlying causes, such as poverty or hunger, that practitioner shows concern in a way that dominates the one seeking treatment, who will no more be able to help herself next time than now. Heidegger (1996) describes this dominating form of concern as "leaping in" for the other. In this mode, because the other's own care is taken over and taken away, "the other can become one who is dependent and dominated even if this domination is a tacit one and remains hidden from him" (p. 114).

As an alternative to this mode of concern, Heidegger (1996) offers "the possibility of a concern which does not so much leap in for the other as *leap ahead* of him, not in order to take 'care' away from him, but first to give it back to him as such." This concern, or authentic care, "helps the other to become transparent to himself *in* his care and *free for* it" (p. 115). When Kavanagh calls for healthcare practitioners to turn their attention to problematic structures and systems that surround, limit, and perhaps endanger the individuals in their care, she is advocating this *leaping ahead* rather than the simpler but dominating *leaping in*. She insists that healthcare practitioners "are ethically bound to respond to societal-level concerns" (p. 250). Through such a response, practitioners can aim toward restoring autonomy, freedom, and *possibilities* to those who may find little or none in the current system.

We cannot ignore, however, the fact that the current societal and governmental structures and systems, both nationally and globally, are well-rooted and may be quite difficult to change. Some systemic problems may even be hard to *see* in the first place, or to recognize as changeable. Richard Rorty (1999) seeks a pragmatic solution to these problems; to help himself and others gain perspective on systemic problems, he adopts a fictional "looking back" from 100 years later to comment on our current situation. From this perspective, he writes:

Just as twentieth-century Americans had trouble imagining how their pre-Civil War ancestors could have stomached slavery, so we at the end of the twenty-first century have trouble imagining how our great-grandparents could have legally permitted a CEO to get 20 times more than her lowest paid employees. We cannot understand how Americans a hundred years ago could have tolerated the horrific contrast between a childhood spent in the suburbs and one spent in the ghettos. Such inequalities seem to us evident moral abominations, but the vast majority of our ancestors took them to be regrettable necessities. (p. 243)

These regrettable necessities of which Rorty speaks surround us every day in our experiences as social beings and are particularly troubling for healthcare practitioners dealing with the constraints of managed care, the repercussions of poverty, or the complications of treating patients living in the country illegally.

Margaret Jane Radin (1990), whose feminist philosophy overlaps significantly, she acknowledges, with the pragmatism that Rorty advocates, finds that these underlying systemic problems often leave would-be improvers of society in a double bind. Radin is primarily concerned with the role of legislators, but her views are equally applicable to the situations currently imposed on healthcare professionals. For instance, nurses in a clinic may find that some of their patients, in order to afford an essential medication, are going without other necessary medicine or perhaps even adequate food. However, if these nurses give the medicine to these patients without charge, the clinic will no longer be able to afford its operating costs, and it will be of no help to any patients if it has to close its doors. Radin's solution to this sort of double bind "is not to solve but to dissolve it: remove the oppressive circumstances" (p. 1700).

Following Radin's advice, nurses in the above situation would realize that there *is* no solution to their problem until they and others can change the conditions that caused it in the first place. This realization, of course, does not help the nurses decide what to do now, in these circumstances. To this end, Radin suggests we learn to think at once both about "an ideal world, the best world that we can now conceive," and the nonideal world in which we now live (p. 1700). Next we should ask ourselves, "Given where we now find ourselves, what is the better decision? In making this decision, we think about what actions can bring us closer to" the ideal world we've envisioned (p. 1700). The double bind is always a problem situated in a nonideal world, and Radin believes the "only solution can be pragmatic. There is no general solution; there are only piecemeal, temporary solutions" (p. 1701). These temporary solutions aim toward a larger goal, though. Nonideal solutions are our means of making progress toward the ideal world we have envisioned and are reenvisioning every day.

Radin is particularly concerned with hierarchies and dominant paradigms that constitute the framework of our current nonideal world. Kavanagh, with Moss, focuses on this concern as well, recommending a deconstruction of ideas in order to "systematically displace such conceptual hierarchies as male/female, black/white, lower class/working class/middle class" (p. 260). It is likely that a displacement of these hierarchies would offer a voice to those who currently have none. A person previously dismissed because of the group to which he was assigned by others might now be able to speak simply as a human being, like all other human beings, rather than as a member of a particular group. But oppression can breed silence, and recovering from years of silence may not be an easy task. For people in such a situation, Radin (1990) recommends that others with similar experiences of oppression—a group in which she places most women—help through consciousness raising, which can make communication possible.

As great thinkers from Socrates to King have emphasized, each of us is a member of society at least as much as she is an individual. No matter how much we want to make that society better, though, we may feel trapped in a hopelessly flawed and unjust system. No matter how much we want to help an individual and "leap ahead" of him in our concern, we may feel forced to "leap in" instead, because of the limits on his capacity or the restrictions of our own practice and laws. Kavanagh is well aware of the problems of the current structures of society, but her study is a call to think beyond the boundaries of our flawed system, to open our minds to possibilities opened by the world's constantly increasing diversity, to look beyond ourselves and our individualism to the importance and opportunity of community in all its richness and complexity.

References

Heidegger, M. (1996). *Being and Time* (J. Stambaugh, Trans.). Albany: State University of New York.

King, M. (1963). *Letter from Birmingham jail.* Retrieved May 1, 2005, from http://www.nobelprizes.com/nobel/peace/MLK-jail.html.

Radin, M. (1990). The Pragmatist and the feminist. *Southern California Law Review, 63,* 1699–1711.

Rorty, R. (1999). *Philosophy and social hope.* London: Penguin.

7

An Ethics of Diversity

Listening in Thin Places

JEANNE M. SORRELL and
CHRISTINE S. DINKINS

Celtic traditions describe the concept of a "thin place," an in-between place that merges the natural and sacred worlds, where the ordinary and non-ordinary mingle, where the seen and the unseen share common ground. Gomes (1996) suggests that these thin places are likely to be found where there is greatest suffering, among the marginalized and excluded.

If one burrows down through the theoretical and philosophical perspectives of ethics, it may be argued that, at bottom, ethics is concerned with the suffering humans cause one another and the related capacity of humans to recognize and address this suffering through the empathetic virtues of sympathy, compassion, and caring (Roberts, 1996). Much suffering throughout history can be related to the problem of "unacceptable" diversity among individuals or groups. Remembering the cruelties of the Nazi exterminations of Jews, slavery in the United States, and discrimination against homosexuals jolts us to awareness of the suffering of those who are "different." A task of ethics, then, is to include, rather than exclude (Post, 1995). One approach to an ethics of diversity for healthcare professionals is a call for intimate listening to the stories of those who are different, who may be unseen, marginalized, and excluded in our healthcare systems. Unless we listen to these voices of diversity, we are likely to remain oblivious to the harm being done in healthcare through unwitting oppression of minorities.

As reflected in stories in this volume, 21st-century healthcare has fueled new questioning about how we want to live and interact with others. Cook (2003) notes that "diversity" has many definitions, including gender, cultural, spiritual, biological/physical, social, environmental, moral, ethical, economical, educational, political, and ethnic differences. All of these diversities affect healthcare practices and beliefs and may lead to further disparities in healthcare. Thus, it is important to explore diversity from an ethical perspective and come to know how to move through our worlds of differences so that we can grow, understand, and care.

Listening to stories of diversity can help healthcare practitioners understand the potential for oppression built into the structure of our language, our social institutions, and, especially, our healthcare systems. These stories are all around us if we only choose to listen. As editors, we share a few personal stories with you: A young professional told of being humiliated by her female gynecologist when she wanted to discuss her lesbian sexual practices. A nursing student confided that her instructor did not allow her to miss clinical practicum to attend the funeral of a friend with AIDS because he was not "family." A Saudi nursing student on the hospital elevator listened as a passenger told an acquaintance that Saudis should have no rights in American hospitals. An African American nursing student told how his patient assumed he was the maintenance man for the hospital.

Those who dominate by class, ethnicity, age, or gender may be unaware of the invisibility of privilege within our society (Roberts, 1996). For members of a dominant group in society, their particular identity is transparent, in other words, not perceived by them as a specific identity. They may be oblivious to how they first attained membership in groups and the significance of group membership that is not "other." For nondominant groups, however, their identity is always experienced as particular, as specific to them as members of the group. To help bridge these two worlds of the dominant and nondominant, we need to listen to narratives of those experiencing the lived realities of diversity so that the often-muffled voices of these individuals are heard.

Intimate Listening in Thin Places

Thin places in the healthcare system may be found within stories of diversity. Stories embody a personal way of knowing that is unique, as relationships between the narrative and narrated events uncover meaning. Harvey (1999) suggests that we need to learn to listen to stories of diverse places, landscapes, others, and ourselves as we explore new relationships. The sharing of stories opens up possibilities for new conversations and understandings between narrator and listener. As we listen, intimately, to someone's story, we are drawn into the unique reality of that individual, helping us to see the world through experience, rather than through theorizing.

An ethics of diversity can be developed not merely through philosophically based reasoning and traditional ethical principles, but through active listening to persons of the "other" groups. Canales (1997) suggested that healthcare practitioners often assume an understanding of ethnic minority women from stereotypes and myths evoked by their appearance. As a result, ethnic minority women may experience double jeopardy from a society that devalues both women and members of specific racial or ethnic groups. Research helps us to understand that clients' stories are never just their stories—they connect the listener with larger cultural narratives of shared meanings (Emden, 1998). For example, Draucker (1998) explored storytelling as an intervention with women who had experienced repeated sexual violence and abuse. These women were encouraged to discuss moments of strength, autonomy, and emotional vitality that were hidden in their life stories—stories that were otherwise filled with suffering and oppression. Results of the research study suggest that storytelling may help women to find ways to construct new, empowering life narratives.

Through listening to personal stories of diverse clients interacting with the healthcare system, we can better understand the unique healthcare needs of these individuals (Evans & Severtsen, 2001). When a life is viewed through narratives, embedded values, goals, and concerns become connected with these narratives and contribute to understanding of the individual's personal identity as well as to the shared identity of a person with his/her culture. Healthcare practitioners can facilitate life narratives through intimate listening in thin places.

Conclusion

Karl (2002) notes that cultures have dominant narratives that we internalize, using them as the lens through which we construct reality.

He warns, however, that dominant stories do not cover all of reality. "Pushed to the margins are other experiences that contain rich, lived, local experience" (p. 33). These marginal experiences may not yet be shaped into stories because they may be seen as lacking value for a legitimate voice. Karl asks: "How do we care for the soul of what we do?" (p. 30). He encourages us to remember and pay attention to core values and meaning in our work settings. In the beginning of this volume, Nancy Moules shared her surprise that "somehow I forgot that stories lie here in this topic of ethics" (p. 7). Authors in this volume have given voice to some of these whispered stories. Listening to the whispers from the margins of healthcare alongside the shouts and cries from its central arenas can help us to create an ethics of diversity in which we explore the thin places where suffering lies hidden. If we do not listen and if we do not start listening *right now*, the shouts and cries will remain unanswered, and the whispers may fade into silence.

(Adapted from Sorrell, J. M. [August, 2003]. The ethics of diversity: A call for intimate listening in thin places. *Online Journal of Issues in Nursing.* Available from http://www.nursingworld.org/ojin/ethicol/ethics_13.htm). Reprinted with permission.)

References

Canales, M. (1997). Narrative interaction: Creating a space for therapeutic communication. *Issues in Mental Health Nursing, 18*(5), 477–494.

Cook, C. (2003, January 31). The many faces of diversity: Overview and summary. *Online Journal of Issues in Nursing, 8*(1). Retrieved April 19, 2003, from http://nursingworld.org/ojin/topic20/tpc20ntr.htm.

Draucker, C. B. (1998). Narrative therapy for women who have lived with violence. *Archives of Psychiatric Nursing, 12*(3), 162–168.

Emden, C. (1998). Theoretical perspectives of narrative inquiry. *Collegian: Journal of Royal College of Nursing, Australia, 5*(2), 30–35.

Evans, B. C., & Severtsen, G. M. (2001). Storytelling as cultural assessment. *Nursing and Health Care Perspectives, 22*(4), 180–183.

Gomes, P. (1996). Words for the heart. Retrieved March 20, 2003, from http://www.pbs.org/newshour/gergen/december96/gomes_12–24.html.

Harvey, M. (1999). Intimate listening: Stories, the marketplace, and imagination. *Celtic Well E-Journal.* Retrieved March 20, 2003, from http://www.applewarrior.com/celticwell/ejournal.lughnasa/storytelling.htm.

Karl, J. C. (2002). Caring for the stories that come to us: Work narratives and their sacred promise. *The Journal of Pastoral Care and Counseling, 56*(1), 29–40.

Post, S. G. (1995). *The moral challenge of Alzheimer Disease.* Baltimore: Johns Hopkins University.

Roberts, L. (1996). Teaching the ethics of diversity or getting to the heart of the matter. Proceedings of Conference on Values in Higher Education, April 11–13, 1996, at the University of Tennessee at Knoxville. Retrieved March 20, 2003, from http://oregon state.edu/Dept/philosophy/rob.html.

Contributors

Christine S. Dinkins received her BA with Honors in philosophy from Wake Forest University and her MA and PhD in philosophy from Johns Hopkins University. She is an assistant professor in the Philosophy Department at Wofford College in Spartanburg, SC, where she teaches courses in Ancient Greek philosophy, 19th- and 20th-century German philosophy, philosophy of law, and philosophy through literature. Dr. Dinkins's primary interests are the philosophical methods of Plato and Heidegger. Her current research includes employing Heideggerian hermeneutics in a nondoctrinal contextual interpretation of Plato's works. She is also exploring hermeneutics in music, and her chief hobby is composing choral music, both sacred and secular. In her work with undergraduates, Dr. Dinkins encourages philosophy students to engage in interdisciplinary research with students in other humanities fields and the sciences.

Bruce H. Greenfield, PT, PhD, OCS, is an assistant professor in the Department of Rehabilitation Medicine, Division of Physical Therapy, at Emory University School of Medicine, where he is an active teacher, clinician, and researcher. Dr. Greenfield's current research uses qualitative methods to examine aspects of the psychobiological model of patient care, including moral orientation and ethical decision making of physical therapists during delivery of patient care. He is collaborating with other faculty members in the Emory Department of Rehabilitation Medicine in a pilot study that qualitatively examines subjects' perceptions of their research experience. He is also collaborating with colleagues at the Atlanta Veterans Administration Hospital in a qualitative study of patients' perception of informed decision making. Dr. Greenfield has received the Breg Award from the Sports Section of the American Physical Therapy Association for the best sports research article published in 1992. He currently serves on the Research Committee of the Physical Therapy Association of Georgia and is currently on the Editorial Review Board for the *Journal of Orthopedic and Sports Physical Therapy*.

Kathryn H. Kavanagh, BSN, MS (Nursing), MA (Anthropology), PhD, is a medical anthropologist who has taught for many years in the University of Maryland system. Her interest in cross-cultural aspects of healthcare led her to conduct a series of summer field schools on the Pine Ridge Reservation in South Dakota, where students worked with Oglala-Lakota health initiatives. She also taught at Northern Arizona University, where she directed a baccalaureate program on the Navajo and Hopi Reservations. She currently teaches courses in medical anthropology, indigenous healing traditions, and American Indian cultures for the University of Maryland and other schools in the Baltimore area. Widely published in cultural aspects of healthcare, she continues to write on diversity-related topics.

Simon J. Craddock Lee, MPH, PhD, is a cancer prevention fellow in the ethics of prevention and public health at the National Cancer Institute, Division of Cancer Control and Population Sciences, Behavioral Research Program, Basic and Bio-behavioral Research Branch. A medical anthropologist, he is developing a critical theory analysis of cancer disparities research and policy. He completed his MPH at the University of California, Berkeley before earning a PhD from the joint program between UC-San Francisco and UC-Berkeley in 2003. He currently serves as cochair for the Culture and Qualitative Research Interest Group, a group of intramural and extramural scientists sponsored by the National Institutes of Health.

Nancy J. Moules, PhD, RN, is an associate professor in the Faculty of Nursing at the University of Calgary. Her research and clinical interests lie in the areas of grief, families, therapeutic conversations, and Family Systems Nursing. Her areas of teaching expertise include graduate program qualitative research methods and hermeneutic inquiry. She is currently involved in programs of research using hermeneutic inquiry to examine grief and therapeutic interventions around grief, therapeutic conversations with families who are experiencing suffering in their lives and relationships, and family nursing relational practices in cardiac and oncology settings. Her various publications are in the areas of grief, postmodernism and spirituality, hermeneutic research, pediatric oncology, therapeutic letters, and the teaching of family nursing.

Tobie H. Olsan, PhD, RN, CNAA, BC is an associate professor of Clinical Nursing, Director of Education Research, and Director of the Leadership in Health Care Systems program at the University of Rochester School of Nursing. She has held a variety of executive positions in healthcare organizations and nursing education, and in 2004 was selected as a Fuld Fellow in Academic Leadership at the American Association of Colleges of Nursing. She brings interests in professional activism, institutional ethics, and education reform to the courses she teaches in health policy, politics, technology, leadership, and professional issues in nursing. She has published on the nursing shortage, ethics and managed care, and the value of service learning for helping RN-BS students develop political skills for advancing health policy. Her community service work is dedicated to persons infected with and affected by HIV/AIDS.

John Paul Slosar, MA, PhD, is the Director of Ethics for Ascension Health in St. Louis, MO. Dr. Slosar has a Master's Degree in Moral Philosophy and a PhD in Healthcare Ethics from Saint Louis University. He began his career with Ascension Health in 1999, where his responsibilities include ethics consultation, research and education, coordinating the five Ethics Networks of Ascension Health, and cochairing a task force on ethical issues raised by the future of genomic medicine. He has authored and coauthored articles in numerous journals, including, the *Hastings Center Report,* the *American Journal of Bioethics,* the *National Catholic Bioethics Quarterly, Health Progress, Ethics & Medics,* and *Healthcare Ethics USA.* He is also currently a member and vice-chair of the Gateway Catholic Ethics Network, which serves Catholic hospitals and health systems in the greater metropolitan St. Louis area. His professional research interests include moral theory and method, clinical decision making at the end of life, healthcare reform and genomics.

Jeanne M. Sorrell, PhD, RN, FAAN, is a professor in the School of Nursing at George Mason University. She earned a BSN from the University of Michigan, a MSN from the University of Wisconsin, and a PhD from George Mason University. Her scholarly interests focus on philosophical inquiry, writing across the curriculum, qualitative research, and ethical considerations for patients with chronic illness. Her current research uses interpretive phenomenology to explore ethical concerns in the lived experience of patients and caregivers with Alzheimer's Disease. Based on this research, she facilitated production of an educational video through the Office of Health Care Ethics at George Mason University. The video, *Quality Lives: Ethics in the Care of Persons with Alzheimer's,* received a Sigma Theta Tau International Award for Nursing Electronic Media.

Index

Interpretive Studies in Healthcare and the Human Sciences

Series Editor

Nancy L. Diekelmann, PhD, RN, FAAN, Helen Denne Schulte Professor
Emerita, School of Nursing, University of Wisconsin–Madison

Series Associate Editor

Pamela M. Ironside, PhD, RN, Assistant Professor, School of Nursing,
University of Wisconsin–Madison